# WAR AND PUBLIC HEALTH

## A HANDBOOK

Dr Pierre Perrin

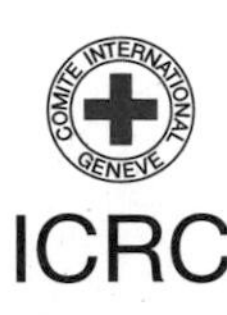


ICRC

International Committee of the Red Cross
19 Avenue de la Paix
1202 Geneva, Switzerland
**T** +41 22 734 60 01 **F** +41 22 733 20 57
**E**-mail: shop.gva@icrc.org
**www**.icrc.org

The author would like to thank Mr Jean Philippe Lavoyer for his assistance in reviewing the chapter on Protecting the Victims of Armed Conflicts, and Frederick Burkle, Professor of Public Health, University of Hawaii, School of Public Health, and Gilbert Burnham, Department of International Health, School of Hygiene and Public Health, Johns Hopkins University, Baltimore, for their review of the rest of the text.

The Center of Excellence in Disaster Management and Humanitarian Assistance — University of Hawaii — supports the publication of this text.

*Translated from the French by Martha Grenzeback.*
*Tables and diagrams are by the author.*

ISBN 2-88145-077-6

# TABLE OF CONTENTS



## Chapter 1

## GENERAL PRINCIPLES OF PLANNING



## Chapter 2

## FOOD AND NUTRITION

# Chapter 3

# WATER AND ENVIRONMENTAL HEALTH

# Chapter 4

# COMMUNICABLE DISEASES

## Chapter 5

## MEDICAL AND SURGICAL CARE

# Chapter 6

# EPIDEMIOLOGY

# Chapter 7

# THE HEALTH-CARE SYSTEM

# Chapter 8

# DISASTERS AND DEVELOPMENT

# Chapter 9

# PROTECTING THE VICTIMS OF ARMED CONFLICTS

# Chapter 10

# INTRODUCTION TO HUMANITARIAN ETHICS

# FOREWORD

Training health personnel has always been a priority for the International Committee of the Red Cross (ICRC). In 1986, together with the World Health Organization and the University of Geneva Faculty of Medicine, the ICRC Medical Division organized the first H.E.L.P. (Health Emergencies in Large Populations) course.

Since then, the course has been given each year in Geneva and has developed along two lines. First and foremost, it has been decentralized. The course is now also given in Latin America (in Costa Rica and Mexico), Asia (in Hong Kong, the Philippines and Thailand), North America (in Canada and the USA), Europe (in Hungary and Sweden, as well as in Switzerland) and Africa (in Ethiopia, South Africa and Togo). The course has also become part of the curriculum at the Johns Hopkins University School of Hygiene and Public Health (Baltimore, Maryland, USA), the Nordic School of Public Health (Göteborg, Sweden), the University of Montreal (Canada), the University of Pretoria School of Health Systems and Public Health (South Africa) and the National Institute of Public Health (Cuernavaca, Mexico); this is in line with the long-term objective of promoting humanitarian issues from within academic institutions. So far, the course has been given over 60 times, to some 1,300 participants in all.

This *Handbook* contains the concepts, ideas and views needed by health personnel who take public health decisions as part of their humanitarian work. The technical considerations involved in decision-making are considered in light of the constraints inherent in emergency situations, especially armed conflicts, where implementing a public health policy is often a real challenge.

The *Handbook*'s aim is to provide health personnel with guidelines on how to react to specific health problems arising from given situations; it does not propose any universally applicable solutions.

It is hoped that the *Handbook* will contribute to improvements in health care in humanitarian operations and, ultimately, to more effective protection for the victims of war and other disasters.

**Yves Etienne**
Head of the Health
and Relief Division

# INTRODUCTION

The people caught up in armed conflicts constitute a permanent challenge for health personnel. Medical care — treating the wounded and sick — is of course important, but it is incomplete if it is not backed up by preventive health care. Hence, when armed conflicts arise, the obvious medical and surgical problems are compounded by health problems in the broad sense, including access to food, water supplies and measles control campaigns. Such an approach to humanitarian operations calls for in-depth knowledge of the public health tools used to set priorities, plan health programmes and assess their impact.

The *Handbook* refuses to come up with easy "health remedies"; rather it aims to develop a method for examining health problems and suggest different ways of handling them. It relies on ingenuity rather than on learning alone.

Our hope is that by adopting a rational approach to health problems, staff will be able to confront the challenges they meet daily in the field and come up with appropriate solutions.

Familiarity with public health tools is not enough to resolve health problems during armed conflicts. Health personnel must bear in mind the political background and the frequently impoverished social and economic context in the countries where humanitarian work is necessary. Their knowledge must encompass these factors, and include a grasp of the legal and ethical concepts enabling them to have a better understanding of the environment in which they work.

Each of the ten chapters in the *Handbook* covers a specific area:

- general principles of planning,
- food and nutrition,
- water and environmental health,
- communicable diseases,
- medical and surgical care,
- epidemiology,
- the health-care system,
- disasters and development,
- international humanitarian law (protecting the victims of armed conflict),
- humanitarian ethics.

## General Principles of Planning

The complexity of armed conflicts calls for a rational approach to health problems.

This chapter discusses the following points:
- problem identification,
- identification of difficulties,
- establishing priorities,
- determining objectives and strategies,
- planning activities,
- assessing the results obtained.

This chapter also clarifies the terminology used in the planning process.

## Food and Nutrition

It is essential in any armed conflict to have an overall view of the food supply system so as to identify any weak points. From this starting point appropriate help can be organized, for instance food distribution and nutritional rehabilitation programmes.

## Water and Environmental Health

Health personnel are not always familiar with the very close link between the environment and people's health. This factor is absolutely crucial in emergency situations because of increased risks connected with poor hygiene: unsafe water, overpopulation, inadequate shelter, etc.

## Communicable Diseases

This chapter does not claim to review fully all infectious diseases, tropical ones in particular. Its purpose is to help those trying to control a limited number of communicable diseases, chosen for their frequent incidence in emergency situations (diarrhoeal diseases, measles, tuberculosis, malaria and meningitis), decide how best to do so.

## Medical and Surgical Care

Armed conflicts require major medical facilities. This chapter deals with the assessment of existing health systems and the organization of a health infrastructure to meet the medical and surgical needs caused by armed conflicts.

## Epidemiology

Epidemiology is the overriding key to public health. It has a three-fold application in situations of armed conflict:

- initial assessments to identify problems and criteria so as to determine priorities;
- monitoring and systematic evaluation of progress in health work, including results;
- analysis of an epidemic.

## The Health-Care System

There must be a standard approach to health problems, in particular combining prevention and cure. The general rule whereby all health programmes must be an integral part of a proper health system applies equally in times of armed conflict. This chapter reviews some of the principles to be followed when setting up a health system.

## Disasters and Development

By their very nature, disasters imply emergency aid. Although the intervention methods and policy are quite clear, emphasis should be placed on renewing the link with development activities which existed before the conflict, or on creating the conditions for a smooth transition from humanitarian aid to a development process which will move into high gear once peace has returned.

## International Humanitarian Law

International humanitarian law applicable in situations of armed conflict comes within the ambit of health-care strategies. This chapter outlines the specific regulations for health-care personnel, for instance: the rules protecting non-combatants, the rights and duties of health-care personnel, respect for the red cross/red crescent emblem.

## Introduction to Humanitarian Ethics

Humanitarian ethics are normally in line with the rules governing humanitarian operations. Thus, respect for the traditions and beliefs of the victims, and the implementation of programmes corresponding to the needs of the victims rather than of the humanitarian agency concerned, are considerations which health personnel in the field must constantly bear in mind.

In order to focus more clearly on humanitarian ethics, this chapter concentrates on outlining the limitations of ethical considerations by referring back to the planning procedures described in Chapter 1.

# Chapter 1

# GENERAL PRINCIPLES OF PLANNING

***This first chapter is intended to define the elementary principles of planning, which will be illustrated throughout the rest of the handbook. No health programme can be set up unless these elementary principles have been mastered.***

# 1. Outlining a Plan

There may seem to be little point in planning a relief operation, since obviously the constraints of an emergency situation will necessitate constant changes in any plan of action. Yet, in fact, the more complex the situation is, the more a rational approach becomes imperative; otherwise, the operation is apt to flounder in the midst of confusion. Although most emergency relief organizations recognize this, we need only read a few mission reports to see how badly assimilated the terminology is, and to what extent the different planning stages are lumped together.

The organizers of relief operations are also commonly advised to assess the operation's achievements. Yet they cannot do this unless the objectives of the operation were laid down at the outset.

Many planning blueprints exist already; some of them are very complex, others use a jargon that medical personnel unaccustomed to the planning process find difficult to follow. Bearing in mind the problems inherent in emergency situations (shortage of time, difficulty of identifying health problems in the absence of reliable information), I will define a simple, easily assimilated planning procedure that strikes a balance between the necessity of planning operations and the need to act quickly in situations where plans cannot be tested in advance.

## 1.1 Definition of the Planning Process

*"A continued process of anticipating the resources and services required to achieve objectives determined according to an order of priority that permits the selection of the optimal solution or solutions from among several alternatives; these choices take account of the context of internal and external constraints, whether already known or foreseeable in the future."* [1]

*"The core of planning...is the analysis of alternative means of moving toward identified...goals in the light of specified priorities and existing constraints."* [2]

---

1 R. Pineault, *La planification de la santé* (1986), p. 35.
2 W. Reinke, *Health Aspects, Overview of the Planning Process* (1972), p. 63.

Empirically, we can establish a plan containing all the elements mentioned in these two definitions by asking a series of questions in a logical order.

## 1.2 Defining the Plan

### What Is Happening?

The raw data that flow in during a disaster are often imprecise and contradictory, and are certainly an inadequate basis for deciding whether action should be taken, and, if so, in what form. The first requirement, then, is to make an initial assessment of the situation.

### What Is Important?

The initial assessment will bring into focus a set of problems, some of them more important than others. The task here is to identify the problems of highest priority.

### What Can Be Done?

Pinpointing the most urgent problems does not mean they can be solved. At this point, the constraints of the situation help establish priorities for action.

### What Will Be Done?

To decide what should be done, planners must take note of existing norms and the constraints of the situation. This will allow them to define the limits of what can be realistically attempted — in other words, to set objectives.

### How Will It Be Done?

To achieve a particular objective, planners can choose between several types of activities. Initially, they must define all the activities that can be undertaken to accomplish a specific objective, and then decide which will actually be carried out and in what order — in short, determine a strategy.

### With What Will It Be Done?

Implementing the activities chosen will require the use of resources (human, material, financial, etc.), so resources must be planned.

### Implementation

The activities are carried out.

## What Was Done?

The evaluation of what has been done should cover not only the quantities of resources used, but the entire planning process (quality of services provided, impact on the victims' health, and so on). This is known as evaluation and surveillance.

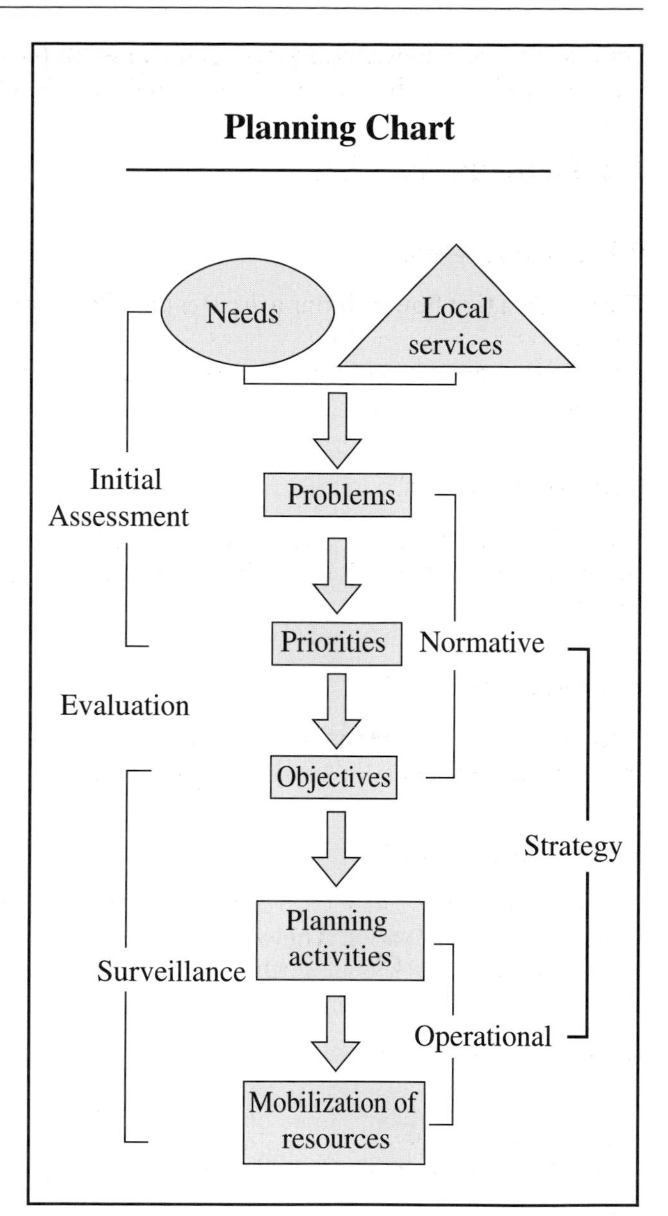


All these aspects, when listed one after the other, together define a planning sequence, as follows:

- identify the problems
- establish priorities for action
- set objectives
- plan activities
- mobilize resources
- supervise

All these stages can also be grouped under three broad headings:

- initial assessment of problems and priorities
- program design
- evaluation and surveillance of the operation

# 2. Initial Assessment

## 2.1 Concept

The aim here is not to try to memorize lists of questions that can be found in every manual on emergency relief, but rather to define the general principles underlying an initial assessment. To make such an assessment correctly, the first requirement is to know what information to look for. Finding it is then a simple matter.

Two principles are fundamental:

1. An emergency situation is defined in relation to a "normal" situation, which is characterized by a certain equilibrium between the needs of a population and the services designed to meet those needs. If, for one reason or another, these services are no longer able to fulfill the population's needs, the result is an imbalance which, depending on its magnitude and seriousness, may lead to real catastrophe.

Thus, the problems that relief planners try to identify derive from an evident imbalance between the victims' needs and local resources. This means assessing not only the victims' status (health, nutrition, employment, etc.), but also the state of the local services (agriculture, market, health services, etc.). The assessor may note, for example, the coexistence of:

- a large number of wounded and an absence of surgical facilities;
- a high rate of severe malnutrition and crop destruction;
- widespread diarrheal illnesses and consumption of polluted water.

2. An emergency situation is not simply a photograph taken at a given moment. It follows a dynamic made up of two elements: the causes of imbalance and the potential evolution of that imbalance in the short and medium terms.

- The initial assessment should help planners decide on priorities for action. These priorities must take causes as well as consequences into account.
- The initial assessment should provide information on the future evolution of the situation, in order to limit as much as possible the hazards of "risky" decisions — always a feature of situations of this type.

## 2.2 Problems

### Defining the Problems

The degree of imbalance between the needs (psychological, social, security, etc.) of a population and the local services available to meet them should be measured. The role of international aid derives from the concept of imbalance between the two.

It is commonly said that every situation is different. Nonetheless, every major type of disaster involves certain standard problems which must be understood before they can be correctly identified in the field. These problems also necessitate familiarization with the use of certain measuring techniques (quantitative assessment of a hospital, anthropometric assessment, etc.).[3]

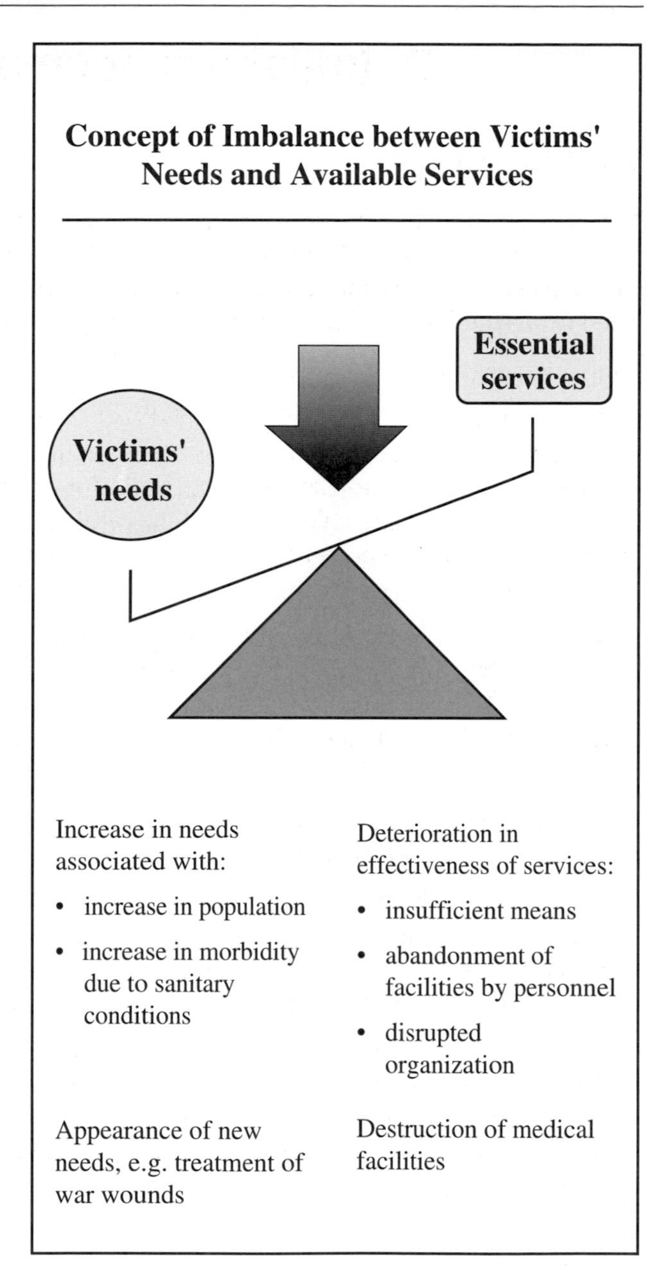


## Collecting Data

To define problems, the planner must rely on a set of data describing the populations involved and their environment.[4] Numerous ready-made assessment questionnaires are available, in which the evaluator need only check the correct box for each question. Such forms are useful in that they force the evaluator to collect data systematically. They should not, however, be allowed to obscure the fact that collecting information is not an end in itself, but rather

3 These methods will be studied in the relevant chapters.
4 The word "environment" should be understood in the broad sense, including — in addition to the physical and climatic environment — social (health services), economic (access to food resources), and other conditions.

a means of identifying the health problems directly or indirectly linked to the disaster.

### Synthesizing the Data

The sheer mass of data may make interpretation difficult, so the genuinely important facts must be singled out and then put in simple and schematic order.

### Analyzing the Data

Simply identifying problems is not enough. An assessment team should analyze health problems with the following points in mind:

- *the determining factors:*
  Severe malnutrition may be due to lack of access to food, but it may also be related to infectious diseases, an unhealthy environment, or social and cultural taboos. Moreover, a high rate of malnutrition that began abruptly does not have the same significance as one that is the result of a long process of deterioration. Familiarity with the previous living conditions of the population in question is therefore an essential counterbalance in any analysis of the population's current health problems.

- *the extent of the problems:*
  Simply perceiving problems is not enough. An attempt must be made to quantify them (extent of the problem, number of people affected).

- *the context:*
  The problems perceived have a particular context (ecological, economic, sociocultural, and political) that should also be analyzed during an initial assessment. This is the point at which planners encounter most of the constraints that will ultimately limit their options for action.

## 2.3 Establishing Priorities

Every emergency situation comprises a multitude of problems that cannot be addressed simultaneously. Consequently, priorities must be established, on the basis of precise criteria rather than the mood of the moment.

### Selection Criteria

There are two key factors in establishing priorities: the extent of the problems and their urgency. These factors can be measured by means of data on the number of victims, the degree to which local services have deteriorated, mortality, and morbidity. A problem should not become a priority for action, however, unless intervention is actually possible. Accordingly, planners must analyze:

- *the feasibility of a technical solution:*
  Technical effectiveness is judged on the basis of recognized terms of reference or identical experiences in similar situations.

- *the magnitude of the constraints:*

a) Political constraints:
   - Difficult access to the victims is a constant in conflict situations. It may result from security factors which prevent access to the conflict zone, or reasons of state, in the name of which access to the victims is prohibited.

b) Logistic constraints:
   - Pitfalls lie everywhere in the logistical chain, from the purchase of supplies to their distribution to the victims, and include:
   - storage difficulties;
   - transport delays (very substantial in the case of goods transported by boat);
   - communication lines may prove inoperable due to weather or security conditions.

c) Administrative "red tape" does not constitute a formal constraint, but it slows down the aid process (relief supplies may be held up by customs officials in the target country).

d) Organizational constraints, involving essentially:
   - administrative disorganization of local services. It is sometimes difficult to find people with the authority to make decisions or willing to do so (to authorize passage for aid, to authorize the use of local resources, etc.).
   - population instability. Conflict situations are characterized by frequently unpredictable population movements.
   - the medical personnel's inexperience with unusual situations (both expatriate and local personnel).

**Examples of Constraints**

1. POLITICAL CONSTRAINTS
   - Reasons of State
   - The sovereignty of the State
   - Disinformation
   - Lack of security
2. LOGISTICAL CONSTRAINTS
   - Shipping delays
   - Customs formalities
   - Storage problems
   - Communication problems
3. ORGANIZATIONAL CONSTRAINTS
   - Mobility of the victims
   - The number of victims
   - Administrative disorganization
   - Inexperience of professional health-care workers
4. FINANCIAL CONSTRAINTS
   - The high cost of relief operations
   - The channeling of financial resources towards certain types of situations to the detriment of others

– budgetary restrictions, which limit the response to problems.

### Establishing Priorities

The establishment of priorities is a function of technical feasibility and the constraints encountered in the field. Thus, it may be necessary to concentrate on certain problems, certain population groups, or certain geographical areas. Such restrictions, however, should not be considered definitive. For example, where lack of security makes a satisfactory aid response impossible, relief coordinators should negotiate with the competent authorities to find a solution to the problem. The first priority is negotiation, which, if successful, will be followed by the appropriate technical intervention.

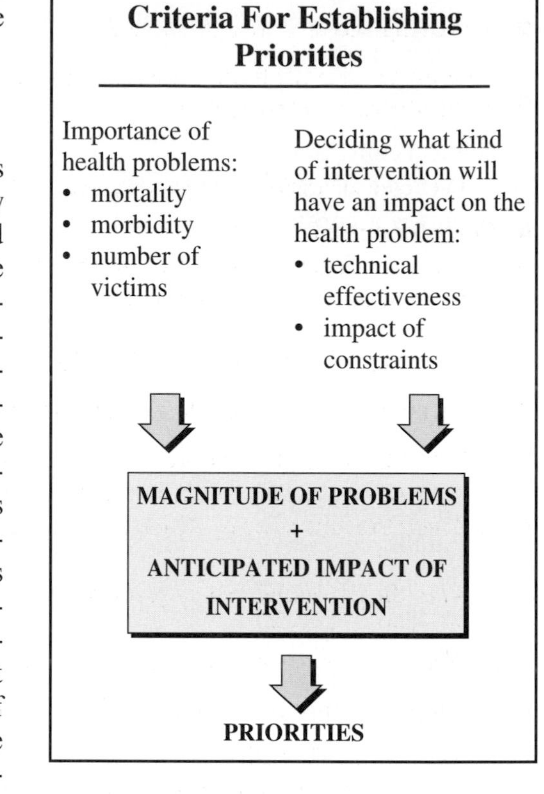


# 3. Conceiving a Program

## 3.1 Establishing Objectives

Establishing objectives is the most difficult stage of the planning process. Basically, it consists in translating an idea — usually a very general one — into specific activities.

The purpose of a relief operation in the health field is to improve and/or to maintain a population's health status. A pious wish indeed — but one which provides absolutely no clue as to how the deed can be done. To come to any practical conclusions regarding the actions to be taken, planners must break down objectives into increasingly specific elements. Thus, improving the health status of a particular population might involve, for example:

- covering food needs;

- reducing the rate of communicable diseases;
- improving access to health services.

The definition of objectives is governed by certain rules, the aim being to move from the abstract to the concrete.

### *An Objective Should Always Be Expressed by an Active Verb*

- *Cover* food needs;
- *Reduce* the incidence of communicable diseases;
- *Improve* access to health services.

### *An Objective Should Be Stated in Descriptive and Quantified Terms*

"An objective [...] must include a specification of:

- *1. What:* the nature of the situation or condition to be attained;
- *2. Extent:* the quantity or amount of the situation or condition to be attained;
- *3. When:* the time at or by which the desired situation or condition is intended to exist;
- *4. Who:* the particular group of people or portion of the environment in which attainment is desired;
- *5. Where:* the geographical area to be included in the program."[5]

More simply, an objective can be broken down as follows:

- a statement of the action to be undertaken;
- the target: a population group, a group of services, etc.;
- the expected results;
- the expected duration of the operation.

### *Stating the Action: What Is to Be Done?*

In the example of malaria control, the following goals would serve as the basis for a combination of different activities:

- Reduce the transmission of malaria.
- Reduce deaths linked to malaria.

In the first case, the main activity would be controlling malaria vectors, while in the second, treatment of clinical cases would take precedence.

In emergency situations, most health objectives will aim, at least initially, at reducing mortality and morbidity.

---

5 W. Reinke, *Health Planning, Overview of the Planning Process* (1972), pp. 63-64.

### *The Target*

The tendency is to confuse "target" with "target population." Obviously, in discussing health operations, people think first of population groups, as in this objective, for example:

– Reduce the incidence of measles in children aged nine months to five years.

Nonetheless, it may often be necessary, particularly during emergencies, to set objectives for groups of facilities:

– Maintain the supply of medicines to dispensaries in a given geographical area.

### *Anticipated Outcome*

The statement of anticipated outcome should take two factors into account:

– *Generally accepted standards.* For example, the rule for supplying water is 20 liters per person per day, while a basic food ration is 2,200-2,500 kilocalories (kcal) per person per day.
– *The context of a given situation.* For example, in a situation where water is scarce, relief providers may be obliged to moderate their ambitions and furnish perhaps only 10 liters of water a day. Care must be taken, however, not to fall below the minimum threshold of effectiveness. To provide 2 liters of water per person per day, when the temperature outside is 40°C (104°F), is akin to manslaughter. Similarly, distributing basic food rations that furnish only 1,000 kcal will not help reduce the mortality rate.

**Characteristics of a Health Objective**

An objective should incorporate:

1. Statement of the health problem.
2. Definition of the population targeted by the relief program.
3. Statement of the results expected from the operation.
4. Estimated length of time necessary to attain the expected result.

### *When Can the Desired Outcome Be Expected?*

In emergency situations, it is very difficult to estimate the length of time a program will have to run in order to achieve the desired result. In conflict situations, the numerous constraints — mostly political — make estimates unreliable. Nevertheless, precision is still desirable, even if obstacles to the operation must be taken into account in the interpretation of results.

## Formulating Objectives

The formulation of an objective should include all four elements listed above — for example, "reduce the rate of malnutrition from 20% to 5% among children under the age of five within three months."

Defining objectives is often considered to be an intellectual exercise of no practical value, when in fact it is a key element of the planning process. Defining objectives obliges planners to determine what action is possible and realistic in a given context, and to adopt some sort of yardstick by which to assess the results of a program.

Once the general objectives have been defined, the same principle should be used to define increasingly precise goals. For example, the general objective of reducing deaths attributable to malaria[6] can be broken down as follows:

- treat clinical cases;
- identify 80% of the malaria cases appearing in health facilities;
- establish procedures for the treatment of all malaria cases;
- supply health facilities with anti-malarial drugs;
- train health-care personnel.

## Moving from Objectives to Action

The idea here is to slide imperceptibly from the general objectives to concrete measures; paring objectives down to some extent allows planners to define practical activities[7] — for example, "to supply medical facilities with essential medicines." We know what we are actually supposed to do.

## Moving from Activities to Specific Tasks

It is a good idea to take the planning process still further and break down activities into specific tasks. The activity mentioned in the preceding section, for example — "supply medical facilities with essential medicines" — can be broken down as follows:

- decide what medicines to provide;
- decide which dispensaries to assist;
- purchase medicines;

---

[6] Only a single objective is analyzed here as an example. All the measures used to control malaria will be studied in the chapter on communicable diseases.

[7] R. Pineault, *La planification de la santé* (1986), p. 345.

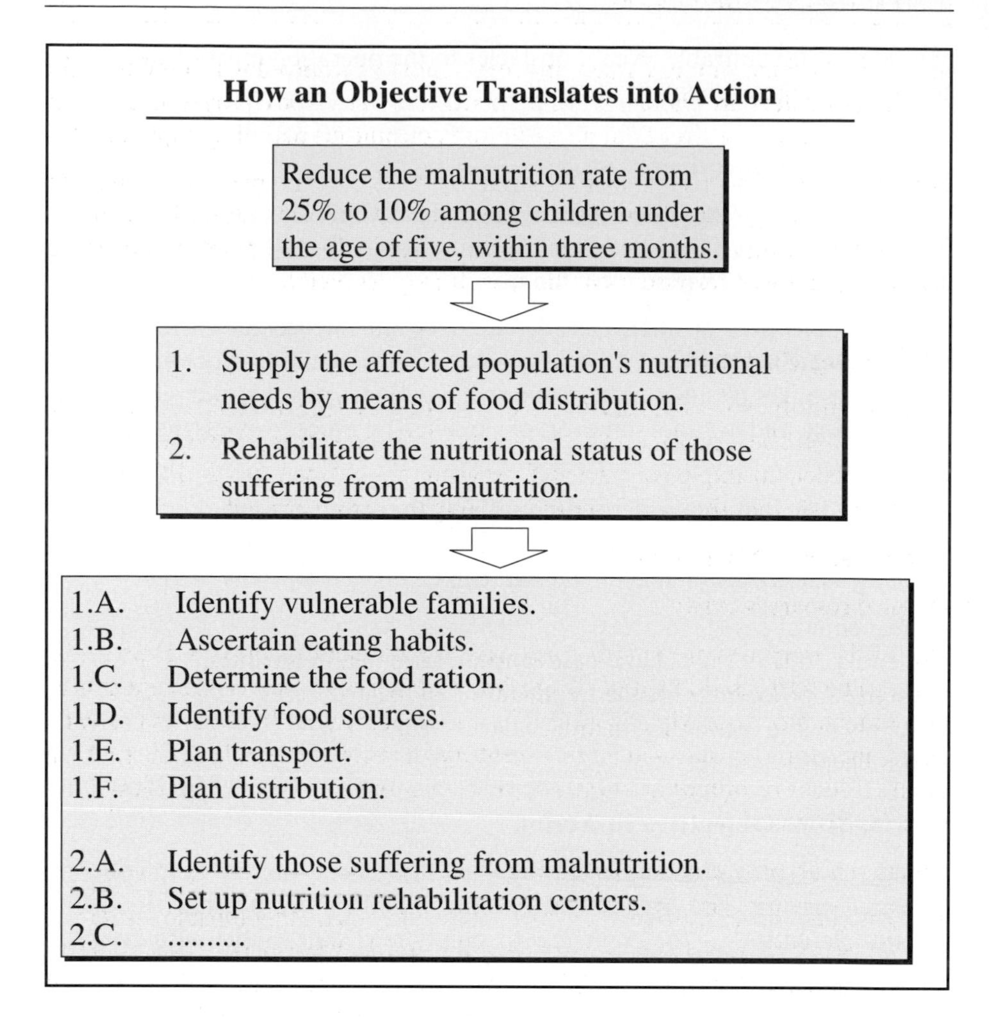


- transport medicines;
- distribute medicines;
- evaluate the use of the medicines.

Pinpointing specific tasks makes it easy to determine the resources necessary to carry them out:

- to purchase medicines > financial resources;
- to transport medicines > vehicles;
- to choose, transport, and distribute medicines > manpower.

Breaking down an activity into tasks may be a never-ending process, since each task in turn can be broken down still further. In emergency situations, tasks must be well defined so that everyone knows what he or she is supposed to do; but care should be taken not to err on the side of an administrative overemphasis on meticulous planning. For one thing, too much perfectionism is apt to take up a great deal of time, whereas urgent problems must be resolved without delay; for another, disasters are characterized by frequent and drastic changes in the basic circumstances of the situation, necessitating continuous planning adjustments.

Different activities may involve similar tasks. For example, food must be transported for general food distribution, for nutrition rehabilitation centers, and to feed hospital patients. Tasks should therefore be coordinated in order to optimize the use of resources (in this case, transport facilities).

## Mobilizing Resources

To carry out the tasks described above, a set of human, material, and financial resources must be mobilized. A fundamental decision at this point is whether the means needed to implement a relief program should be mustered from local sources or whether they will have to be brought in from abroad.

Two questions are paramount:

**Do local resources exist?**

One of the purposes of the initial assessment is to highlight any local potential that can be harnessed in aid of the victims of a disaster. This assessment can be made much more quickly and easily if a contingency plan for disasters already exists, including, in particular, an inventory of resources available in such an event. If local resources are nonexistent or insufficient, then international aid must be mobilized.

**Do the victims have access to local resources?**

The existence of local resources does not necessarily mean that outside assistance is of no value. In some cases — essentially for political reasons — the victims do not have access to local services. This is the case, for example, when the victims of a conflict live in an area cut off from regular health-care services, or when refugees do not have access to the services of the host country.

The role of international agencies — particularly the International Committee of the Red Cross (ICRC) — in situations of armed conflict is to guarantee access to routine services. When such access cannot be protected, a decision must be made as to whether international material aid will be necessary.

International aid must correspond to the real needs of the victims, and it must arrive in time. Aid that is not suited to local customs or that is disproportionate to the requirements of the situation should definitely be avoided.

Resources can be divided into four categories:

- *Human resources:*
  Local personnel are better acquainted with the victims' problems and sociocultural environment than expatriates are. The human resources in developing countries, however, are often insufficient. Mobilizing them in time

of disaster may tend to disrupt normal activities. Moreover, in situations of conflict, expatriate personnel often have easier access to the victims than local personnel, for security reasons.

- *Material resources:*
  The choice of material resources used during exceptional situations depends on various criteria:
  - compatibility with local customs;
  - rapid mobilization;
  - easy storage;
  - easy distribution.

To meet all these conditions, the choice of material resources must be considered in advance. There are numerous standard lists of supplies and equipment (drugs, medical supplies, food, water supplies, etc.) which offer a satisfactory compromise in this respect.

- *Transport facilities:*
  Transport is essential for the proper functioning of a relief operation, especially during the urgent phase, when speed is of the essence for the success of the operation. It should be noted, however, that air transport is very expensive, and is reserved for extreme cases.

- *Financial resources:*
  Compared to the usual relief actions, emergency operations are generally very expensive, for several reasons:
  - resources are mobilized from abroad;
  - resources have to be mobilized rapidly (the cost becomes exorbitant if air transport is necessary);
  - autonomous facilities are constructed (hospitals, dispensaries, etc.).
    Naturally, every effort should be made to implement relief programs as cheaply as possible, but the cost-effectiveness factor is very relative in emergency situations. The humanitarian ethic is based, above all, on the principle of assisting victims who are in immediate need; and this type of operation is costly. Lack of resources, however, may lead relief coordinators to modify their objectives.

## 3.2 Determining a Strategy

Traditionally, the word "strategy" is used to define the order of priorities and objectives (normative planning), while the word "tactics" defines the order of operational goals, the activities deriving from them, and the mobilization of resources to carry out those activities (structural planning). To avoid terminological overload, I will use only the word "strategy" here, specifying its application.

## Applying the Strategy to General Objectives

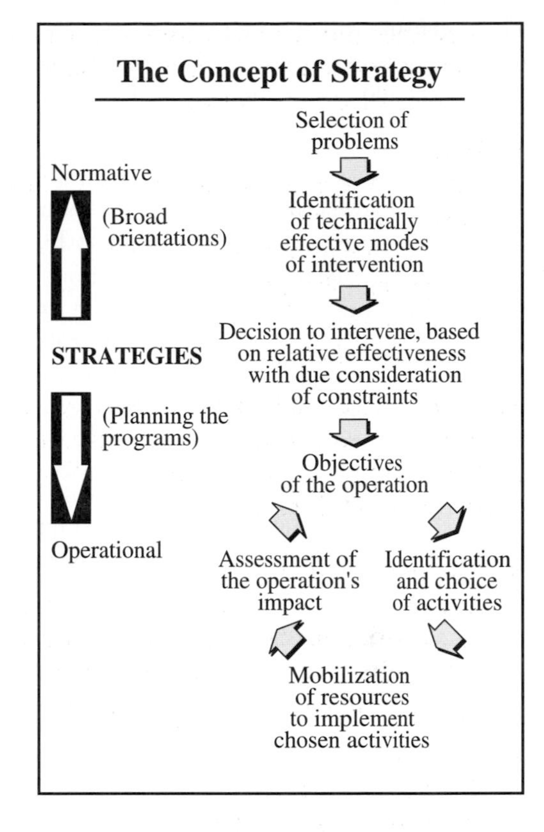


General objectives concern the broad orientations that will be adopted — for example:

- insure that all patients have access to medical care;
- prevent the appearance of communicable diseases;
- guarantee a supply of clean water for the entire population.

The first strategic level consists in selecting the most urgent objectives and/or deciding in what order they should be pursued. In the example above, this means deciding whether to emphasize prevention and assign priority to the last two objectives; or, alternatively, choosing a curative orientation — that is, exclusively the first objective. In emergency situations, organizations will occasionally concentrate on caring for the sick, without bothering to take necessary preventive measures for the general population. Yet it is difficult to treat diarrhea without taking account of the water supply and personal and family hygiene.

A strategic error made at the beginning of an operation may have dramatic consequences for the future.

## Applying the Strategy to Activities and Specific Objectives

This approach has the merit of being systematic. Planners are obliged to review all conceivable measures, knowing they will have to settle for the more realistic ones and to respect the rules needed to establish a coherent program.

To achieve a specific operational objective, planners may be able to choose between several types or combinations of activities. Defining their strategy will consist in deciding which activities are most appropriate, not only in terms of technical effectiveness, but also in terms of the local sociocultural context and the political and logistical constraints that condition the situation.

Thus, in order to supply a population with water within a time limit of 24 hours, relief workers may resort to distributing drinking water by means of tank trucks for the first days of the operation. This solution, though quickly implemented, is costly; but it gives planners time to organize a less expensive, autonomous supply system.

The technical effectiveness of an operation should not be judged merely on the basis of its short-term effects, but also by its possible long-term impact. For example, the distribution of food may effect a rapid improvement in a population's nutritional status; but in the long run it may also help turn beneficiaries into chronic aid recipients, totally dependent on external assistance. Accordingly, planners of food relief schemes should consider from the outset alternative measures that, in the medium term, could make the populations concerned self-sufficient.

In this case, the strategy for action would be a combination of two types of activity, both with the same purpose — namely, to give a population access to food resources — but with different, complementary timeframes.

## Applying the Strategy to Task Implementation and Resource Mobilization

At this stage, strategy does not affect the choice between tasks, since it derives from activities that have already been selected. It affects rather the order in which tasks will be performed and in which the necessary resources will be mobilized. For example, there is no point in selecting essential drugs to supply to dispensaries without first collecting data on the dominant pathologies, local habits, and so on. Similarly, transport should not be mobilized if the supplies to be transported are not available. Here, strategy must be combined with common sense.[8]

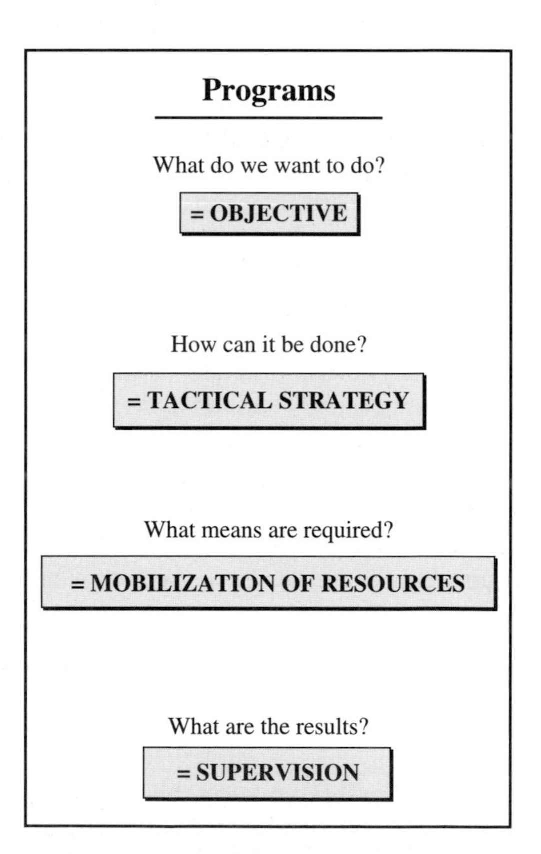


[8] Contrary to popular belief, common sense is not the world's best distributed asset.

**Health programs are often empirically conceived and based on the idea that they are indispensable in a given context, and no analytical effort is made to ascertain whether they are necessary, coherent, and amenable to integration with other programs. The method I propose for designing them may therefore seem complex, even finicky. Nonetheless, it calls for a rigorous analysis of what the operation is supposed to do, which is essential for a correct preliminary conception and evaluation of outcome.**

# 4. Evaluation and Surveillance

This last stage in the planning process is often neglected, owing to a tendency to consider emergency operations as essentially concrete actions to benefit needy victims. In this context, setting up a system to supervise programs and assess their impact on health is considered a secondary activity, or, indeed, a waste of time. Nonetheless, there is currently a trend towards better supervision of aid programs, thanks to the increasing involvement of epidemiologists in relief operations.

## 4.1 Definition of the Concept

P. Fournier defines the evaluation process as follows:

*"Very schematically, programmatic planning has consisted in defining a problem and then in describing the ways of addressing it. The program in question is applied in inverse sequence: Resources are mobilized to produce activities leading to results that must correspond to the stated objectives."* [9]

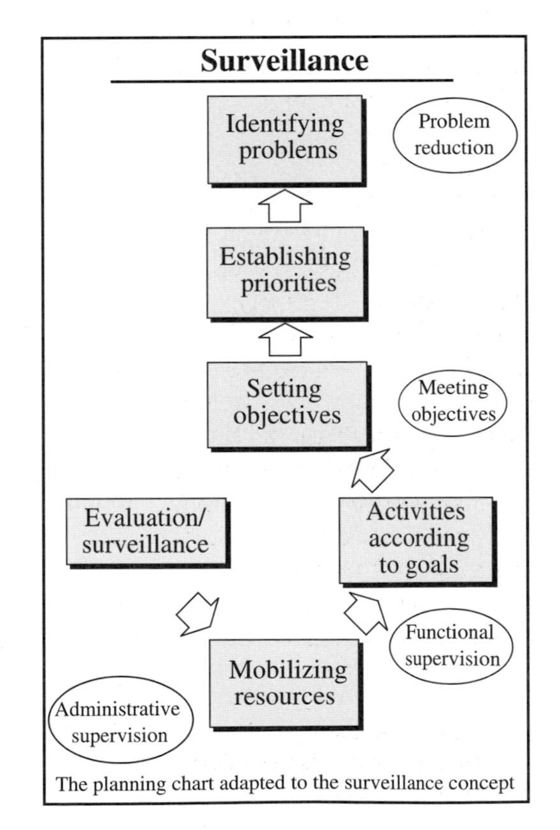


The planning chart adapted to the surveillance concept

9 P. Fournier, "Généralités sur le processus de planification," in A. Rougement and J. Brunet-Jailly, eds., *La santé dans les pays tropicaux* (Paris: Doin Editeurs, 1989), p. 105.

Taking the planning process in reverse offers a simple means of identifying levels of reference for a surveillance system:

- resources used (mobilization, appropriateness);
- services provided (quality, quantity);
- victims' health status (impact).

## 4.2 Analysis of Surveillance Levels[10]

### Analysis of Resources Used (Input)

Input analysis is both qualitative and quantitative.

- *Qualitative analysis*: This type of analysis is concerned with whether the medicines sent corresponded to the real needs of the victims, whether the food distributed suited the dietary habits of the beneficiaries, whether the means of transport used were adapted to the communication routes, whether the personnel employed had the appropriate training for the tasks demanded of them.

- *Quantitative analysis*: The purpose of quantitative analysis is to monitor the quantities of resources used and the ends to which they are put.

### Analysis of Services Provided (Output)

- *Qualitative analysis*: Did the services provided (medical consultation, distribution of food rations, provision of water) correspond to the norms defined in the objectives, to local habits, and to technical standards of effectiveness? Did the criteria followed during an immunization campaign conform to the standards proposed by the agency and/or the health ministry of the country?
  Objective analysis of the quality of services may prove difficult — for example, evaluating the quality of medical care offered in the course of an outpatient consultation.

- *Quantitative analysis*: Does the number of food rations distributed correspond to the total quantity of food sent? Does the number of vaccines dispatched[11] match the number of children immunized?

---

[10] These levels can also be defined as follows:
– Input (IP) = resources
– Output (OP) = services provided
– Outcome (OC) = impact on health status.

[11] Taking into account a certain rate of loss.

### Analysis of Impact on Victims' Health Status (Outcome)

Analyzing the operation's impact on the victims' health status is by far the most important part of the evaluation, since its purpose is to determine whether the relief operation has effectively assisted the disaster victims (effectiveness). Measures of effectiveness which are grouped can reveal a trend. To assess a program's impact, we must compare its results with the operational objectives established at the beginning of the intervention.

In practical terms, the following conditions are necessary:

- the objectives must specify the health problem, the target population, and the expected outcome of the operation;
- the objective must be composed of measurable elements;
- the measuring methods must be reproducible.

Thus, the evaluator might ascertain, for example:

- whether the rate of malnutrition has fallen from 15% to 5%, as specified in the original objective (effectiveness);
- whether any cases of measles have been diagnosed in the immunized groups (utility);
- whether the incidence of diarrheal illnesses has been reduced by 75% following the implementation of sanitation measures.

## 4.3 Analysis of Interaction between Levels

The relations between levels are also the subject of analysis — for example:

- evaluation of the quality and quantity of services provided in relation to the resources mobilized for that purpose. It is possible to determine the "cost" of a hospital patient, a child in a nutrition rehabilitation center, etc.
- evaluation of the appropriateness of the activities set up in relation to the problems identified at the outset.
  - Has the provision of water contributed to reducing the rate of diarrheal illnesses?
  - Have medical examinations decreased the number of deaths linked to malaria?
- evaluation of service coverage, meaning the ratio between the number of people benefiting from the program and the total number of people targeted by it.[12]

[12] A distinction must be made between different levels of coverage:
- Appropriate coverage, which corresponds to the number of people who have used the services as a percentage of those who should have used them;
- Effective coverage, which corresponds to the proportion of the population affected by the services who actually benefited from an efficacious service.

This idea is the basis, for example, for the entire analysis of immunization program effectiveness, which looks at the number of measles cases among those immunized versus the number of cases among the non-immunized population.

An evaluation should not be considered simply as a way of measuring the performances of an intervention after the fact, but also as a navigational guide to be used while the intervention is in progress. Repeated during the operation itself, it permits planners to modify their orientation if interim evaluations reveal obvious gaps in the program. Moreover, this type of evaluation is essential for learning lessons that can be applied in subsequent operations, and is a basis for operations research.

**Concept of Surveillance**

Regular gathering of information to obtain objective elements making it possible to:

- define tendencies
- detect epidemics
- reorient a program
- stop a program

Global evaluation of a situation to obtain an overall view of it that can be compared with the initial situation.

**The concepts covered in the chapter on planning may seem theoretical. Nevertheless, they are essential in order to give all course participants a common methodology and vocabulary which will allow them to address jointly and rationally the practical problems discussed further on.**

**Naturally, emergency situations involve major constraints with regard to time, security, and communication — constraints which make strict adherence to this sort of planning procedure difficult. The absence of a plan, however, can only increase chaos in an already confused situation.**

Chapter 2

# FOOD AND NUTRITION

***Access to food is vital for every population; understandably, then, it is always an issue in emergency situations. Nonetheless, it should not be confused with food aid; and the simplest way to avoid that mistake is to examine the basic principles governing the satisfaction of a population's food needs. It will then be easier to understand the mechanisms underlying food emergencies and, consequently, to determine the measures required to deal with them.***

# 1. General Principles

To underline the complexity of the feeding problems that arise in emergency situations, I will begin with the basic principles underlying the concept of food access, namely:

- nutritional needs;
- food resources;
- factors balancing nutritional needs and food resources;
- levels of imbalance.

## 1. Nutritional Needs

*"Nutritional needs represent the average quantity of nutrients a person needs every day to remain in good physical and mental health, taking account of his or her physiological condition, sex, weight, age, environment, and physical activity."* [1]

The issue of quantifying nutritional requirements in the context of an emergency situation has aroused much controversy. Everyone, of course, agrees as to what those requirements are, as determined on the basis of the factors mentioned above. Differences arise, however, when it comes to deciding whether the coverage of nutritional requirements must conform as far as possible to conventional norms, or whether these norms can be adapted to the constraints of an emergency situation, in order to keep victims alive until they regain access to a regular food supply.

To provide a solid basis for discussion, a brief review of physiological nutritional requirements may be useful here.

1 A.M. Masse-Rainbault, "L'alimentation et la nutrition des populations," in Rougemont and Brunet-Jailly, eds., *Santé dans les pays tropicaux*, p. 671.

## 1.1 Classification by Type of Requirement

Nutritional requirements can be divided into four categories.

- *Energy requirements*, to maintain:
  - basal metabolic rate (BMR) — There are tables providing a breakdown of the specific needs of each organ (liver, heart, muscles, etc.). This rate can be calculated according to weight, gender, and age — for example:
    - for a 25-year-old man, BMR = 15.3 x weight in kg + 679
    - for a 45-year-old woman, BMR = 8.7 x weight in kg + 829
  - growth — Energy supply is particularly important for children, since it is a major contributor to healthy growth. The energy "cost" of growth is 5-10% of the total energy requirement.
  - physical activity — The magnitude of food energy needs depends directly on the types of physical activities undertaken; available tables show average values[2] based on the individual's activity level and gender.
  - response to cold — In emergency situations, victims often lack shelter, blankets, and clothing; this exposure to the cold increases energy needs.[3]
- *Protein requirements*
  Protein is necessary for cell growth and renewal. It is also essential for the synthesis of hormones and enzymes. This is not the place for a biochemical discussion of the protein values of different foods, but the following points should be noted:
  - Proteins of animal origin are better digested than plant proteins (digestibility coefficients are, respectively, 95% and 85%).
  - Proteins of plant origin are deficient in certain essential amino acids — cereals lack lysine, and legumes lack methionine.[4]
  - The level of protein utilization depends on energy intake: energy supplied by protein must be 10-12% of total intake.

---

[2] These values are usually expressed in terms of BMR values. Thus, a very active man would need an energy supply of BMR x 2.10, while a moderately active woman would need BMR x 1.64.

[3] "We call the temperature at which a rise of metabolic rate is evident the lower critical temperature (LCT: 25°)... During 1969, we measured the temperature in Nile, Western Ethiopia, in an area roughly analogous to the area where the Wollo famine occurred, and found that some 15 hours a day the temperature was below the LCT. The extra food demand imposed on men with light clothing and with no shelter would have been in excess of 1,000 Kcal per day or 300 gr. of cereals." J. Rivers, "Physiological Aspects of Shelter Deprivation," *Disasters* 3 (1): 21.

[4] These facts are important to remember when putting together a food ration. A basic ration can be constituted from foods of plant origin if cereals and legumes are combined to compensate for their respective deficits in essential amino acids.

– *Vitamin[5] and mineral requirements*

The necessity of furnishing a balanced vitamin intake — long underestimated in emergency relief operations — was largely demonstrated by recent experiences in Ethiopia and Sudan.[6]

Studies done in Indonesia[7] and in India[8] have shown that vitamin A supplements reduce mortality among preschool-age children (vitamin A plays an important role in the maintenance of mucous membranes, thus enhancing local resistance to penetration of viruses and bacteria). This finding has direct implications for emergency situations, since the food rations traditionally supplied in relief operations are low in vitamins, particularly vitamins A and C.[9]

In October, 1991, one of the conclusions reached by a conference entitled "Ending Hidden Hunger" was that vitamin and mineral deficiencies could have dramatic effects, and that governments should prepare intervention programs as quickly as possible. The possibility of furnishing vitamins and minerals by the vehicle of expanded programs of immunization (EPI) was suggested.

**WHY THE BODY NEEDS FOOD**

**AS A SOURCE OF ENERGY FOR:**

Basic metabolism
Growth
Physical activities
Maintaining body heat

**AS A SOURCE OF PROTEIN FOR:**

Growth
Maintenance
Production of enzymes
Production of hormones

**AS A SOURCE OF VITAMINS:**

Vitamin A
Vitamin $B_1$
Vitamin C

---

5 Vitamin A plays a role in vision, the immune system, and the maintenance of the mucous membranes. Vitamin C is instrumental in the maintenance of connective tissue and enhances iron absorption.

6 During the great famines between 1984 and 1988, widespread vitamin deficiencies were noted in Sudan and Ethiopia, particularly for vitamins A and C.

7 "Impact of Vitamin A Supplementation on Childhood Mortality," *The Lancet* (24 May 1986): 1170.

8 L. Rahmathullah *et al.*, "Reduced Mortality among Children in Southern India Receiving a Small Weekly Dose of Vitamin A," *The New England Journal of Medicine* 323, No. 14 (4 Oct. 1991).

9 "Many relief rations are more or less deficient in vitamins A, B complex, C, and in iron and zinc. There have been large outbreaks of scurvy and pellagra in some places." J. Seaman, "Management of Nutrition Relief for Famine-Affected and Displaced Populations," *Tropical Doctor*, Supplement 1 (1991): 39.

## 1.2 Classification by Age and Gender

A person's energy needs depend on his or her body weight. Although in absolute terms a child's requirements are lower than those of an adult, it must be remembered a child needs foods of high nutritive quality to satisfy nutritional needs, a quality which depends on the ratio of the food's weight to the amount of energy it provides, the presence of essential amino acids, etc. Pregnant and nursing women have increased energy needs.[10] All these factors must be taken into account in the composition of the food ration.

## 1.3 Average Nutritional Requirements

Average nutritional requirements can be established by the calculation of each individual's specific needs and the proportion of each category of persons in the population (children, adults, pregnant women, and nursing mothers). In 1971, a study published by the Swedish Nutrition Foundation proposed a subsistence ration of 1,220 kcal for a tropical environment.[11] Recommendations have evolved considerably since then, though the levels proposed by the different humanitarian organizations furnishing emergency food aid still vary widely. The ICRC suggests a ration providing 2,400 kcal and 70 grams of protein.[12]

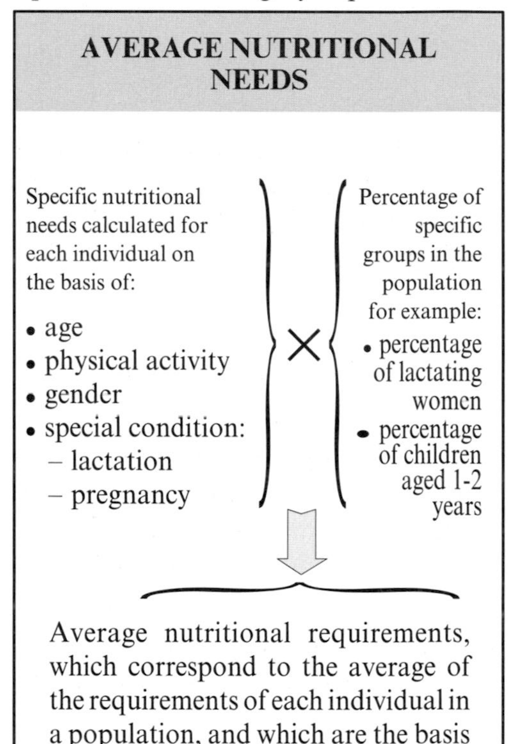


In general, the accepted level is in the neighborhood of 2,200 kcal. Obviously, this figure has no validity for a specific individual, since nutritional requirements are affected by age, sex, degree of physical activity, and other factors; yet the concept of average

---

10 The increase is approximately 350 kcal for women in the third month of pregnancy and 550 kcal for nursing mothers.

11 According to G.B. Masefield, this would be enough to maintain life for one month, though weight loss would be inevitable and no work could be expected of anyone subsisting on such a ration. See G.B. Masefield, "Nutrition and Relief Operations in Times of Disaster," in The Swedish Nutrition Foundation and the Swedish International Development Authority, *Famine* (1971), p. 170.

12 A. Mourey, *Nutritional Aspects of ICRC Assistance in Conflict Situations* (ICRC, 1988), p. 13.

needs is essential nonetheless, as an aid to understanding the mechanics of designing a food ration (which will be discussed in the context of food distributions). Moreover, for practical reasons, rations cannot be calculated individually for each recipient.

## 2. Food Resources

The selection of food resources should take various factors into account.

### *Nutrient Value*

All books on nutrition contain various tables classifying foods by nutritional value (calories, protein, vitamins, trace elements).

### *Origin*

The foods found in a given environment may have been produced locally, bought on the regional or national level, or imported from abroad. A description of local foods is important — not only the most common ones, but also those eaten during periods of crisis, which are not necessarily the same products consumed normally.

### *Acceptability to the Population*

Every population has its own food preferences. Most people are familiar with certain general preferences: Asians eat rice, Central Americans eat corn, and Africans eat wheat or corn. In addition, certain regional preferences may have important consequences for a population's nutritional status — for example, the consumption of cassava, polished rice, etc.

Thus, each population group has its own traditional diet. Since food has no nutritional value unless it is actually consumed, taking food preferences into account is imperative in emergency situations.

### *Degree of Processing*

The extent to which foods have been processed is important in emergency situations. Processed food products are often sent for emergency relief, since they are easier to use. Such products include precooked foods, mixtures of several foods in one product — for example, corn, soya, and milk (CSM), and food enriched with vitamins. Although such foods offer the theoretical advantage of being easy to use in the field, they may be unsuited to traditional eating habits and are subject to misuse.

# 3. The Food System

Analyzing the food system is a complex exercise. For the sake of simplicity, two aspects will be considered separately:

- the components of the food chain;
- the factors influencing the links of the food chain.

## 3.1 The Food Chain

The food chain can be defined as all the stages food products pass through in the process from production to consumption by individuals.

These stages may be defined as follows:

- *food production*, including local, regional, and national production. Imports are not included here; food aid, which is not, strictly speaking, production, enters through the distribution system.
- *food distribution*, meaning the way food resources circulate within a population.
- *food availability*. If production and distribution are satisfactory, food resources will be available in the population's immediate environment.
- *food consumption*. Availability does not mean food is uniformly distributed on the basis of the dietary needs of all the subgroups making up a population. Economic level, social origin, and political affiliation may affect an individual's access to food resources.
- *biological utilization*. Physical access to food (availability of food) and economic access (ability to buy what is available) are no guarantee of a uniform coverage of nutritional needs.

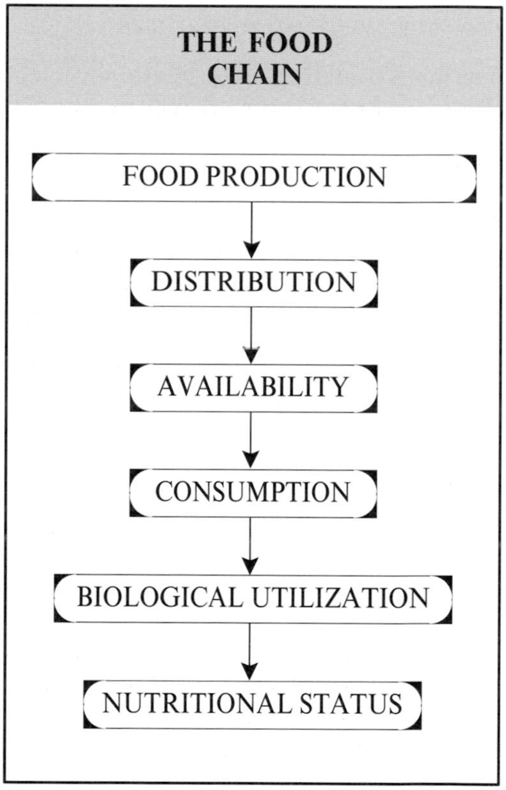

**THE FOOD CHAIN**

FOOD PRODUCTION
↓
DISTRIBUTION
↓
AVAILABILITY
↓
CONSUMPTION
↓
BIOLOGICAL UTILIZATION
↓
NUTRITIONAL STATUS

## 3.2 Parameters Normally Influencing Each Link of the Food Chain

Representing the food system in linear form reflects its progression, but not its complexity. Each stage is actually influenced by several factors, which must be studied if we are to have any real idea of the food system. It may be helpful to take as a typical example the food chain of a rural population in a developing country, and to identify the factors that come into play at each of the levels represented above.

### *3.2.1 Production*

The level of production depends on:

- *structural factors*
  - available arable land
  - quality of arable land (degree of soil erosion)
  - agricultural techniques
  - available equipment
  - ownership of land
- *circumstantial factors*
  - climate (period of drought)[13]
  - economic environment (access to seeds, tools, fertilizer, etc.)

The type of production also depends on many factors:

- *tradition*
- *the impact of national agricultural policies*, which may change production habits considerably — for example, they may encourage a shift from the cultivation of products intended for consumption as food (grains) to the cultivation of inedible agricultural products (cotton).
- *recourse to imports*, a measure that does not permit a long-term solution of the food deficit problem.

### *3.2.2 Distribution*

Distribution may be more or less complex, depending on various factors.

#### *The Existing Economic System*

If the country has a centrally planned economic system, the population's food resources are the food it produces and the food available in the local market. The control of goods, exchanged through a central system, guarantees a certain price stability, but does not encourage production. This type of system is gradually disappearing.

---

[13] According to E. Kennedy, a study carried out in Kenya on the 1984 drought showed that corn production had been 60% lower than in a normal year (1986). "The Impact of Drought on Production, Consumption and Nutrition in Southwestern Kenya," *Disasters* 16, No. 1 (March 1992): 11.

If the country has a liberal economic system, food products are bought and sold freely. This exchange mechanism, however, is governed by the laws of the market (prices fluctuate according to the quantity of goods available).

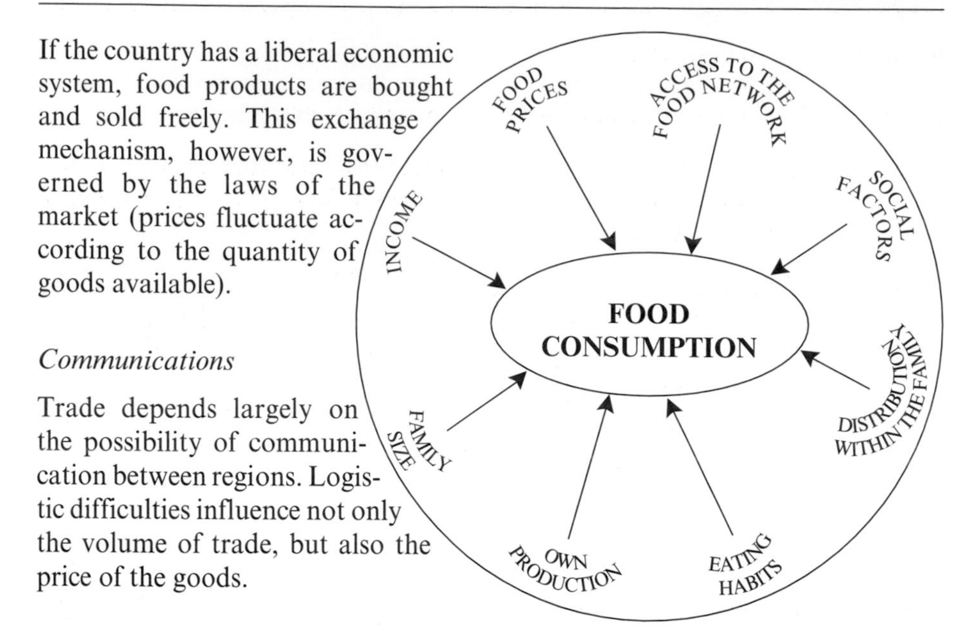


*Communications*

Trade depends largely on the possibility of communication between regions. Logistic difficulties influence not only the volume of trade, but also the price of the goods.

*The Social Fabric*

The way a population is organized socially also influences trade, particularly of agricultural resources. According to D. Rahmato,

*"peasants also attend markets to meet relatives and friends, to exchange information (about agricultural conditions, seasonal employment opportunities, etc.), to discuss exchange arrangements (livestock, loans, land renting, and the like), to make social deals (marriages, etc.)..."* [14]

The social aspect is particularly important when conditions become difficult and people fear a serious crisis that will disrupt access to food. At this point, local mechanisms of mutual assistance come into play. Thus, in societies that recognize the concept of the extended family, needy individuals are taken care of by relatives who have preserved their livelihood.

### *3.2.3 Availability of Food Resources*

Although food may be available in a population's environment, not all the population necessarily has access to it. Within a given population, the economic or social vulnerability, ethnic origin, or political affiliation of certain groups restricts their access to food resources. The distribution of food within a population can be studied by assessing food consumption at the subgroup or family level.

---

[14] D. Rahmato, "Peasant Survival Strategies in Ethiopia," *Disasters* 12, No. 4 (1988): 334.

### *3.2.4 Food Consumption*

The level of food consumption depends on various factors:

- **purchasing power**. This index is more representative than income, which does not take into account the very rapid fluctuations in food prices that may occur in certain exceptional circumstances.

- **agricultural production** for the producer's own consumption (especially common among rural populations living in some degree of autarky).

- **family size**. The accepted dogma is that large families are more vulnerable, but in emergency situations it has been noted that isolated persons, such as unaccompanied children and old people, are often prevented from reaching food.

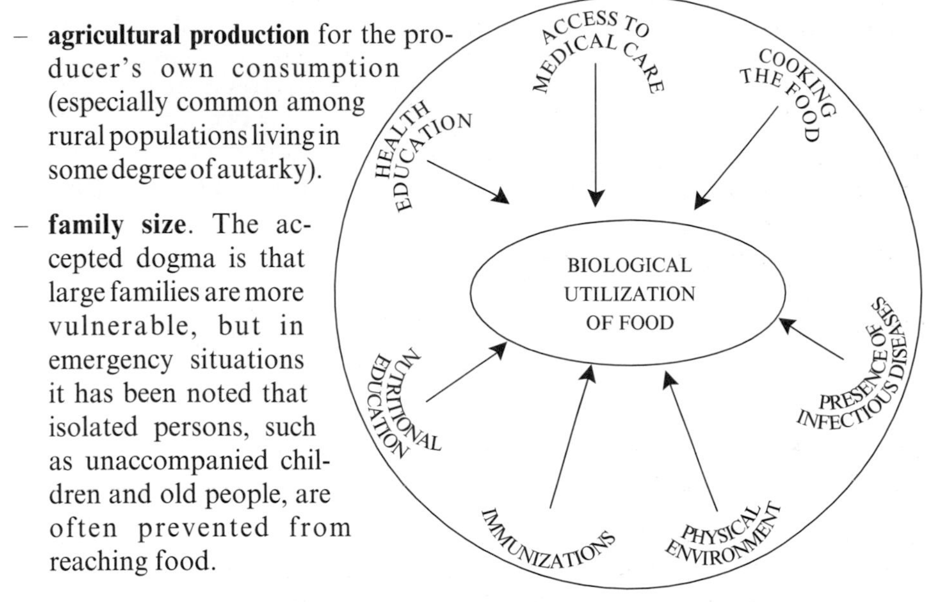


- **food distribution within the family**. A family's access to food resources does not guarantee an absence of malnutrition. Within the family, food is allocated according to culturally dictated principles. Although some cultures tend to favor the children, others give priority to the strongest members, those whose activity — work — insures the survival of the social group.

### *3.2.5 Biological Utilization of Food*

Consumption of food by an individual does not mean that the problems of food access have been resolved. Certain facts must be determined:

- whether the foods eaten supply the calories, protein, and vitamins needed by the organism. Certain foods — such as cassava, which is used as a staple food — do not cover the same spectrum of nutritional needs as cereals; and certain population groups traditionally reduce food intake during illness, a time when in fact nutritional needs are increased by fever, etc.

- whether the organism is able to absorb and digest the food adequately to extract the maximum nutritional value from it. Food absorption may be hindered by diarrheal illnesses and intestinal parasites.

This, then, is the outline of the food system, its central framework corresponding to the various links of the food chain, and its main branches corresponding to a series of factors affecting production, distribution, consumption, and so forth.

Yet this is still only a bare outline. Each main branch is itself influenced by other parameters. We can take the last link of the food chain, the biological utilization of food, as an example. It has been noted that disease (measles, diarrheal illnesses, intestinal parasitic infestations) affects the biological utilization of food consumed. If we trace these diseases back to their causes, we find poor hygiene, no immunization program, and a lack of clean water.

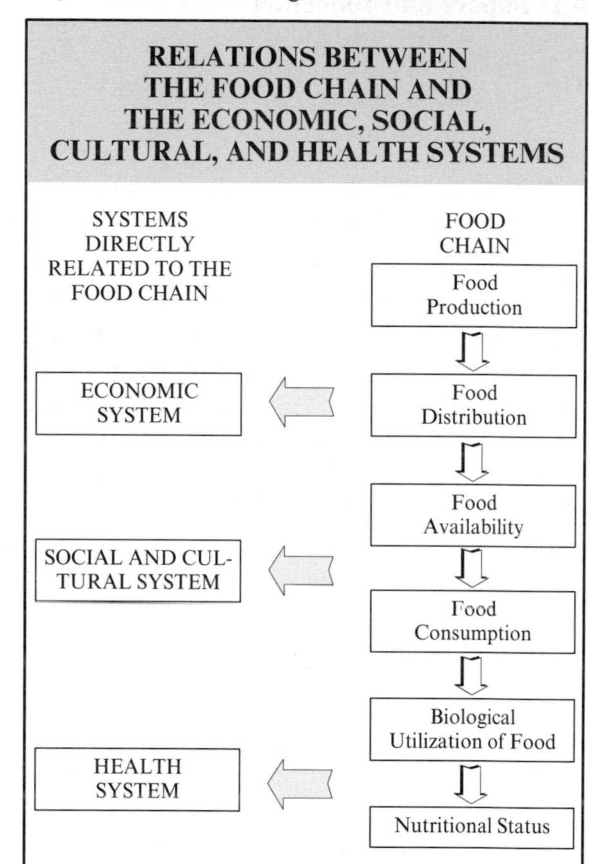


By following the branches of the food system in this way, we come to the health system. We could just as easily have taken the example of food consumption and ended up at the social system (production and distribution), which in turn leads into the economic and political systems. This chapter, however, will not discuss the relations between systems; that subject will be examined in Chapter 8 ("Disasters and Development").

## 4. The Impact of a Shock to the Food System and the Local Way of Life

We will not examine all the possible misfortunes that may affect the food system, but as an example we can take the impact of a drought or conflict on the essential links of the food system[15] in a rural population. The way the system adapts to the

[15] The complete exercise would be to define the impact of these calamities throughout the food system, including all its branches. The purpose of this lesson, however, is not to demonstrate the complexity of the food system, but rather to provide students with a tool to help them grasp its essential elements.

problem must be defined, as well as the disruptions that occur when the normal adaptation mechanisms are overwhelmed. Such disruptions may engender a true disaster, and are not limited to the food system, but have ramifications in the social, economic, and — sometimes — political systems as well. This section will discuss only local disruptions, leaving aside the subject of their repercussions for the entire country.

## 4.1 Impact on Production

Populations respond to crisis by means of various kinds of adaptations. Threatened by drought, for example, farmers can modify their production system — by increasing the area of land under cultivation to offset low yield, for example.[16] They can also vary the kinds of crops they grow, increasing cultivation of food crops at the expense of cash crops. Hungry populations may even seek out food products that they do not normally consume.[17]

However, disruptions occur when the adaptive mechanisms are inadequate to compensate for the lack of production. For example, a sedentary rural population may no longer be able to produce enough food for its own consumption needs following the destruction or confiscation of its crops, a major restriction of land,[18] or else the absence of alternative food resources. Similarly, the difficulty of obtaining seeds, tools, and draft animals to prepare for the new agricultural season is the beginning of a vicious circle in which the lack of means of subsistence and the lack of production means perpetuate each other.

These upsets have repercussions on the second link of the food chain.

---

[16] "The proportion of total areas planted to food crops was also higher in the drought period (49.2 percent) than non-drought periods (37 percent) across all household types as well." See E. Kennedy, "The Impact of Drought in Southwestern Kenya," *Disasters* 6, No. 1 (March 1992): 11.

[17] For example, D. Rahmato notes: "Generally speaking, berries like agam (clarissa edule) and quegga (rosa Abyssinica) are consumed, particularly by youngsters, in normal times as a snack or a treat. In distress conditions these berries are systematically collected and consumed in the family." "Peasant Survival Strategies in Ethiopia," *Disasters* 12, No. 4: 333. Similarly, J. Cekan has remarked: "Villagers responded to the food and income shortages by increasing outmigration. Across much of northern Mali, villagers rely on remittances from migrants to survive between February and June. The old and the young are left behind in the villages, while stronger family members find work elsewhere, often far away. But one should not underestimate the contribution made by those who remain in the villages to their own self-provisioning by, for example, producing and selling mats and soaps. They also supplement reserves by foraging for edible wild foods (roots, berries, insects) and selling firewood." See "Seasonal Coping Strategies in Central Mali: Five Villages During the Soudure," *Disasters* 16, No. 1: 67.

[18] The use of anti-personnel mines in rural areas can reduce the area of arable land considerably, since they force farmers to choose between reducing production or risking their lives among the landmines. Angola is a typical example of this situation.

## 4.2 Impact on Distribution

Problems in distribution may be due to a deficit in production, or they may occur even though production is normal. For example, the routine circulation of goods may no longer be possible. The consequences will be generally similar in both cases.

Adaptations may take place in the local economy or in the circulation of food. In the local economy, the scarcity of food leads to an increase in the prices of cereal products. Under these circumstances, farmers will maintain their purchasing power by selling their cattle. This move is succeeded by a flood of secondary effects, the main one being a drop in the price of cattle due to the surplus supply in the market. Alternatively, the economy may move towards a barter system, or financial reserves may be mobilized.[19] Yet another way that farmers may maintain purchasing power is by borrowing grain or money.[20]

Adaptation in the circulation of food operates through the mechanism of increased prices, which may promote the circulation of foodstuffs from producing regions to needy regions.

All these adaptation mechanisms rapidly reach their limits. Financial reserves dry up quickly as a result of the inflationary rise in cereal prices,[21] while the possibility of borrowing is greatly limited by the chronic insolvency of rural populations — a problem exacerbated by the circumstances of the disaster.[22]

Meanwhile, price increases are apt to give rise to speculation: merchants stockpile food, keeping it off the market until prices have reached the maximum. In addition, a conflict in the area may seriously impede the circulation of foodstuffs, since it can give rise to a blockade of the region or unsafe communication routes. In this case, the extent of the risk traders are willing to take to deliver food supplies will depend on the price they expect to get.

## 4.3 Impact on Availability of Food Resources

Lack of production[23] and/or dysfunctional distribution[24] affect the availability of food resources. Social adjustments are the main response. An initial

---

19 In the Sahelian countries, certain population groups may have substantial financial holdings.

20 G. Maddox, "Famine, Impoverishment and the Creation of a Labor Reserve in Central Tanzania," *Disasters* 15, No. 1: 37.

21 R. Hogg has described this problem: "Over the last year, high inflation in Somalia has reduced the value of the Somali shilling against the Ethiopian birr, reducing purchasing power for Ethiopian goods. Once the supply of goods from Somalia dried up — in particular grain and other goods denominated in Somali shillings — at the end of last year, pastoralists have been left with shillings and/or livestock which they are unable to exchange at reasonable rates to buy needed goods." See "Famine in the Ogaden," *Disasters* 15, No. 3: 272.

22 "There is reason to believe that rural money-lending dries up in times of serious food shortages, as the risks of lending are very high." D. Rahmato, "Peasant Survival Strategies in Ethiopia," p. 329.

23 Most common in cases of drought.

24 Most common in cases of conflict.

adjustment is the migration of laborers to regions where they can expect to find work.[25] In addition, families lacking food are sometimes assisted by relatives who are unaffected by the food shortage.

When purchasing power cannot be maintained, however, major social upheavals ensue as entire populations pick up and go elsewhere.

## 4.4 Impact on Food Consumption

Whether people have begun to migrate or whether they are still living in their original homes, the shortage of food will change the eating habits of both families and individuals. One way of adapting to the shortage is by eating uncustomary foods — for example, seeds intended for sowing. Another way is by restricting food intake.[26] Similarly, displaced people must adapt their diet to the foods they find in their new environment, particularly when they must rely on emergency food-aid rations.

The normal distribution of food within the family may be disrupted, with priority being given to those who can insure the survival of the household or group. However, the normal mechanisms are usually respected even in emergencies.[27]

## 4.5 Impact on the Nutritional Status of Individuals

Individual adaptation to lack of food is completely relative. If the individual is obese to begin with, the loss of weight due to food restriction is a positive adaptation. Reducing physical activity is another kind of adaptation; but the reduction of physical activity will also reduce work output, necessary for the production and distribution of food resources. In this way a vicious circle is created.

At a more advanced stage, malnutrition begins. It has already been shown that many factors influence nutritional status. During a disaster, the lack of food combined with poor hygiene (common in camps for displaced persons) or infections may result in a state of malnutrition.

---

[25] See J. Drèze: "Perhaps what struck me most was the fact that, for many people, life went on more or less as usual during the drought period. This applies particularly to wage labourers. Not only were they protected from starvation, they were also able to earn their living in a dignified way, to take their wage home and cook their own food." "Famine Prevention," *Disasters* 15, No. 3: 266.

[26] "This is where a peasant household's resource management system is put to its severest test as the needs of the family have to be carefully balanced with the available food resources, which have to be used frugally to make them last as long as possible. Resource management here also involves sharply altering the mix of food items normally consumed in the family as well as reducing their variety and quality." D. Rahmato, "Peasant Survival Strategies in Ethiopia," p. 329.

[27] J. Drèze wrote in connection with the state of Gujarat, India, "there are no indications that intra-familial distribution has severely worsened during the drought. Informal surveys suggest that children were probably protected, rather than neglected." *Op. cit.*, p. 266.

Malnutrition does not affect all individuals to the same degree, however. This can be attributed to a number of factors which increase the vulnerability of certain individuals or groups.

- Nutritional vulnerability linked to age:
  Children under the age of five years[28] are the most vulnerable nutritionally. This is because their food intake must respond to specific growth needs, because they are the most susceptible to infectious diseases, and, finally, because they may be subject to the detrimental effects of certain feeding practices.
- Vulnerability linked to physiological condition:
  Pregnant and breastfeeding women are more vulnerable to lack of food owing to their increased needs.
- Vulnerability linked to environmental conditions:
  - Physical environment
    It is recognized that environmental conditions play a predominant role in child development; a lack of clean water, regular contact with human refuse, and unhealthy living conditions are a few of the factors that interfere with normal development.
  - Cultural environment
    Certain feeding practices can have a devastating effect on nutritional status — for example, the custom of not feeding sick children.
  - Political environment
    The insecurity that prevails in most conflict situations tends to break up the family unit and separate family members, as well as straining family ties (disrupting the mother-child relationship, for example); this increased family vulnerability most affects children.
- Vulnerability linked to disease:
  A malnourished body is prone to infection; infectious diseases, in turn, may be the first step towards malnutrition. Generally speaking, sick people are particularly vulnerable to shortages of food appropriate for their condition.

[28] Current studies seem to indicate that the vulnerable period is from six months to three years rather than six months to five years.

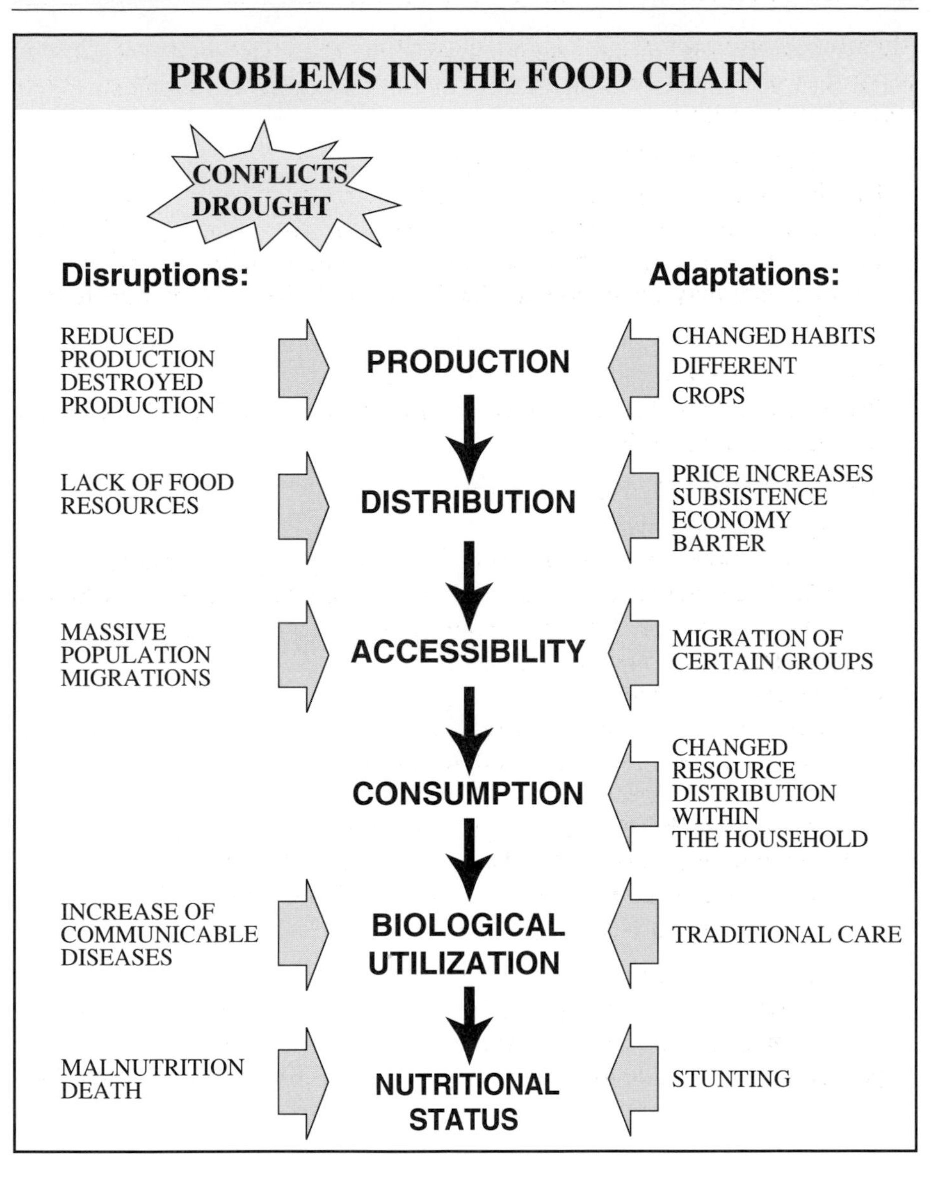


# II. Assessment of Food-Related Problems

## 1. Principles

The assessment of nutritional needs is a constant in most emergency situations. First, however, the concept of "needs" must be defined. This term has already been used to define nutritional norms. In standard usage, the expression "assessment of needs" means determining whether there is a "need" for aid. This sense, then, is completely different from that of nutritional requirements.

A food system can be assessed from the top or from the bottom. An assessment of nutritional status and the collateral factors apt to influence it tries to analyze the consequences of a crisis, without seeking out its causes in the upper levels of the food system. Many organizations used this approach up to around 1985, although studies indicated the necessity of a more comprehensive assessment. The danger, of course, is that relief agencies will confine themselves to implementing palliative programs with no lasting effects.

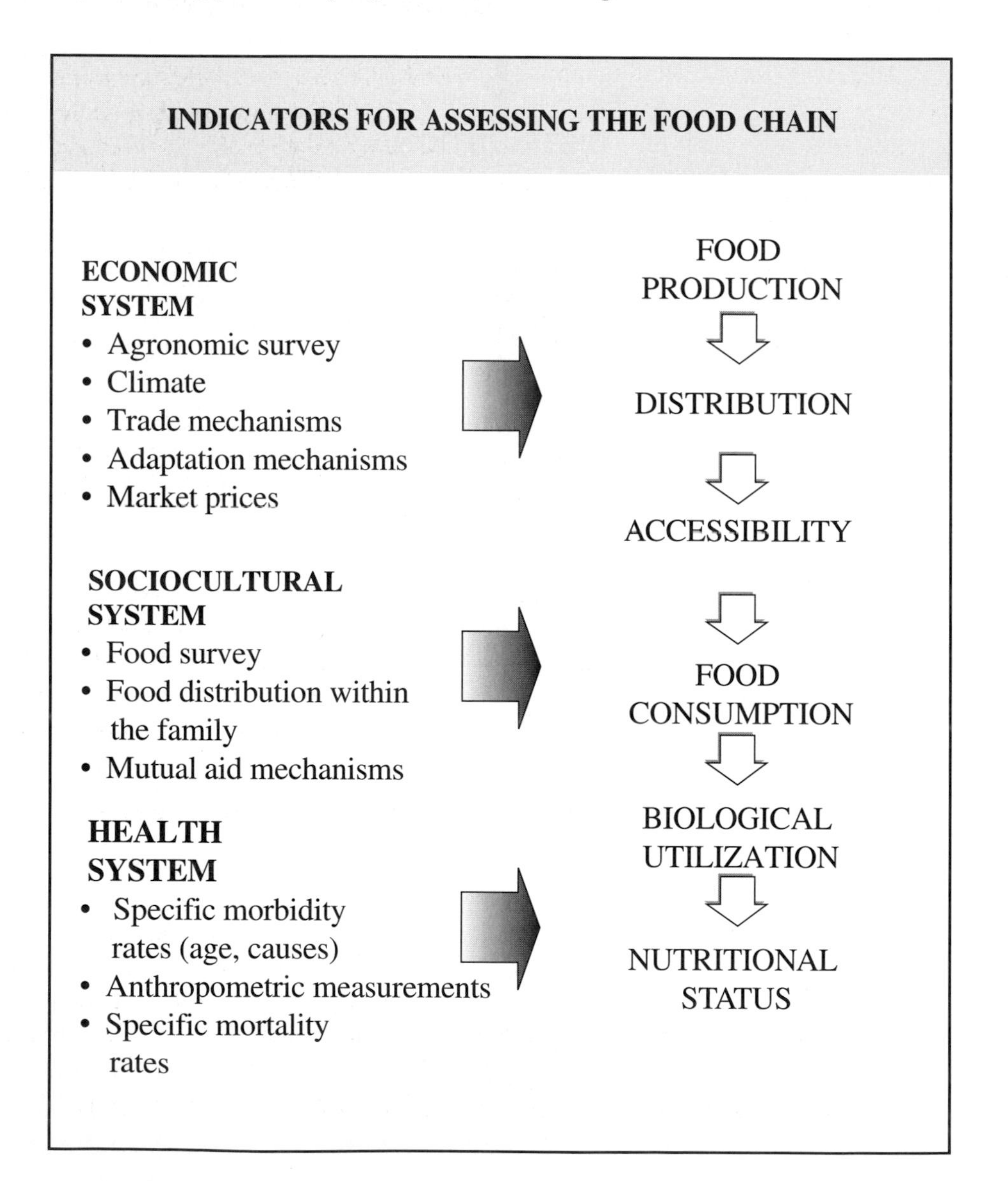

The alternative approach is to start from the top of the food system, with an analysis of production and distribution that will provide information on the factors and mechanisms that gave rise to the crisis. This approach is the more logical, as long as it does not get off the track into an elaborate macroeconomic study, and as long as the analyst does not neglect the use of nutritional assessment to detect those urgent problems requiring rapid intervention.

**The principle stages of the food chain must be assessed with the help of collateral data, every time there are signs of blockage at a given level.**

## 2. Methods

The epidemiological techniques used for assessments — defining indicators, determining sample size, statistical interpretation of results — will be examined in Chapter 6 ("Epidemiology").[29]

The food system is assessed on the basis of a set of data that can be classified according to the following criteria:

- food-chain level: production, distribution, consumption, etc.
- source: ministries, organizations, reports, population, etc.
- type: ecological, economic, political, social, cultural, health, nutritional, etc.
- the way the data are collected: formally or informally.[30]

For each situation, indicators covering the main stages of the food system must be defined. P. Autier[31] proposed the following nine indicators for assessing the nutritional status of displaced populations in Chad following a drought:

- cause of displacement
- number of displaced people
- type of displaced people
- mortality
- nutritional status
- homogeneity of families
- type of foods consumed
- family food reserves
- existence of vitamin deficiencies

---

[29] Since these techniques are applicable to all the topics covered in this book, it is logical to group them together.

[30] When Oxfam intervened in Kordofan, in Sudan, it collected socioeconomic data both during meetings with the local people and by means of questionnaires. See J. Shoham and E. Clay, "The Role of Socio-Economic Data in Foods Needs Assessment and Monitoring," *Disasters* 13, No. 1: 50.

[31] P. Autier, "Nutrition Assessment through the Use of a Nutritional Scoring System," *Disasters* 12, No. 1: 71-72.

Each item of information is sought for a specific purpose. An informal approach to measuring malnutrition does not permit a correct analysis of a population's nutritional status. Assessing difficulties in agricultural production and the distribution system, in contrast, requires a less structured approach involving cross-checks of data obtained from different sources.

## 2.1 Assessment of Food Availability

To measure the availability of food resources, it is essential to assess the two factors that control food availability: production and distribution. This involves collecting data on:

- ecological conditions — type of soil, vegetation, etc.,
- way of life — whether the population is sedentary or nomadic, rural or urban,
- climatic conditions — rainfall trends,
- agricultural policy — agrarian structure, loans, subsidies, etc.,
- agricultural techniques — types of seed, use of fertilizer,
- type of social organization — division of labor,
- distribution mechanisms,
- prices of available foods,
- food aid.

Some of these data can be measured by simple means such as market price, agricultural yield, and pluviometry, while others need only be estimated. For example, to assess the food available to a rural population, the assessor will use the RRA method ("rapid rural appraisal"), which is based on semi-structured interviews with local inhabitants. Clearly, this method, being centered on talks with the people directly concerned, has the advantage of quickly identifying problems, as long as the cultural differences between the assessors and the populations studied do not lead to misunderstandings over words, concepts, and problems.[32]

## 2.2 Assessment of Family Food Consumption

The facts needed to assess family food security fall into three categories:

- economic — purchasing power, management of the family budget, etc.;
- social — which groups are needier than others, food distribution within the family;
- political — whether a blockade is preventing access to food resources, etc.

[32] "The informal interview is an important way of furthering our understanding of the lives of rural people, but it needs to be understood by its practitioners." J. Mitchell and H. Slim, "Listening to Rural People in Africa: The Semi-Structured Interview in Rapid Rural Appraisal," *Disasters* 15, No. 1: 68.

These facts can be obtained by means of informal interviews regarding family income and surveys of household food consumption.

## 2.3 Assessment of Nutritional Status

### *The Role of Nutritional Assessment*

Nutritional assessment is often assigned particular importance, because in many emergencies malnutrition is a serious problem that tends to be the focus of attention.

Clearly, however, in the context of the food system, the importance of nutritional status is relative, since it is only the last stage of a complex process. This is more than a simple statement of fact; it challenges the entire approach to emergency relief. Either we measure nutritional status and wait until it deteriorates enough for us to intervene; or else we assess the food system in order to take early action when the preliminary signs of inadequate access to food first appear — *before* nutritional status deteriorates. Thus, this idea calls into question the whole philosophy of emergency food aid.[33]

This said, the assessment of nutritional status must nevertheless be given its due; it does allow relief organizations to assess the urgency of a situation, and it helps them to monitor food programs already in operation. The emotional impact that the malnutrition rate has on donors is also something to consider. Nonetheless, any interpretation of the malnutrition rate must also take into account such variables as the child mortality rate, the periods of harvest, and population movements.

### *Choice of Methods*

Health personnel commonly choose between different methods, which will not be discussed in detail here. Emphasis will be laid, however, on the role of nutritional assessments in the food system. *In this respect, it should be noted that in emergency situations the focus is on* ***acute*** *malnutrition.*[34] *The effects of chronic malnutrition are of less concern.*[35] Certainly, acute malnutrition represents an immediate vital risk for the children who suffer from it, especially when it is combined with infectious diseases. It should not be assumed, however, that the different forms of chronic malnutrition present no danger. Studies examining long-term mortality (two years) associated with the two types of malnutrition are enlightening in this respect, since they indicate that the risk of death among growth-retarded

---

33 This problem will be covered in more detail in the section on intervention strategies.

34 Characterized by substantial weight loss.

35 Characterized by growth retardation.

(stunted) children is three times higher than that for children who show no growth retardation. Similarly, the risk of death among acutely malnourished (wasted) children is 2.8 times higher than for children who are not acutely malnourished. The risk of death to children who are both stunted and wasted is 6.8 times greater than for children showing no form of malnutrition.[36] At the beginning of an emergency, of course, relief workers will give priority to identifying the forms of acute malnutrition which present an immediate risk; but the other types of malnutrition must be taken into consideration as well.

The assessment of nutritional status is based on the measurement of two types of indicators, anthropometric and clinical.

### 2.3.1 *Anthropometric Indicators*

A number of anthropometric measurements may be used to assess nutritional status:

- weight relative to height
- arm circumference relative to height
- arm circumference
- weight for age
- height for age

The method chosen will depend on the nutritional problem being screened for, the method's epidemiological value for identifying that problem, and the type of decision that will be made on the basis of the results obtained.

*Nutritional Problem Screened for*

Acute malnutrition is measured by one of the first three methods, while stunting is measured by height relative to age. The weight-for-age method is very widely used, especially by health ministries, but it does not clearly distinguish acute malnutrition from chronic malnutrition. Moreover, age-based methods are hindered by the practical difficulty of determining age. Consequently, our discussion will focus on the first three methods, which are sufficiently valid indicators of acute malnutrition.

*Epidemiological Value of the Method*

Numerous comparative studies have examined the epidemiological value of these anthropometric methods. The differences between the various methods in terms of sensitivity and specificity have been studied,[37] as well as in their positive

---

[36] See L.C. Chen, "Anthropometric Assessment of Energy Protein Malnutrition and Subsequent Risk of Mortality among Pre-School children," *American Journal of Clinical Nutrition* 33 (1980).

[37] H. Van Loon *et al.*, "Screening for Marasmus: A Discriminant Analysis as a Guide to Choose the Anthropometric Variables," *American Journal of Clinical Nutrition* 45 (1987): 488-493.

predictive value. Naturally, it is important to choose a reliable method; but reliability depends most of all on non-statistical epidemiological criteria, such as:

- *the accuracy of the measurements taken.* Gross errors in measuring (weight, arm circumference, and height) invalidate any statistical discussion of the results.
- *the sampling technique.* Is the sample representative?
- *comparison with previously taken measurements.* If the aim is to measure an indicator relative to a previous situation for which measurements obtained by the same method for the same type of problem are available, the local method should be used — particularly since personnel can be found locally to carry out the assessment using the familiar method.
- *comparison with a given standard.* The use of international references has often been questioned, the preference being for local references.[38] In an emergency, constraints of time and personnel limit the opportunities to assess a control population. One way of getting around this difficulty is to use international norms, but to adjust the cut-off points.[39]

These factors are more significant criteria for choosing a method than statistical comparisons between the different techniques.

### *Type of Decisions to Be Made on the Basis of the Results*

The purpose of taking anthropometric measurements must be considered. Is the aim to select malnourished children for participation in a nutritional program? Or is the assessment part of a more comprehensive evaluation designed to determine the nutritional problems of an entire population?

In the first case, the method of choice will be the one that identifies the greatest number of malnutrition cases (high sensitivity), even though a certain number of normal children will be mistakenly included among the malnourished ones (weak specificity). If the prevalence of the problem is high, the method's positive predictive value will remain acceptable. The health team can always take another series of measurements later, using a more specific method for the group of children selected with the first method.

In the second case, the health team may not necessarily have the opportunity to take a second series of measurements to clarify the results obtained by another system. In this case, the method chosen should be both sensitive and specific.

The choice is difficult, but in an emergency, relief teams should seek the best compromise between accuracy and simplicity of use. In this respect, the

[38] "The problem of the local standard can be solved by using a local survey. This reference has to be updated regularly in order to follow secular changes." *Ibid.*: 493.

[39] D. Nabarro, *The Assessment of the Nutritional Status of the Individual Child* (1982).

measurement of arm circumference would be ideal,[40] if it were not flawed by weak specificity. Arm circumference for height is also a quick,[41] simple, and accurate indicator. The weight-for-height method is more time-consuming, but previous references are expressed in this form, permitting useful comparisons.

#### *2.3.2 Clinical Indicators*

*Clinical Indicators Directly Linked to Nutritional Disorders*

- The presence of edema permits a diagnosis of kwashiorkor;[42] these cases can be classed from the outset in the category of severe malnutrition.
- Signs of vitamin A, C, and $B_1$ deficiencies. It is important to detect vitamin A deficiency, since it damages the eyes.
- Clinical signs indicating mineral deficiencies (notably iron).

*Clinical Indicators Reflecting Particular Risk*

Signs of infectious diseases, such as diarrhea or pulmonary infections, must be weighed together with the anthropometric values obtained. For example, a child suffering from moderate malnutrition combined with a pulmonary infection should receive the care normally reserved for cases of severe malnutrition.

## 3. Data Analysis

### 3.1 The Principle

The goal in analyzing data is to integrate enough reliable information to gain a coherent view of the situation and to discover whether victims have enough food to cover their essential needs. In short, the aim is to determine the victims' degree of food security by population group or, more precisely, by family unit. A family's food security can be judged by whether the family has access to the food that meets its nutritional needs and is culturally acceptable, and whether the family is able to maintain that access over the long term.[43] This definition comprises two important principles:

---

[40] "The use of arm circumference < 12.5 cm as a screening method has the advantage of being very simple and can be implemented at very low costs (personnel, training). Applied to the same data this method yields a PPV [positive predictive value] (5.6%) similar to that from common selection procedures, although with a very high sensitivity (97.5%)." H. Van Loon *et al.*, *op. cit.*: 493.

[41] An important factor when little time is available for carrying out a nutritional assessment.

[42] Although edema may, of course, be caused by other factors (renal insufficiency, for example), in an environment where nutritional deficiencies are common, edema in a child should be considered *a priori* as a sign of kwashiorkor.

[43] ACC/SCN, "Nutrition-Relevant Actions," State of the Art Series, Nutrition Policy Discussion Paper, No. 10, p. 30.

- *Access to food.* This idea connects with a topic already discussed — namely, the availability of food resources. In certain situations, food resources do, in fact, exist, but are not accessible for various reasons (prohibitive cost, political blockade). In other cases, food resources are available, but certain population groups have no access to them. Thus, the responses to these problems must take circumstances into account, balancing economic, political, and social factors as well as possible.
- *Permanence of access.* Any assessment of family food security must take into account potential developments in the current situation. If at the time of the assessment the families surveyed have access to food but this access is believed likely to be interrupted in the days, weeks, or months to come, the assessment of the current situation must take this into account. This sort of prospective analysis may ultimately prompt a decision to intervene before access to food is broken off. This approach introduces the idea of "preventive" intervention, which will be discussed in the context of action strategies.

The idea of food security encompasses essentially two aspects of the food system: the availability of food and its consumption. An analysis of food security must also address the causes of food insecurity (production, distribution) and its consequences (migration, malnutrition). It should be balanced by consideration of a set of factors which help to place the problem in its socioeconomic and political context.

## 3.2 Factors to Consider

- *The level of development*:

  In societies where food production, distribution, and consumption are precariously balanced, the upheaval caused by a major shock will lead to a sudden and severe imbalance, most affecting those whose access to food is problematic at the best of times.

- *The time of year*:

  The vulnerability of rural populations follows the rhythm of the seasons. Populations are much more vulnerable during the period when family food stocks are at their lowest, the critical period before the harvest. This is an important point, because it can influence the way that a relief operation will be conducted. Moreover, these fluctuations in food availability affect nutritional status.

- *The pace of events*:

  The seriousness of a disaster is also determined by the speed with which the food imbalance has developed, by the extent to which access to food is interrupted, and by the number of individuals affected.

- *Evolution over time*:
  The purpose of an assessment is to provide a picture of the situation that will serve as a basis for making decisions. Obviously, decisions will also depend on what is likely to happen in the future.

### 3.3 Types of Analysis

There is a tendency to focus on the interpretation of malnutrition rates. This sort of analysis has little value unless it also integrates other elements of the food system. The rate of malnutrition does reflect the seriousness of the situation. However, taken as an isolated figure, that rate does not indicate whether the problem is a habitual, temporary phenomenon — the transition period between harvests, for example — whether the mechanisms of socioeconomic adaptation are at work, or whether the crisis will resolve itself with the next harvest.

Conversely, a macroeconomic analysis of the national production and distribution system does not reveal a disaster's effects on family food security. A country's overall production may be satisfactory, while individual regions are seriously affected by a disaster.

In an emergency situation, an analysis of food security[44] allows relief agencies to "plug into" the middle of the food system. They can then work backward to the causes of any food insecurity, and forward to its consequences: migrations and an abnormally high rate of malnutrition. This approach involves "scanning" the food system, while maintaining a level of analysis compatible with making immediately operational decisions.

# III. Intervention Strategies in Cases of Food Insecurity

## 1. Objective of Interventions and Food Security

*"A family's food security is judged by its capacity for access to the food it needs to maintain a healthy life for all its members (in terms of quality, quantity, safety, and cultural acceptability), and when it runs no risk of loosing that access."*[45]

This objective can be broken down into a set of operational goals, as follows:

---

[44] For example, the assessment system established by Caritas and *Médecins Sans Frontières* (MSF) in Angola to monitor population movements and to gain an idea of the food security of these populations.

[45] ACC/SCN, "Nutrition-Relevant Actions," State of the Art Series, Nutrition Policy Discussion Paper, No. 10, p. 30.

1. Develop or restore the country's potential
   a. Increase production capacity
      i. Reform agrarian structure
      ii. Develop new agricultural techniques
   b. Restore production capacity
      i. Distribute seeds
      ii. Distribute tools
      iii. Restore access to agricultural land
   c. Increase distribution capacity
      i. Increase transport capacity
      ii. Increase storage capacity
   d. Restore distribution capacity
      i. Restore transportation routes
      ii. Reestablish free passage of food products on transportation routes
2. Guarantee family food security
   a. Restore families' usual food consumption level
      i. Distribute food to impoverished families
      ii. Provide financial support for impoverished families
      iii. Distribute food
   b. Modify family food consumption
      i. Introduce the use of new food products
      ii. Change behaviors within the family
3. Insure food security for the most vulnerable individuals
   a. Prevent malnutrition with a supplementary feeding program
   b. Develop a program for nutritional rehabilitation at home
   c. Set up a program for nutritional rehabilitation in a therapeutic feeding center.
      i. Build a nutrition rehabilitation center
      ii. Identify beneficiaries

These objectives may be rearranged and broken down as desired. Of course, in any given situation, relief workers will not undertake all the activities listed above. Strategy consists in selecting objectives and the activities deriving from them according to the problems and constraints inherent in each case.

## 2. Strategies

This concept should be explained, since any confusion in this respect poses a danger of serious mistakes.

## 2.1 Factors Influencing a Strategy of Action

### *Prevention*

The earlier intervention in the food system takes place, the greater the chances of preventing food and nutritional problems. If stocks of food for emergencies are laid in and efficient distribution channels are set up, food availability is preserved. If food aid is distributed as soon as family food security is in danger but before any nutritional damage occurs, then malnutrition will not increase beyond the usual rate.

### *Agency Mandate and Means*

Depending on their mandates and their means, aid institutions orient their activities within a specific field, such as immediate aid, nutritional rehabilitation, etc.

### *Media Coverage*

The mobilization of the international community and the financing of humanitarian operations are often related to the media impact of the crisis. The less a crisis is publicized, the more likely its victims will not be assisted; or else they will be helped at a late stage, when the situation is tragic enough to take the number-one spot in the media.

However, media pressure may also "impose" attitudes that do not conform to reality — for example, encouraging the dispatch of non-essentials, or food products that are difficult or even dangerous to use in emergency situations, such as powdered milk.[46]

### *Urgency*

When rural populations have lost everything and they have no immediate access to food, teaching them new agricultural techniques is not the first priority.

### *Constraints*

Constraints are what most often determines the form that intervention will take. If food production is normal but, for political reasons, food is not accessible to certain population groups, and negotiations to restore access meet with a flat refusal, relief organizations may be "forced" to assist these groups.

---

[46] Powdered milk is difficult to use in emergency situations for several reasons, notably the absence of clean water — which makes the reconstitution of the milk an exercise in microbiological culture — and ignorance concerning the correct proportions of powder and water.

*Interaction Between Factors*

Media interest in a situation may facilitate the implementation of measures intended to prevent problems before it becomes necessary to solve them. Urgency and drama are often synonymous with financial support. Local authorities sometimes use access to food resources as a weapon to achieve political purposes such as encouraging populations to leave or cutting the enemy off from its sources of food.

## 2.2 Errors

The most common error relief agencies make is to use a group of malnourished people as the basis for determining a strategy of action. Of course, it has been shown that mortality is directly related to the severity of malnutrition. In an emergency, then, the malnourished members of the population merit particular attention. Today's nutritional rehabilitation programs are well-organized and capable of achieving good results quickly. Without a broader strategy encompassing the maintenance of family food security, however, rehabilitated children will find themselves back in a dysfunctional food system where families' basic needs are not covered. Such children will inevitably slip back into their previous malnourished condition, with its attendant risk of death.[47]

The second common error is not to plan for a long-term solution based on self-sufficiency for a population that has already benefited from assistance. Developing a long-term strategy is not an immediate concern in the initial phase of an emergency. But it should be borne in mind that the longer direct food aid is continued (in the form of food distribution), the weaker the likelihood that the assisted population can be made self-sufficient.

The third error concerns the mechanics of the aid. Once the necessity of food distribution has been clearly established, it should be remembered that the way such distributions are carried out can have a considerable influence on the future of the assisted population. Efforts must be made to avoid contributing to the creation of displaced-person camps. True, food aid can be more easily arranged in a camp than for a scattered population. But assuming that the strategy for action includes a long-term component, it is clearly much easier to make people self-sufficient in their original homes than in a camp.

To this factor can be added a related concern, the immediate risks involved in the migration of large population groups.[48] This risk was highlighted at a seminar on

---

[47] C. Aall has shown the relation between an estimated 1,300 kcal food ration and the death rate, which may increase sixfold after several months of insufficient food supply. "Disastrous International Relief Failure: A Report on Burmese Refugees in Bangladesh from May to December 1978," *Disasters* 3, No. 4.

[48] The most vulnerable groups have a particularly high death rate when populations migrate to new regions without preparation.

"Famine & War" held in Annecy, France, in March, 1991. Badly planned food aid can help amplify such migrations.

The fourth error involves the economic impact of the food aid. This issue must be seen in its true dimensions, and a distinction must be made between classic international food aid[49] and humanitarian food aid. In the first case, the volume of aid is considerably larger than in the second, and is intended to complement inadequate national production. The risks are many; the main one is that the aid will cease to be a temporary stopgap[50] and simply become a permanent substitute for national production, putting the assisted countries under the political influence of the donors.

The volume of humanitarian food aid is comparatively much smaller, and therefore poses fewer economic risks. Of course, under certain circumstances, food aid may cause a fall in the prices of locally produced foodstuffs,[51] and motivate the assisted populations to concentrate on growing non-food crops. On the other hand, food aid may help revive the local market and also, in some cases, push down market prices.[52]

The fifth error is ignorance of non-food solutions. It may seem paradoxical to propose non-food solutions to food problems; yet during a conflict, the problems are often not because of insufficient production, but rather because people have been cut off from their means of production. The solution is to re-establish access to the latter. Food aid must be considered as a last resort, when negotiations have failed. Similarly, it has been shown that malnutrition is not necessarily attributable to food insecurity, but may also be a consequence of health problems such as infectious diseases. A multifaceted approach is essential.

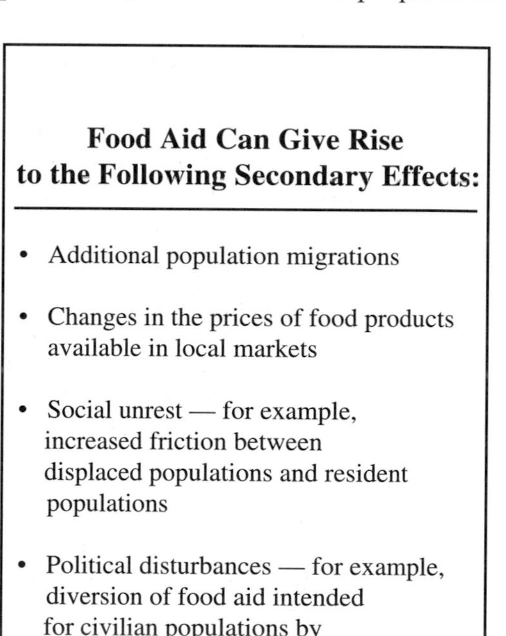

**Food Aid Can Give Rise to the Following Secondary Effects:**

- Additional population migrations
- Changes in the prices of food products available in local markets
- Social unrest — for example, increased friction between displaced populations and resident populations
- Political disturbances — for example, diversion of food aid intended for civilian populations by armed groups

---

49 In other words, regular bilateral food aid between countries.

50 Until national production reaches a level sufficient to meet national needs.

51 As a result of the law of supply and demand.

52 The arrival on the market of food-aid products may discourage food stock-piling for speculative purposes.

The sixth error derives from the first five: food aid is no trifling matter, and its mechanisms must be controlled. This can be done only by setting up an effective surveillance system which provides an overall view of the food system. The tendency has been to concentrate on the measurement of nutritional status as a surveillance tool; but this approach is much too restrictive to allow relief organizations to take steps to prevent malnutrition when access to food is interrupted. It also offers no opportunity to judge the impact of food aid on the local economic system.

## 2.3 Emergency Strategy

Given such a diversity of problems, given the logistical, political, and other constraints, given all the factors that must be integrated into a strategy in order to avoid perverse effects, can an intervention strategy be proposed? Although any strategy must be adapted to the particular circumstances of the situation, certain broad principles may be applied to every emergency intervention.

- *Plan the aid in terms of the food system*
  This approach allows planners to identify problems at the right level and, consequently, to propose appropriate solutions — for example, to respond to a malnutrition problem by providing family food security.

- *Anticipate crises*
  Maintaining food security prevents the development of high rates of malnutrition. Maintaining access to the means of agricultural production and keeping the channels of distribution open prevent the development of food insecurity. On a more general level, it should be noted that economic development (increased food production) gives countries the necessary basis to cope with major ecological problems. Haphazard economic growth, however, obscures the effects of that development. Although the percentage of malnourished children is declining — according to the World Health Organization (WHO) this figure has dropped from 42.6% in 1975 to 34.6% in 1995 — in absolute terms the number of malnourished children has risen, owing to a substantial increase in the population of certain countries, notably in Africa and South-East Asia.[53]

- *Integrate activities*
  In the example of a rural population suffering from a drought, completely lacking food resources, and whose most vulnerable members are already showing evidence of the crisis (malnutrition), the following sequence could be envisaged:

- nutritional rehabilitation;

[53] WHO, 48th General Assembly (28 Feb. 1995).

- food distribution;
- design of an agricultural rehabilitation program, under which production would totally or partially replace food handouts;
- design of economic and social development programs permitting the population to cope with future droughts.

■ *Delegate responsibility*
To exercise control over the distribution of food aid, agencies tend to control all stages of the operation systematically, sometimes going so far as to control food distribution within the family. Oxfam, in contrast, during its operation in Sudan (1985-1986), delegated responsibility for food distribution to the communities themselves.[54]

An example of the philosophy behind the strategy adopted in actions on behalf of the nomads has been described as follows:

*"The need for relief assistance to pastoralists must be identified long before the people collapse from malnutrition. Such assistance should take the form of interventions which sustain the basis of pastoral economy: namely the pastoralist's position as a trader of animals. Interventions should be multifaceted, exploiting the linkages within complex food production systems, to provide the pastoral sector with a respite from abnormal levels of stress."* [55]

# IV. Food Distributions

It should be remembered that the distribution of supplies must be integrated into a global approach to food aid, aimed primarily at re-establishing self-sufficiency as quickly as possible. Food distribution must therefore be considered as a palliative, temporary measure.

## 1. Studying the Food Ration

The nutritional requirements defined earlier will serve as the basis for designing a food ration. Here again, the food ration should be defined by the context of the

---

[54] "In putting bulk food into the hands of the community leaders, Oxfam lost control of deciding which individuals should receive food. This meant that they could not be sure if food aid reached the very needy, the marginal and the voiceless in the community. As such, Oxfam could not target food on their terms which were based on an idea of equity in terms of individuals." H. Slim and J. Mitchell, "Towards Community-Managed Relief: A Case Study from Southern Sudan," *Disasters* 14, No. 3: 268.

[55] P. Walker, "Famine Relief Amongst Pastoralists in Sudan: A Report of Oxfam's Experience," *Disasters* 12, No. 3: 197.

situation. Some populations may have access to some food reserves of their own which are, however, insufficient to cover all their nutritional needs. In this case, the rations distributed will complement the local resources.[56]

This section will examine the composition of complete rations, designed to cover all nutritional needs. They are calculated according to the average of individual needs within the family unit.

A complete ration should furnish:

- 2,200 calories
- 60 grams of protein
- the essential vitamins.

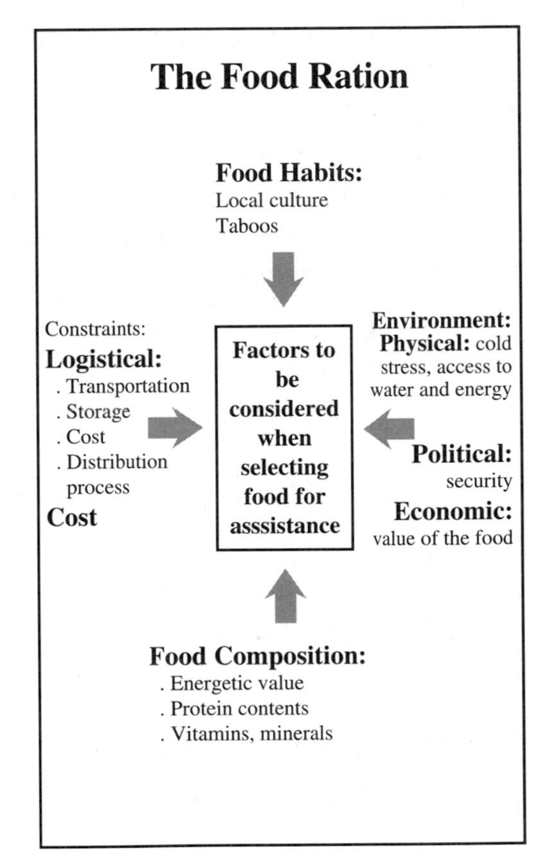


First of all, logistic considerations will dictate the choice of the foods that will be furnished; the difficulties of delivering the food and storage constraints contra-indicate the use of highly perishable goods.

These logistic constraints and nutritional factors reduce the choice of possible foods. The complete basic ration[57] generally consists of:

- cereals = 400 grams
- legumes = 100 grams
- oil = 50 grams

The choice of foods making up a food ration must also, of course, take into consideration the cultural characteristics of the society concerned.

Since a ration of this type does not meet vitamin requirements, additional measures must be contemplated, such as the distribution of vitamin A.

---

56 The terms used for this type of ration vary according to the organization. For the sake of simplicity, they can be called partial rations, to distinguish them from complete rations.

57 The complete basic ration, as defined here, does not take account of supplementary food needs, which are increasingly often integrated in the basic ration.

# 2. Registration of Beneficiaries

A precise census of the potential beneficiaries of a food distribution operation is a key element in the program's success. In refugee camps, where people are geographically concentrated, the computation of beneficiaries is not as easy as it might seem.[58] Elsewhere, the targeted beneficiaries may be scattered far and wide, so that estimating their numbers is much more difficult. Moreover, displaced people are often mixed in with resident populations, making census-taking problematic.

The results of censuses taken during conflicts are very unreliable, since political instability can rapidly change the number of potential beneficiaries. Thus, the number of people to be helped should be constantly re-evaluated.

# 3. Logistics

Food distribution programs provide a useful framework in which to examine a few basic elements of logistics.

## 3.1 Source of the Food Distributed

The food to be distributed may be obtained locally, nationally, or internationally.

- *Local or regional sources*: Food bought in the local market has the advantage of being preferred by the beneficiaries (cultural acceptability). Care must be taken, however, to avoid creating price inflation by increasing demand.
- *National sources* : If certain regions have a food surplus while others are in want, a redistribution of resources — in accordance with the rules of the market — is a possible solution.
- *International sources:* Importing humanitarian food aid involves a rather long waiting period,[59] unless the food can be obtained from neighboring countries.

The criteria for choosing one source of supply rather than another are as follows:

- cultural acceptability

---

[58] R.S. Stephenson and P.C. Romanosky have noted the following problems:
- Multiple registration for the same family
- Inflation of family size
- Registration of people who do not meet the criteria for aid
- Sale of documents granting access to food assistance. *Disasters* 11, No. 3 (1987).

[59] Relief agencies can expect to wait for a period of up to three months between the moment they decide to import food from Europe and North America and the moment it arrives in the country.

- availability
- urgency of the situation
- period required for delivery
- economic impact on the local market in the case of mass purchases
- quality of the goods
- cost — purchases or donations
- transport facilities
- customs problems, if the food is bought abroad.

## 3.2 Food Transport and Storage

The issues involved in transporting food concern the entire period from the time the food leaves its source (whether it is purchased or donated) until it is used by the disaster victims.

If the food must be imported and transported by boat — the usual case — consideration should be given to the fact that delivery periods in the country where the operation is being conducted may be on the order of several months. Consequently, the urgency of the situation will be a prime factor in deciding whether the delivery period is acceptable, or whether different supply sources and/or means of transport need to be adopted to get the food to its destination more rapidly.

Transport within a country is generally by means of trucks. For security reasons, however, in some cases only air transport may be possible, meaning a considerable increase in cost.[60]

Moreover, the delivery of large quantities of food creates storage problems. Large-capacity warehouses must be found in which the food will be safe from bad weather, insects, rodents, and theft.

Nor do the problems of transport and storage cease with the distribution of the food. Consideration must be given to the fact that the aid recipients must transport the food to their homes and store it.

All these factors, together with the risk run by victims in conflict situations of having to "participate in the war effort" of one of the adversaries,[61] may influence the quantity of food given out at any one time.

---

[60] A truck has more or less the same capacity as a plane of the Hercules type; but the cost of using the latter is 500 times greater.

[61] Victims may be forced to "give" part of the food they receive to the combatants who control the region where the victims live.

# 4. The Practical Organization of a Food Distribution

## 4.1 Managing Crowds of Beneficiaries

Large-scale food distribution requires extremely careful organization; otherwise complete chaos is apt to ensue, hurting mostly the weakest, who are unable to demand their right to food aid.

Normally food is distributed in the form of family rations. The relief organization registers each family, giving the head of the family a card indicating the number of family members. While food is being handed out, the crowd must be carefully controlled to insure that distribution is equitable[62] and swift.

## 4.2 Managing the Food to Be Distributed

Plans should be made in advance for transport and on-site storage of the food, in order to avoid any interruption of supply in the course of distribution. Each family should receive a family ration calculated on the basis of the standard ration and the number of people in the family.

## 4.3 Managing Support Systems

Large-scale food distribution is accompanied by accessory measures such as the provision of drinking water and basic medical services.

## 4.4 Planning the Distribution Site

The distribution point must be rationally organized according to certain criteria:

- extensive open space;
- separate routes for the flow of food and the flow of beneficiaries;
- possibility of setting up support activities.

## 4.5 Distribution Mechanism

Where possible, victims should be assisted near their homes. However, when dispersion of the population or political constraints preclude this, relief workers are obliged to used the technique of the "landbridge" — a distribution point where people come to collect their rations, which they then take back home with them.

[62] Food distributions are often the scene of manipulative attempts. Some beneficiaries may try to collect food several times during a single distribution.

In all cases, efforts should be made to avoid creating displaced-person or refugee camps — unless, of course, security conditions do not allow victims to remain in their homes.

## 5. Surveillance

The surveillance of a food-distribution program is normally integrated in the general surveillance program. Only a few particular aspects will be mentioned here.

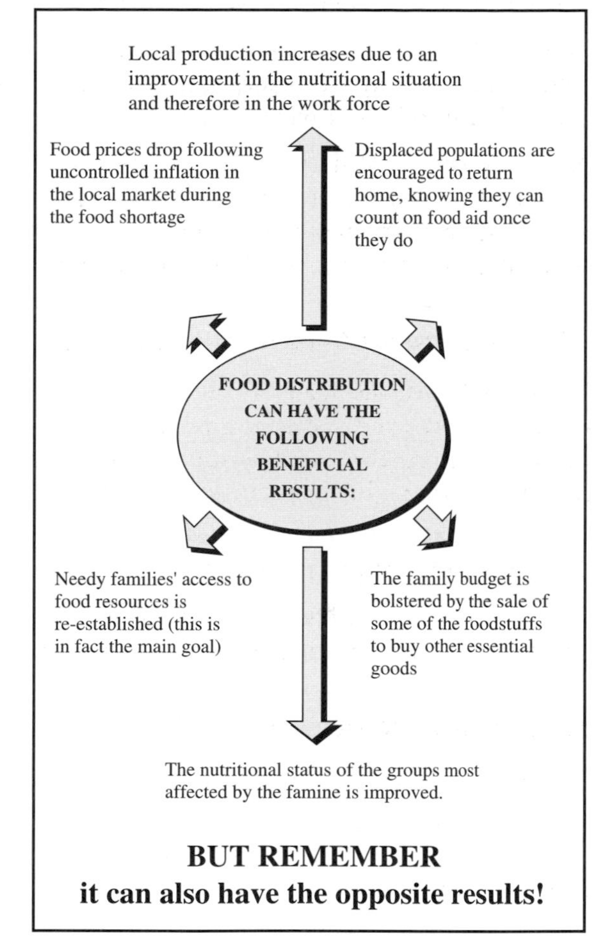


Surveillance of a food-distribution program entails monitoring food stocks, the distribution itself,[63] and the impact of the food aid on the beneficiaries' nutritional status. The last item is the most important part of the surveillance process, since it shows whether the distribution program is indeed achieving the desired result. The tool of surveillance is studied in detail in Chapter 6 ("Epidemiology"). Nonetheless, emphasis should be placed on the indicators that must be monitored, particularly:

- nutritional status
- intra-familial distribution of food aid
- market prices
- population movements.

This sort of surveillance also provides the information necessary in order to decide when food distribution can be stopped.

[63] Monitoring is necessary not only at the moment of distribution, but also afterwards, to make sure, first, that the beneficiaries are not robbed of their food rations, and second, that the goods received are not systematically resold on the local market by the beneficiaries themselves.

# V. Supplementary Feeding

## 1. Definition

The terminology used to define supplementary feeding is not standardized. For example, in the UNICEF manual *Assisting in Emergencies,* supplementary feeding is defined as:

*"the need...to ensure that young and moderately malnourished children, pregnant and lactating women receive adequate and suitable food [...] The best strategy for ensuring appropriate food for these 'vulnerable groups' must be decided locally in each case on the basis of a thorough assessment of the causes of their nutritional vulnerability and the practical possibilities for reducing that vulnerability."* [64]

More specifically, the procedure is described thus:

*"Additional food is given to selected, nutritionally vulnerable individuals to compensate for specific deficiencies — in energy, protein, vitamins and minerals — in the food otherwise available to them. It is intended to be in addition to their normal share of household food, including any general emergency distributions."* [65]

The World Health Organization (WHO) manual *The Management of Nutritional Emergencies in Large Populations* defines the purpose of supplementary feeding as:

*"to supplement deficiencies in energy and/or nutrients, especially protein, in the basic diet of those most vulnerable to malnutrition: children under 5, pregnant or lactating women, medical cases, old people, children selected by a screening method."* [66]

The first definition equates supplementary feeding with nutritional rehabilitation. It is true that in some cases the strategy used to deal with the problem of moderate malnutrition will be the distribution of supplementary rations in addition to the general ration. This approach, however, tends to obscure the fact that supplementary feeding programs are intended for all nutritionally vulnerable groups,[67] not merely the cases of moderate malnutrition.

There may also be confusion with partial feeding, as it was described in connection with general food distribution. In that context, it was defined as a complement to local food resources, provided when the latter do not offer adequate coverage of normal nutritional needs.

---

64 Ron Ockwell, ed., *Assisting in Emergencies* (UNICEF, May 1986), p. 202.

65 *Ibid.*, p. 60.

66 C. de Ville de Goyet *et al.*, *The Management of Nutritional Emergencies in Large Populations* (WHO, 1978), p. 47.

67 The vulnerable groups are the target of every supplementary feeding program. *Ibid.*

This course will use the WHO definition, which tends to equate supplementary feeding with the food that must be supplied to vulnerable groups to cover specific qualitative nutritional needs not covered by the standard basic ration.

On the practical level, the trend is increasingly to supply a supplement to the basic ration distributed to families, consisting of foods chosen to compensate for the specific deficiencies of the basic ration. The resulting increase in the basic ration is essentially intended to respond to the specific nutritional needs of the vulnerable groups, rather than the general quantitative needs of the family.

## 2. Rations

Normally a supplementary ration is supposed to provide approximately 350 kcal and 10-15 grams of protein per day per person in the vulnerable category. The choice of foods for this ration depends mainly on the strategy used in implementing the program. There are two possible options:

- distributing dry supplementary rations to vulnerable groups, in addition to the basic ration;
- feeding vulnerable groups a meal equivalent to the supplementary ration.

In the first case, the foods chosen must meet two kinds of criteria: they must be technically suitable for general distribution (perishability, transport, storage) and they must satisfy the nutritional needs of the beneficiaries. Usually supplementary feeding consists in increasing the proportion of legumes and fats already contained in the basic ration, bringing it to a total of 2,500 kcal and 70-75 grams of protein.

In the second case, more specific foods can be used, such as powdered milk, eggs, etc. These foods are prepared at the feeding center and consumed there by all the vulnerable groups in the form of a daily meal.

## 3. Practical Organization

The organization of supplementary feeding has undergone major changes over the last ten years. At the beginning of the 1980s, the tendency in supplementary feeding was to provide meals at centers constructed specially for that purpose. Various comparative studies on the subject, however, have led to a reconsideration of this method, since the integration of the supplementary energy and protein in the basic ration appears to be preferable to the traditional approach to supplementary feeding.[68]

[68] Nancy Godfrey, "Supplementary Feeding in Refugee Populations: Comprehensive or Selective Feeding Programmes?" *Health Policy and Planning* 1, No. 4 (1986).

The creation of feeding centers also tends to disrupt family life by forcing mothers to go to the centers every day, leaving at home those of their children who are not classified as vulnerable. This is why attendance at such centers is usually sparse.

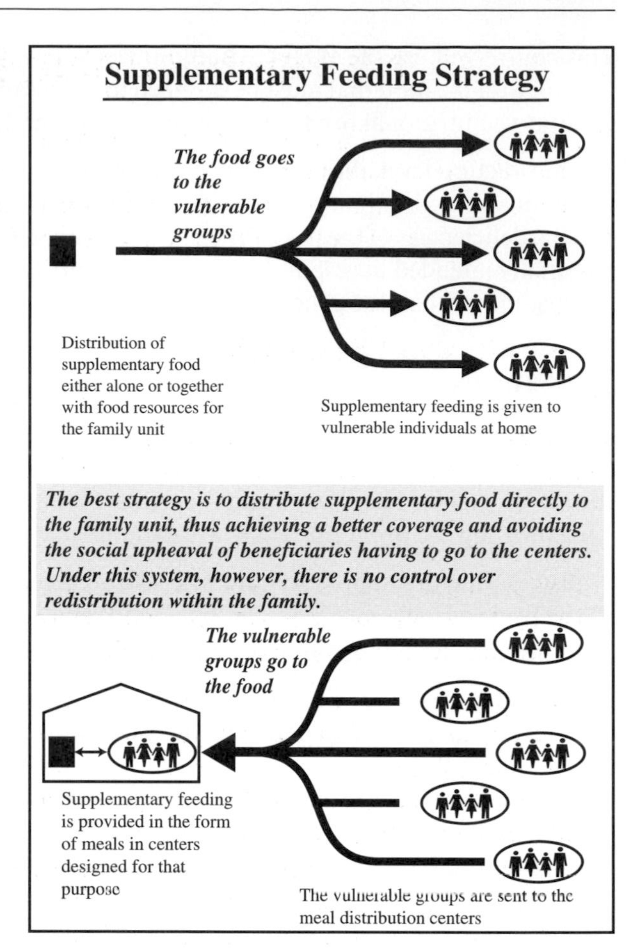


The same study cited above also recommended reinforcing the basic ration, stating that the provision of an adequate basic ration should remain the priority, and that the current emphasis on supplementary feeding programs was in fact a response to the inadequacies of general distribution programs.[69]

**With certain exceptions, today's tendency is to provide supplementary feeding for vulnerable groups by reinforcing the basic ration.**

The logistical problems involved in setting up a supplementary feeding program are the same as for general food distribution.

## 4. Surveillance

Essentially, relief agencies measure the impact of a supplementary feeding program by monitoring the nutritional status of the groups benefiting from it. In emergency situations, it is difficult to differentiate between the results of the supplementary feeding program itself and the impact of concurrent measures, such as an improved water supply and better access to health services.

---

[69] *Ibid.*

# VI. Nutritional Rehabilitation

The purpose of nutrition rehabilitation programs is to restore a normal nutritional status. The tendency is to restrict such programs to intensive feeding regimens for the most severe cases of malnutrition. In this course, however, all the possible ways of responding to the specific needs of the malnourished will be noted.

## 1. Nutritional Deficiencies

The expression "nutritional deficiencies" encompasses various aspects of the nutritional problems that may arise in emergency situations. They can be classified by type, the major category being protein-energy malnutrition. This, in turn, encompasses two main groups:

- *growth retardation (stunting)*
  Stunting reflects an adaptation to environmental stresses such as moderate lack of food and various infections. Children whose growth has been stunted in this manner are of below-normal height.[70]
- *acute malnutrition (wasting)*
  Such malnutrition may be either moderate or severe, depending on the degree of wasting. The moderate forms are characterized by a perceptibly lower body weight than the norm for the person's height. The severe forms can be subdivided into three categories:
  - Marasmus — characterized by a substantial loss of fat and muscle mass
  - Kwashiorkor — characterized by the presence of edema
  - Marasmic kwashiorkor — a combination of the two.

The main vitamin and mineral deficiencies include anemia and deficiencies in vitamins A, C, and $B_1$.

## 2. Nutrition Rehabilitation Programs (NRPs)

### 2.1 General Principles

The first principle of nutritional rehabilitation is that the families involved must be guaranteed access to food. NRPs are established in emergency situations in

[70] "The curve of a child's height is an excellent photograph of the child's previous life, revealing the growth history to date, since a nutritional problem affects the length of the child's body only after a delay of two or three months. If the food deficiency is mainly in energy, and if it persists, growth retardation may be considerable." A.M. Masse-Rimbault, "L'alimentation et la nutrition des populations," in Rougement and Brunet-Jailly, eds., *Santé dans les pays tropicaux*, p. 690.

response to needs which, being urgent and visible, are the focus of media attention. The temptation is strong to concentrate mainly on these groups, disregarding the population as a whole; but if the latter does not have access to food resources, it will continue to "produce" cases of malnutrition. Accordingly, *every nutrition rehabilitation program must also insure that the families of beneficiaries will have some kind of access to basic foodstuffs.*

Exactly what kind of NRP will be implemented is a choice hedged in by constraints. The major ones apply mainly to conflict situations, and will limit the measures that can be taken. Access to nutrition rehabilitation centers, for example, may be hindered by difficulties in getting there, curfews, or insecurity.

The low attendance rates of specific programs are one of the obstacles encountered. In a study of programs in India, Somalia, Sudan, and Thailand, N. Godfrey showed that coverage was between 33% and 67% of malnourished children.[71] This approach, then, should be weighed against the system of integrating supplementary food in the general food distribution.

## 2.2 Supplementary Feeding

As defined earlier, supplementary feeding may be the basis for an NRP in cases of moderate malnutrition. Naturally, certain accessory measures will be required to increase its effectiveness: strict surveillance of the children, a survey of intra-familial food distribution, education of mothers, and the classic measures of hygiene and public health.

With certain exceptions,[72] this type of program should be integrated into the general program of food aid to families.

## 2.3 Specific Nutrition Rehabilitation Programs

There is considerable confusion in the terminology used to designate nutrition rehabilitation programs. They are often equated with therapeutic feeding centers (TFCs), which are specially conceived to implement nutrition rehabilitation programs. It is important to make a clear distinction between NRPs and TFCs. To do this, it may be helpful to go back to square one and ask the following questions:

---

[71] N. Godfrey, *op. cit.*: 291.

[72] For example, a high rate of malnutrition in a population with independent access to food resources. The establishment of a specific NRP may be justified for a short period in order to rehabilitate the nutritional status of the affected subjects. Of course, the cause of the malnutrition must be identified, together with the appropriate solutions.

## *What Is the Problem that Needs to Be Treated?*

NRPs must be able to respond to problems of malnutrition differently according to their degree of severity. Moderate malnutrition is not treated in the same way as very severe malnutrition.

## *What Basic Principles Should Be Applied to the Problem?*

- Feeding should be qualitatively adapted to the level of malnutrition. For moderate forms of malnutrition, a diet based on ordinary foods (those of the basic ration together with eggs, milk, or other foods) is usually adequate. For serious forms of malnutrition, however, a special diet is necessary, based on milk, sugar, and oil.[73]

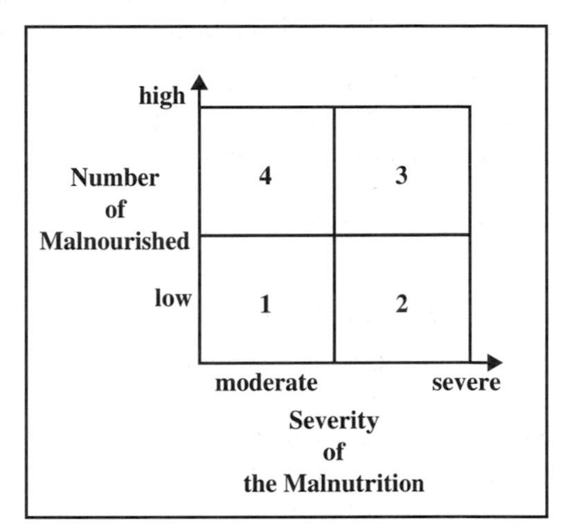


- Feeding should be quantitatively adapted to the level of malnutrition. The more severe the malnutrition, the more frequent feeding must be, if necessary reaching up to eight meals per day in an NRP.
- Medical care should be provided. Malnourished children are particularly vulnerable to infectious agents and, logically, their vulnerability increases with the degree of malnutrition. Access to health services is essential, especially for the most serious cases of malnutrition.

## *What Constraints Might Influence the Organization of NRPs?*

- The political situation may impose restrictions on the organization of the program (curfews, insecurity, etc.)
- Resource requirements (staff, facilities, financing) become heavier as programs become more complex.
- Favorable progress by the program's beneficiaries (which is the aim of the program) creates organizational problems, since the program has to be continually adapted to accommodate that progress (by changes in diet, scheduling of meals, etc.) throughout the patient's stay.

[73] Details concerning the preparation of nutritious foods and mixtures used in nutrition rehabilitation centers are available in many manuals and will not be reviewed here.

- The number of children likely to need the program may pose a problem, since, obviously, the more complex a program is, the fewer the children it will be able to treat.

All these aspects must be taken into account in the planning stage of an NRP.

EXAMPLES OF CHOICES IN NUTRITIONAL REHABILITATION STRATEGY

- **Zone 1**, a few cases of moderate malnutrition: supplementary feeding + hygienic measures to improve the environment.
- **Zone 2 + Zone 4**, a few cases of severe malnutrition and many cases of moderate malnutrition: supplementary feeding, hygienic and environmental sanitation measures, and treatment of severe cases in an existing facility (for example, a hospital).
- **Zone 4 + Zone 3**, many cases of moderate and severe malnutrition: supplementary feeding and environmental hygiene measures for the moderate cases, and treatment of severe cases in therapeutic feeding centers especially designed for that purpose.

### *Classification of NRPs*

Nutrition rehabilitation programs can be classified according to the number of meals beneficiaries receive per day, ranging from four to eight. Experience shows that they can be divided into two categories:

- Category I — This program provides four to six meals a day.
- Category II — This program offers beneficiaries up to eight meals per day, as needed. This constitutes a therapeutic feeding program.

Nutritional programs that offer only two meals a day are inadequate to effect satisfactory cures for the severe forms of malnutrition.

This outline provides a basis for planning the facilities that will be needed. At this point nutrition rehabilitation centers (NRCs) come into the picture.

## 2.4 Nutrition Rehabilitation Centers

### *Under What Circumstances Should an NRC Be Built?*

In deciding whether an NRC will be required, planners should consider two factors: the expected number of beneficiaries and the potential of existing local facilities.

- *Number of local beneficiaries*
  If the problem is limited to a few cases of malnutrition, it is usually possible to have them admitted to a local health facility. Serious nutritional emergencies involving large populations, in contrast, produce a heavy "demand" for nutritional care. In this case, the establishment of facilities designed expressly to meet that demand must be considered.

- *The potential of existing local facilities*
  The degree to which local facilities can meet demand varies from one situation to the next. It should be noted that in most developing countries, the relevant health services, particularly pediatric services, are already overburdened. A massive influx of patients suffering from severe malnutrition and requiring 24-hour care exacerbates an already precarious situation.

When the number of beneficiaries exceeds the capacity of the local facilities, the construction of autonomous NRCs must be contemplated.

### *What Kind of NRC Should Be Built?*

Theoretically, an NRC should be able to provide all the types of NRP that treat the severe forms of malnutrition. For practical reasons, however, the usual procedure is to construct units differently depending on whether the beneficiaries will be treated on a residential or outpatient basis.

- *Day-care NRCs* operate for a limited period of the day. However, since beneficiaries must be given at least four meals a day for effective nutritional rehabilitation, such centers should operate for 8-12 hours a day.

- *24-hour (residential) NRCs* are able to accommodate cases of severe malnutrition which necessitate the implementation of category II NRPs. In terms of organization, they are similar to hospital facilities, with a permanent staff working in three eight-hour shifts, a night nurse, etc.

### *Medical Services in the Centers*

Medical personnel are necessary in all NRCs, although their importance depends on the type of NRP implemented in the center. For category I NRPs, medical services are limited to ambulatory care for the most common medical problems, though provision should be made for referring cases that are beyond the center's medical capacity — either to the closest local hospital or a residential NRC.

For category II NRPs, a greater medical presence is required, owing to the seriousness of the medical problems so often associated with acute malnutrition. Care must be taken, however, not to fall into the trap of pediatric hospitalization, in which the feeding aspect becomes secondary to the purely medical aspect. Here again, the size and level of the medical staff will depend on whether the most serious cases can be referred to the local hospitals.

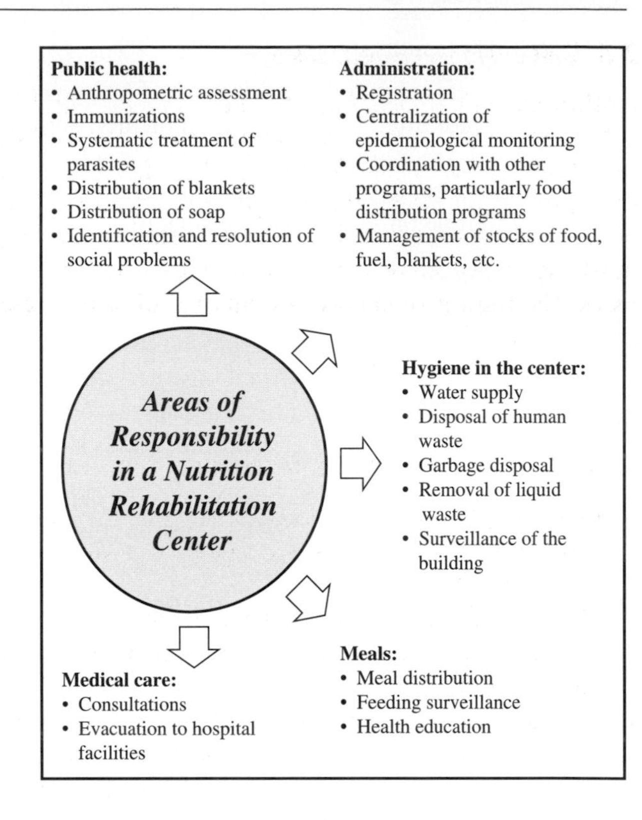


### *Preventive Measures*

- Certain preventive measures are imperative:
  - immunization against measles
  - the systematic administration of vitamin A
  - protection against the cold
  - the organization of health-education meetings for mothers
- Other measures are less important:
  - the systematic treatment of intestinal parasitic infestations (mebendezole, only for children over 12 months of age).
  - immunization against other communicable diseases[74]

### *The Practical Organization of an NRC*

Numerous manuals offer organizational blueprints for setting up an NRC.[75] Some general principles (management of large groups, adaptation of architectural features to activities) will be discussed in Chapter 5 ("Medical and Surgical Care").

---

[74] Health workers should seize the opportunity of easy access to the children under their care to immunize them according to the procedures recommended in the framework of the Expanded Program of Immunization (EPI).

[75] Among the best known are:
C. de Ville de Goyet *et al.*, *The Management of Nutritional Emergencies in Large Populations* (WHO, 1978);
*Oxfam's Practical Guide to Selective Feeding Programmes* (Oxfam, 1984);
Annex 6, "Therapeutic Feeding," in Ron Ockwell, ed., *Assisting in Emergencies* (UNICEF, 1986), p. 260. Médecins sans frontières, Nutrition Guidelines, 1st Edition, 1995.

### 2.5 Selecting Beneficiaries

Anthropometric measurements and a brief clinical examination are usually sufficient to identify those children whose nutritional status warrants treatment in an NRP, to assess their degree of malnutrition and to direct the cases selected to the appropriate NRP. When space in the NRCs is limited, the selection of beneficiaries may at times involve establishing orders of priority. In this case, the most experienced staff members should participate in the selection process, to assess the respective chances of survival of cases preselected according to the standard criteria.

### 2.6 NRP Surveillance

Surveillance of nutrition rehabilitation programs encompasses several aspects.

- First, data on the number of admissions and discharges, the number of deaths, and the number of patients who abandon treatment in mid-course must be collected and analyzed.
- The beneficiaries' nutritional recovery must be evaluated by means of regular anthropometric measurement, and patients who fail to gain weight during the program should be identified.
- Beneficiaries who have completed treatment in an NRP should be followed up after they leave the center by means of regular anthropometric measurement.
- Finally, family food resources must be assessed. This aspect, essential to minimize the risks of a relapse, was discussed in detail in connection with the determination of intervention strategy.

**The persistence of a high rate of malnutrition after an NRP has been operating for several months raises the following questions:**

- **Is the NRP functioning properly?**
- **Do the families of the beneficiaries have access to food resources (to avoid relapses)?**
- **Has the demographic situation changed (new arrivals)?**

# VII. Agricultural Rehabilitation

The principal objective of feeding programs must be *to guarantee food security for the victims*. Food distribution of the kind described previously is one way of achieving this objective, but it must under no circumstances become the objective itself. Moreover, it should remain an exceptional measure, a stopgap to be used until a permanent, less costly, and more reliable solution can be devised.

Food distribution makes beneficiaries totally dependent on an outside food supply. Possible consequences include an abdication of responsibility by the victims[76] and unreliable supply due to political and logistical constraints, which may cut off food aid at any moment.

As soon as possible, then, short- and long-term measures should be taken to re-establish feeding self-sufficiency. These measures may involve:

- rehabilitating the food system by:
  - protecting the means of food production;[77]
  - restoring the means of production, where they have deteriorated during a conflict;
- developing the pre-existing system, in order to make it less vulnerable to the dangers inherent in a conflict;
- developing access to a new food system, where the pre-existing system has become permanently inaccessible.[78] This may entail:
  - developing an agricultural system in a new environment;
  - creating employment for refugees.

This section will examine a few aspects of the rehabilitation measures that may be taken on behalf of rural populations living in their original environment. Ways of developing the existing system and creating new means of subsistence will be dealt with in Chapter 8 ("Disasters and Development").

# 1. Principles

The agricultural systems of developing countries are particularly vulnerable to adversity, whether ecological (drought) or political (conflicts). The consequences of such occurrences are often numerous and intermixed; here we will merely touch on the most visible problems for which rehabilitation solutions exist.

## 1.1 Seeds

Lack of seeds may prevent the resumption of farming. In this case, the distribution of seeds suitable for local conditions is enough to re-establish agricultural production.

## 1.2 Cattle

In very serious crises, draft animals may have been slaughtered or sold in order to buy food. Replacing the cattle helps get agricultural activity restarted.

[76] This is the recognized chronic aid recipients' syndrome, in which beneficiaries come to expect humanitarian organizations to guarantee them long-term food aid.

[77] Article 14 of Protocol II additional to the Geneva Conventions provides a basis in law for this kind of protection. This subject will be discussed in Chapter 9 ("Protecting the Victims of Armed Conflicts"), and studied in greater detail in the "HELP" course.

[78] This is the case of refugees who have settled down permanently in neighboring host countries.

Warfare disrupts the operation of local services, including veterinary services. Where semi-nomadic populations derive their principal food resources from cattle, the rehabilitation of veterinary services contributes directly to the re-establishment of dietary self-sufficiency.

However, reconstituting herds belonging to nomadic peoples whose traditional way of life is based on livestock may come into conflict with a certain historical trend towards a sedentary life style or, worse, extermination. The result is an antagonism[79] between the nomads and the resident population which complicates rehabilitation efforts considerably.

## 1.3 Tools

Distributing basic agricultural tools is also an effective measure, and easy to carry out.

## 1.4 Development of Local Markets

To a certain degree, the presence of humanitarian organizations helps protect the civilian population and may favor the free circulation of people and goods that is the basis of food trade. Of course, this effect is very indirect and difficult to quantify. It has been established that food distribution can discourage local food production, since it increases supply and therefore pushes cereal prices down. In certain circumstances, however, this "indirect control" of market prices may give the poorest people easier access to the local food resources available in the market.

[79] "Because of their way of life, which is not amenable to the organization of services (particularly school), and because they live far from population centers, few cattle-raisers have had any schooling or training. As a result, their representation in governmental bodies is very weak, even non-existent, which both keeps them out of decision-making circles and reduces their chances of pressing their claims. In addition, historical factors tend to exclude certain groups of cattle-breeders from power. In fact, in many Sahelian countries today, administrative and military power is controlled primarily by representatives of ethnic groups with an agricultural tradition. Historically, the nomads of the north exercised a certain dominance over the farmers of the south, whose villages they would come to pillage now and again. This ancestral antagonism is still reflected today, indirectly, in the relations between different ethnic groups, and sometimes makes contacts between them difficult." L. Loutan, "Les problèmes de santé dans les zones nomades," in Rougemont and Brunet-Jailly, eds. *Santé dans les pays tropicaux,* p. 232.

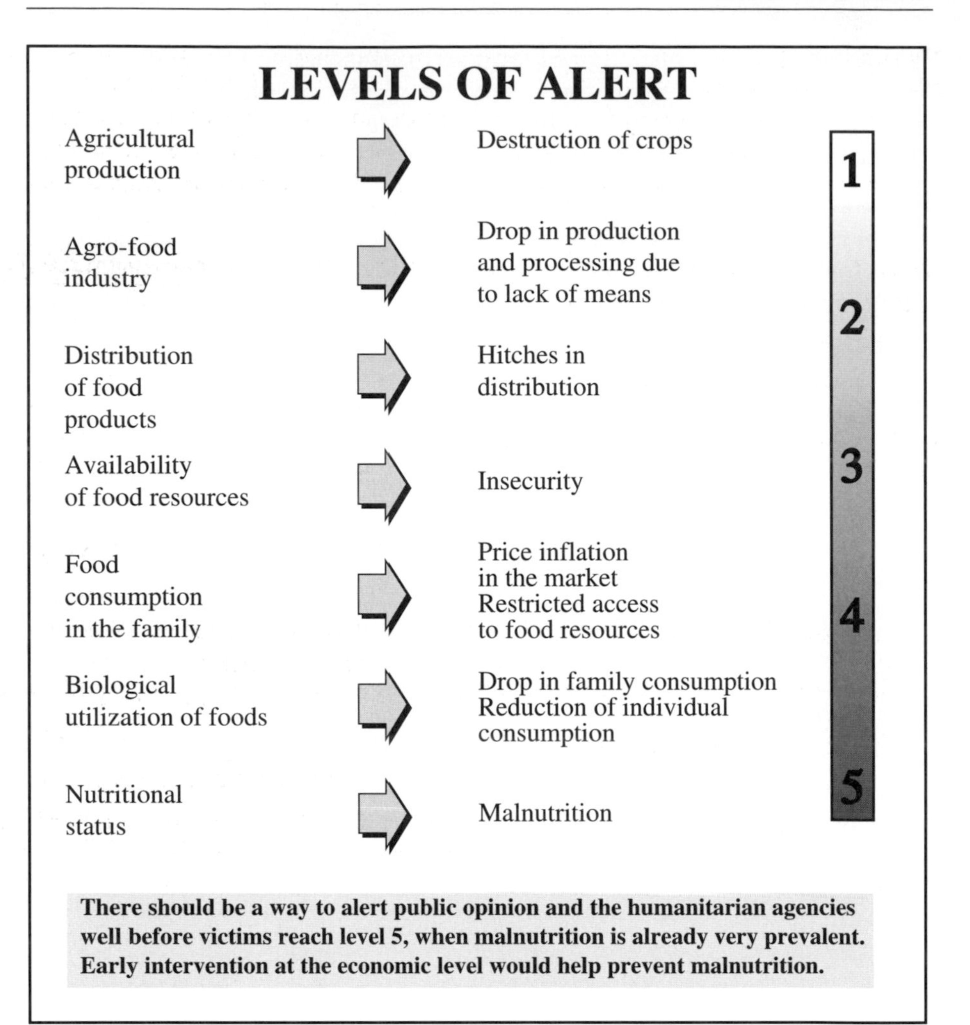


# VIII. Financial Support

Although food donations have always been a symbol of the humanitarian act, cash donations are still rather taboo in this field. In 1986, the Emergency Relief Desk (ERD)[80] made financial contributions directly to the Eritrean Relief Association (ERA) and the Relief Society of Tigray (REST) to cover the cost of buying and transporting food supplies to the two Ethiopian provinces concerned. The reasons given were that:

---

[80] The Emergency Relief Desk is a group of non-governmental organizations whose identity is confidential (taboos again!). See B. Hendrie, "Cross-Border Relief Operations in Eritrea and Tigray," *Disasters* 13, No. 4: 354.

*"[...]inputs of cash to REST for the purchase of (mainly) sorghum has given farmers incentive to increase production; prices are set at market value and REST prohibits merchants from setting a minimum on the amount of grain purchased from local growers. Similarly, small traders have increased their activity and are expanding purchasing and transport networks into areas previously unserved by an integrated market."*[81]

This is not yet one of the "classic" approaches to food aid; nevertheless, relief workers should know that it exists.

Generally speaking, when a food problem arises during an emergency, the entire socioeconomic system should be analyzed before a decision can be made regarding the appropriateness of distributing food. An early-warning system based on this type of analysis would permit preventive intervention well before the populations suffering from armed conflict or other disasters reached a significant level of malnutrition.

**Food aid is a complex issue for several reasons, notably:**

- **It affects the economic, social (including social and health-care organization), and political systems.**
- **In conflict situations, food aid has a strong political connotation (the risk of "feeding the enemy") which tends to paralyze its implementation.**

**A global comprehension of the issue of food aid is indispensable, even if dealing with it remains a complicated business.**

[81] *Ibid.*, pp. 356-357.

Chapter 3

# WATER AND ENVIRONMENTAL HEALTH

***The purpose of this chapter is not to train sanitation engineers able to carry out complex technical operations to improve water quality, for example, or to supply energy to a displaced population. The aim is, rather, to teach participants to do the following:***
***– first, to identify those health problems that have some connection with environmental problems;***
***– second, to recognize those situations where a sanitation specialist is needed to determine and implement the appropriate technical measures;***
***– finally, if necessary, to take responsibility for the technical follow-up of the measures taken, and to evaluate their impact on the beneficiaries' health status.***
***This field is relatively unfamiliar to health-care personnel, since it is not part of the standard curriculum of medical courses;[1] it may therefore be useful to describe very generally the interaction between a population and its environment, as well as the factors that influence that interaction.***

**In terms of health, environmental interventions revolve around three key concepts: Survival Minimization of Risks Prevention**

# I. General Principles

Whatever approach is adopted to address health problems must take into account the relations between a given population and its physical environment. In developed countries, the environment usually goes unnoticed; running water, housing, and sources of energy are all taken for granted. In developing countries, however, all this is much more difficult: water is several kilometers away and of poor quality; housing is flimsy, the environment is infested with communicable-disease vectors, the supply of energy is unreliable. In disaster situations, whatever their cause, mastering the environment becomes more than ever an essential task of the health-care system. Like access to food, access to water is a matter of life and death for populations who have been displaced or cut off from their usual resources. Waste disposal and vector control help considerably to prevent, or at least to reduce, the incidence of communicable diseases.

1 Meaning medical training in the broad sense (doctors, nurses, etc.).

# 1. Interaction Between a Population and its Environment

A list of the environmental factors that influence a population's health status and a parallel list of the human factors that influence environmental hygiene together provide an outline of their reciprocal action.

## 1.1 Types of Interaction

Access to food resources, food hygiene, the quantity and quality of water available, construction material and available sources of energy, the presence of communicable-disease vectors — all these are factors that directly influence health status. At the same time, the population itself helps pollute the environment and exhaust environmental resources by the quantities of solid (garbage, human excreta) and liquid waste it dumps, and by the pressure it exerts on that environment through overpopulation. This interaction has disastrous consequences — for example, the pollution of drinking water by human waste and the exhaustion of energy resources (wood). This process is a vicious circle that should be broken quickly if health is to be preserved.

Moreover, the interaction of population and environment can be very complex. Seldom is only one environmental factor involved in the transmission of communicable diseases. For example, water may be polluted at its source by human waste, or at the point of distribution, by hands soiled with fecal matter. The absence of personal hygiene may itself be a consequence of lack of water.

## 1.2 Technical Implications

It is particularly important to understand the nature of this interaction, which in various ways governs the balance between a population and its environment. Its implication is that no single factor (water, waste, housing) can be grasped without due consideration of the others. The most typical example is technical measures designed to protect sources of potable water. They can be really effective only if other measures are taken at the same time to control human waste and to promote personal hygiene. Practically speaking, an isolated sanitation measure which is not integrated into a comprehensive plan will *a priori* have little impact on a population's health status.

# 2. General Factors Influencing Relations Between the Population and the Environment

Many general factors influence the relationship between a population and its environment. The most important ones are climate and level of development.

Climatic conditions influence the relations between a population and its environment in many ways; they determine the availability of water resources, encourage or discourage the proliferation of specific communicable-disease vectors, and influence the type of housing the population will adopt. Their effects vary, of course, with the changing seasons of the year.

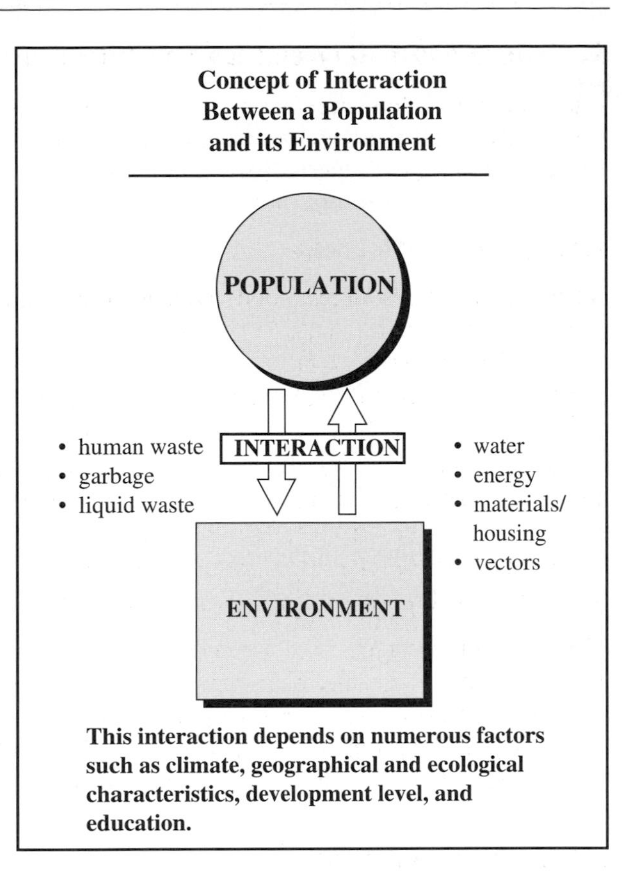


The level of economic, social, and cultural development also conditions the relationship between a population and its environment to a large extent. The use of water depends not only on its availability in the environment, but also on the local level of development. In the industrialized countries, a person might use several hundred liters of water a day, while in rural areas of developing countries a mere dozen liters a day may be the rule. The way available resources are used varies from one culture to another. For example, water has certain ritual uses in the Asian cultures.

## 3. Problems Caused by Exceptional Situations

Exceptional situations radically change the relations between a population and its environment. Such situations involve two essential factors: changes in the environment, and population concentrations.

Environmental changes may be radical. This is the case, for example, when displaced populations or refugees arrive in a new environment, or when a people's movements within its normal geographical environment are restricted. Such restrictions are usually the result of military operations: landmines placed on the roads, for example, tend to reduce access to the usual natural resources, such as water.

Environmental changes usually go together with population movements. Conflict situations are often characterized by population concentrations as people are forced to leave their homes because of dangerous conditions and/or political reasons.[2]

The conjunction of these two factors, environmental change and population concentration, contributes to the overpopulation of a hostile environment,[3] with every conceivable pressure on water, energy, and other reserves, as well as an increase[4] in waste.

The health consequences of this imbalance can be noted at several levels. On the individual level, they contribute, for example, to an increase in the incidence of communicable diseases, attributable to the interaction of numerous factors: lack of water (resulting in inadequate personal hygiene), the contamination of the environment by waste (through contamination of water, or directly from person to person), and the multiplication of disease vectors (since the lack of hygiene encourages the proliferation of flies).

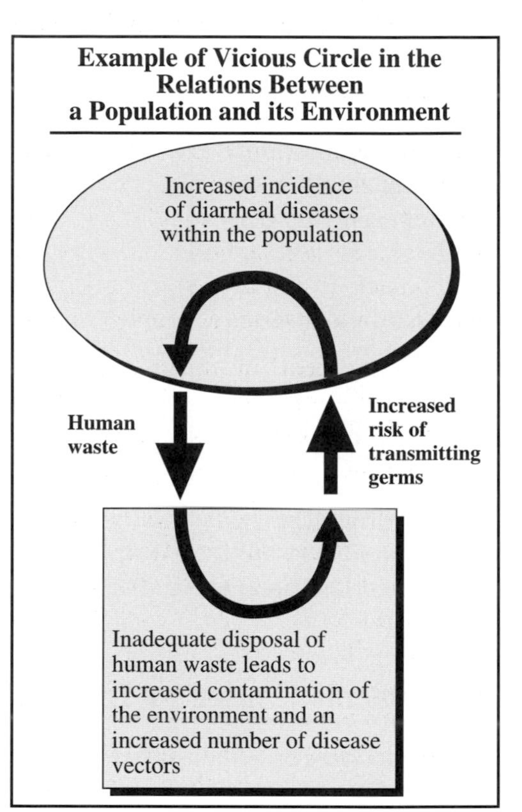


On the social level, the necessity of resorting, in certain situations, to collective living quarters tends to disrupt family life. On the community level, the reduced access to normal resources gives rise to dependence on sources outside the country. This dependence may be politically exploited to keep certain population groups under the tutelage of one of the parties to the conflict. Obviously, whoever controls access to water sources controls the people who depend on them.

This chapter will discuss only the technical aspects of measures designed to optimize the balance between population and environment in situations of acute

---

2 The civil and/or military authorities may force civilian populations to regroup in order to isolate opposition groups from potential support.

3 Hostile, because displaced people do not control the parameters of an unfamiliar environment.

4 The increase is due to the increase in population and the decrease in available space that is often associated with it.

crisis, particularly conflicts. It will not deal with considerations of a more general nature, such as demographic pressure and global warming.

# II. Water

## 1. Water Needs

Everyone knows that water is essential to human survival, to the prevention of many communicable diseases, and to the maintenance of health.

### 1.1 Quantity

People sometimes have a tendency to make a distinction between drinking water and water used for hygienic purposes such as washing and laundering, setting different standards of quality and quantity for each. This distinction is unwarranted, for it assumes that a given population can be provided with two water systems. In most emergency situations, this idea is unrealistic, both logistically and in terms of people's ability to use two networks simultaneously.[5]

Thus, "water needs" means an individual's overall needs. It is tempting to define quantitative norms applicable at all times and in all places, but the reality is completely different: in determining water needs we must take into account physiological, cultural, geographic, and technical factors.

Physiological norms alone indicate that the minimal quantity of water to permit survival would be about 3 liters per person per day in temperate zones, and 6-10 liters in hot climates. Yet water has other uses as well. The use of water for hygienic purposes is particularly important in reducing the incidence of communicable diseases. The general view is that 10-15 liters of water should be supplied per person per day, but this quantity varies considerably from one culture to the next. When determining the quantities of water that should be provided for hygiene, planners must keep in mind that in many cultures water is more of a ritual element than a factor in hygiene.

Climate and geological conditions affect the quantities of water that can be provided. Obviously, in desert regions where water is scarce and therefore precious, it will be doled out parsimoniously, or at least according to the minimum standards.

Finally, the technical characteristics of the water distribution network influence the quantities of water used by a population. Many studies on such factors as the

[5] The two systems become confused: drinking water is used for hygiene and vice versa.

distances between water-supply points and the consumer's home have shown a relation between the quantity of water used and the distance the user needs to go to fetch it. Water use is maximal when it is available within the home. In short, the more ramified the distribution system and the closer it brings the water to the household, the greater the consumption of water. Starting from 20 liters per day, a greater impact on health status can be hoped for; but relief workers must make sure that water sources are adequate, that distribution can be relied on in the long term, and that, in the case of displaced populations, they are not creating a standard different from that imposed on the neighboring local population.

**In general, the standard of 20 liters per day per person can be considered appropriate for emergency situations, with the proviso that this "norm" is very relative and must be adjusted as the situation demands.**

It should be noted that the consumption of water in facilities specifically established for emergency situations (field hospitals, nutrition rehabilitation centers, etc.) is particularly high — an estimated 150-200 liters per patient per day in a hospital, and 30-40 liters per child in a feeding center.

## 1.2 Quality

In general, health personnel are much more aware of the problem of water quality than they are of the quantity required by victims during a disaster.

**What is potable water?**
Potable water is water which contains no elements posing a danger for human consumption or for any domestic use, including personal hygiene.[6]

Such elements may be microbiological, chemical, or physical.

### *Microbiological Quality*

Water may be contaminated by microorganisms (bacteria, viruses, or parasites), usually of fecal origin. The following is a list of some of the water contaminants that have the greatest impact on public health:

- Virus (rotavirus)
- *Escherichia coli*
- *Vibrio cholerae*
- *Shigella*
- *Entamoeba histolytica*
- *Giardia lamblia*
- *Schistosoma*

The presence of fecal coliforms (*E. coli*) is used as an indicator of fecal contamination.

---

6 *Guidelines for Drinking-Water Quality*, 2nd ed. (Geneva: WHO, 1993).

**What are the norms?**

The microbiological quality of drinking water is measured by the presence of *Escherichia coli.*[7] However, an absence of *E. coli* is not always an easily attainable goal in emergency situations; a more realistic target is the WHO-recommended standard for rural areas, which accepts the presence of a few coliforms. The WHO policy, designed essentially for rural areas under normal conditions, has been adopted by UNICEF for emergency situations:

The presence of faecal coliforms indicates that the water has been contaminated by faeces of humans or other warm-blooded animals. Concentrations are usually expressed per 100 ml of water. As a rough guide:

- 0-10 faecal coliforms/100 ml = reasonable quality
- 10-100 faecal coliforms/100 ml = polluted
- 100-1,000 faecal coliforms/100 ml = dangerous
- over 1,000 faecal coliforms/100 ml = very dangerous

*Source:* Ron Ockwell, ed., *Assisting in Emergencies* (UNICEF), p. 327.

## *Chemical Quality*

The presence of toxic substances (arsenic, mercury, lead, nitrates, etc.) or abnormally high levels of trace elements (such as fluoride) in the water poses a risk to the health of the people who consume it. Eliminating such substances requires complex, costly technical measures which are difficult to implement under normal circumstances, and practically impossible during an emergency.

An elevated concentration of salts (chlorides, sulfates) leads to few health problems, since beyond a certain level the water's salty taste deters people from drinking it.[8]

Where chemical contamination presents a danger to health, the only solution is to seek another water-supply source.

## *Physical Quality*

Physical quality concerns the physical attributes of the water, namely taste, smell, and appearance. Water which appears turbid is not necessarily unfit for consumption, if microbiological and chemical criteria are met; but the potential consumers may be disinclined to drink "dirty" water.

---

7 "The most specific of the readily detectable faecal indicators of bacteria and the one present in greatest numbers of faeces is Escherichia coli, and it is therefore recommended as the indicator of choice for drinking water." *Ibid.*, p. 20.

8 The concentration of salts dissolved in water can be estimated by the measurement of electrical conductivity.

## 2. Health Risks

### 2.1 Vital Risk

In certain exceptional situations, a population may be totally deprived of water. This happens mostly in cases where people are besieged in cities or forcibly confined to limited areas which contain no water sources.

Another kind of vital risk is the danger of dying from diarrheal illnesses induced by the consumption of polluted water.

### 2.2 Morbidity

Water plays an important role in transmitting certain infectious diseases, particularly diarrheal illnesses.[9] To avoid memorizing a long, indigestible list of diseases that can be transmitted by water, we can categorize them by the mechanism of transmission.

**Recommendations for Supplying Water**

QUANTITY:
20 liters of water per day and per person

QUALITY:
- Physical characteristics:
  - appearance
  - smell
  - taste
- Microbiological constants:
  - 0-10 E. coli/100 ml
- Chemical constants:
  - arsenic < 0.05 mg/l
  - fluoride < 1.5 mg/l
  - cyanides < 0.1 mg/l
  - mercury < 0.001 mg/l
  - lead < 0.05 mg/l

*Presence of Water*

The mere presence of water favors the proliferation of insects, or water-related vectors, which transmit, for example, the following diseases:

- malaria (mosquitoes)
- yellow fever (mosquitoes)
- dengue fever (mosquitoes)
- arboviruses (mosquitoes)
- sleeping sickness (flies)
- onchocerciasis (flies)

9 It should be kept in mind that water is not an isolated factor, but contributes to disease in combination with other factors: fecal contamination, lack of health education, etc.

### *Contact with Water*

In areas where schistosomiasis is endemic, mere contact with water infested by *cercariae* (the mature larva of the *schistosoma*) is sufficient for the transmission of schistosomiasis.[10]

**Classification of Communicable Diseases by Their Relation to Water**

- consumption of polluted water:
  - cholera
  - amebiasis
- lack of water engendering inadequate personal hygiene:
  - scabies
  - trachoma
- presence in the water of an intermediate host which carries the pathogenic agent:
  - schistosomiasis
- development of communicable-disease vectors in water:
  - malaria
  - yellow fever
- combination of the causes above:
  - amebiasis: polluted water and inadequate personal hygiene

### *Water Quality*

The contamination of drinking water by pathogenic agents causes or increases the incidence of certain diseases, classified as waterborne diseases:

- diarrheal illnesses
- cholera
- amebiasis
- giardiasis
- leptospirosis
- infectious hepatitis

The severity of the disease is related to the quantity of pathogens ingested. This feature has been studied particularly in diarrheal diseases. The quantity varies from one germ to the next.[11]

### *Water Quantity*

The more water people have at their disposal, the greater their ability to maintain standards of hygiene. In practice, this means washing themselves, washing clothes, washing vegetables, and so on. In terms of morbidity, these habits will translate into a reduction in the incidence of water-washed diseases, namely:

---

[10] Transmission of schistosomiasis requires the presence in the water of an intermediate host (snails).

[11] "The results of this review indicate that improvements in one or more components of water supply and sanitation can substantially reduce the rates of morbidity and severity of ascariasis, diarroeal diseases, dracunculiasis, hookworm infection, schistosomiasis and trachoma [...] in addition to reducing the incidence or prevalence of disease, improvements in water and sanitation can be expected to affect other health aspects." S.A. Esrey, J.B. Potash, L. Roberts, and C. Schiff, "Reviews/Analysis: Effects of Improved Water Supply and Sanitation on Ascariasis, Diarrhoea, Dracunculiasis, Hookworm Infection, Schistosomiasis, and Trachoma, *Bulletin of the World Health Organization* 69, No. 5 (1991): 616.

- diarrheal diseases (handwashing)[12]
- ascarids (handwashing)
- ancylostomes (handwashing)
- scabies
- skin infections
- eye infections (trachoma, conjunctivitis)
- diseases transmitted by lice (typhus)
- salmonella infections (food contamination)

## *Interaction of Factors*

To grasp the extent to which the different factors are intertwined, we need only consider the potential impact of the two factors just described, water quantity and quality. Many studies have been carried out to determine the respective importance of each factor in health status, and particularly in the incidence of diarrheal illnesses.

**The general consensus is that the quantity of water takes precedence over the quality:**

*"The impact of water supply and sanitation on diarrhoea, related infections, nutritional status, and mortality is analysed by reviewing 67 studies from 28 countries.*

*The mean reductions in diarrhoea morbidity rates are 22% from all studies and 27% from a few better-designed studies. All studies of the impact on total mortality rates show a median reduction of 21%, while the few better-designed studies give a median reduction of 30%. Improvements in water quality have less of an impact than improvements in water availability or excreta disposal."*[13]

Although quantity is essential, the quality of the water must not, of course, be neglected; it should correspond to the norms defined above. From a practical point of view, if it is necessary to choose between supplying small quantities of pure water or large quantities of water containing a few *coli* bacilli, then the latter option is preferable.

---

[12] The lack of enough water to permit regular handwashing after defecation facilitates direct feco-oral transmission, despite a water supply of reasonably good quality. See Steven A. Esrey and Jean Pierre Habicht: "The provision and use of sufficient water albeit of poor quality, for personal and domestic hygiene could prevent the contamination of food, utensils, and hands and thereby reduce the transmission of the major infectious agents of diarrhea." "Epidemiologic Evidence for Health Benefits from Improved Water and Sanitation in Developing Countries," *Epidemiologic Reviews* 8 (1986): 118.

[13] S.A. Esrey, R.G. Feachem, and J.M. Hughes, "Interventions for the Control of Diarrhoeal Diseases among Young Children: Improving Water Supplies and Excreta Disposal Facilities," *Bulletin of the World Health Organization* 63, No. 4 (1985): 757.

## 2.3 Malnutrition

The impact of water supply on nutritional status shows quite clearly that water quantity and quality are closely linked. A study carried out in Madras,[14] for example, shows that for children under the age of three years, water quality is relatively more important, while quantity is more significant for children over that age.

The main thing to remember is that water, through its role in the transmission of diarrheal diseases, has an impact on nutritional status.

At this point, we know the norms for supplying water and the risks we run by deviating from them. We are also familiar with the principle of integrating the different sanitation measures, with each other and with health-education activities. This subject will not be discussed further in this chapter, but will be raised again in connection with diarrheal illnesses (Chapter 4, "Communicable Diseases").
The next section will cover the technical principles involved in a water-supply system.

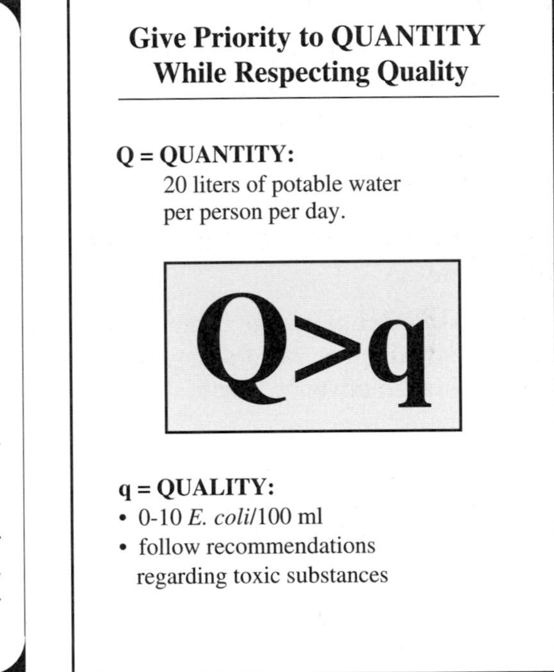


# 3. Water-Supply Techniques

In disaster situations, water-supply systems are often partially destroyed, or the materials necessary to maintain them are lacking. In such cases, relief workers must determine to what extent the missing elements can be replaced.

When, due to an exceptional situation, populations are displaced, they occasionally find refuge in an area containing no infrastructure for providing water. In such cases, a water system furnishing the minimum quantity of water consistent with the norms described earlier must be put together quickly.

---

[14] J.R. Hebert, "Effects of Water Quality and Water Quantity on Nutritional Status: Findings from a South Indian Community," *Bulletin of the World Health Organization* 63, No. 1 (1985): 143-155.

We will take this type of situation as our primary example in studying basic water-supply techniques. This study will follow a logical progression, from the identification of potential water sources up to the moment the water is consumed by the individual.

## 3.1 Water Sources

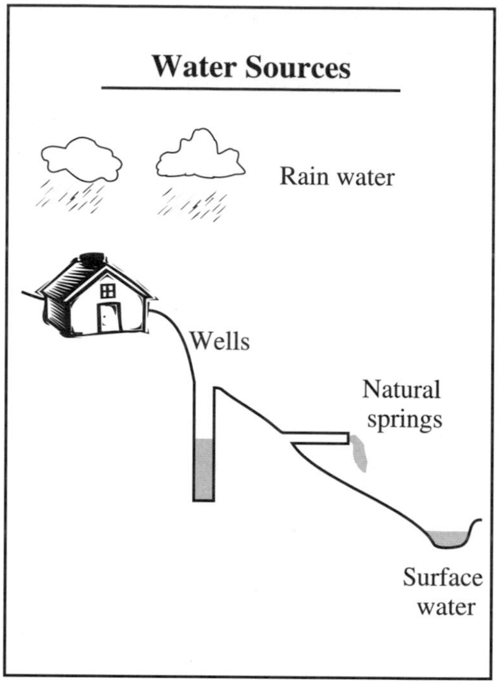

**Water Sources**

Rain water

Wells

Natural springs

Surface water

### *Evaluation of Water Sources*

The purpose of evaluating water sources is to determine the best source of water supply in a given situation. As shown in the diagram, water may fall from the sky (rain), lie on the earth's surface (rivers, lakes, swamps), or be contained within the earth (ground water).

A certain number of criteria can be used to judge the value of a water source in advance. These criteria are:

- *the quantity of water that the source can provide*. The techniques used to estimate this quantity vary according to the type of source:
  - rain — quantity is measured by the volume of precipitation and the surface on which it falls;
  - well — the quantity is measured by the time the well takes to refill after depletion. In addition, the impact that well construction can be expected to have on the water table is assessed,[15] as is the effectiveness of the well's protection.
  - spring, river — the rate of flow is measured.
- *reliability in different seasons*. This criterion is obvious in the case of rain water, but it is also relevant for the other types of water source, in which the flow may vary considerably between the dry and wet seasons.
- *accessibility*: There are two kinds of accessibility:

[15] The impact a well is likely to have on the water table must be carefully assessed. Uncontrolled exploitation may lead to a rapid depletion of the ground water, and drilling in coastal areas may result in saltwater seeping into the borehole.

- physical — The distance between the water source and the people who use it may signify two things:
  a) that consumers will have a longer or a shorter distance to walk in order to fetch water;
  b) that it may be necessary to construct a long water conveyance network to carry the water close to the living quarters of the population.
- political — In conflict situations, access to water sources may be controlled by one of the parties to the conflict; or it may present dangers to the population owing to the presence of landmines or fighting on the road.

– *quality of the untreated water*. Rain water and ground water are potable by definition,[16] whereas surface water is by definition non-potable. This statement must, of course, be qualified; lakes containing pure

[16] Ground water is potable because it is filtered through the geological strata. However, the nature of the soil must be taken into account, as well as possible fractures through which contamination may penetrate.

**Assessment of a Water Supply Point (ICRC Assessment Form)**

**I. Site:**
City, village
Locality
Province

**II. Type of supply point:**
a. Spring:
- approximate flow
- development
- protection

b. Well:
- dug by hand/ by drill/ by machine
- year of construction
- depth
- present level of water (from the ground)

Ask users these questions:
- maximum level observed / when?
- minimum level observed / when?
- amount of water pumped each day
- protection (cover, external slab, etc.)
- type of soil (clay, sand, humus, gravel, etc.)
- nature of the aquifer (layer containing the water)

c. Surface:
- description (stream, river, lake, etc.)
- in use all year? (dry season)
- volume of water taken out each day (estimation)

**III. Equipment:**
a. Existence of a pump: manual or motorized
- type: brand:
- year of installation
- maximum possible flow
- if immersed, depth within well

b. Existence of a reservoir:
- volume: distance from water-supply point
- difference in altitude between water-supply point and reservoir

c. Pipes: material: diameter: condition:

**IV. Use:**
- number of people served
- length of waiting time
- quality of water: smell/ taste/ color

**V. Remarks:**

water can be found, as can polluted ground water. Nevertheless, the principle can be used as a basis for discussion during the process of selecting a water source.

The microbiological analysis of water is a technique used to identify the presence of *E. coli*, which is considered a good indicator of fecal contamination. A sample of the water to be analyzed is put into an appropriate culture medium for 48 hours. *E. coli* grows in colonies, the number of which indicates the degree of contamination. This analysis can be carried out in the field with the aid of a simple, portable kit.

- *engineering*. This criterion covers all the work necessary to make the source usable. Usually a combination of measures is required: extraction of ground water, treatment of surface water, establishment of a water carrier and distribution network, etc. The engineering aspect influences both the cost of the project and the time needed to implement it. The latter is crucial in emergency situations, when safe water must be obtained quickly.

The process of assessment must take all these criteria into account. Ready-made assessment forms are available for this purpose.[17]

### *Selecting a Source of Water*

Merely filling out an assessment form does not in itself solve the problem of choosing a water source, especially where various options exist. The evaluator must examine the data collected in terms of each criterion, with the understanding that the value of each may vary according to the factors that influence it, notably:

- *the sociocultural context*. The engineering technology used must be appropriate to the local economic level — so that it can be maintained in the long term — and to the local culture — so that the water source will be used.
- *the political context*. The exploitation of water resources for a displaced population must take the resident population into account.
- *the size of the population*. The sources chosen must be adequate to meet the needs of the consumer population (quantity criterion) with no danger that they will run dry or that access to them will be denied (criteria of reliability and political accessibility).
- *the degree of urgency*. The speed of intervention may necessitate the use of expensive techniques (engineering and cost criteria).

[17] ICRC, "Feuille d'évaluation des points d'eau."

- *the medium-term view.* Different approaches can be combined, as in emergency situations, when there is a choice between two sources; one can be quickly put to use with the help of intensive technical means, while the other requires long labor but is inexpensive. The second option would take over from the first in the medium term.

Here again, forms synthesizing all these factors can be obtained.[18] Organized as flow charts, they permit the decision-maker to judge which water source is the most suitable in a given context.

**Criteria for Selecting a Water Source**

- Quantity of water:
  - immediate capacity
  - reliability over time (dry season)
- Quality of water:
  - present quality
  - risk of pollution
- Technology required for exploitation:
  - type of technology required
    - to put it in use
    - to maintain it
  - acceptability to local consumers
- Accessibility:
  - geographical
  - social
  - financial (i.e., whether payment is required)
  - safe access in conflict zones

The choice of a source is not as simple as it might seem at first. Not only is an evaluation of the source itself required, but also an estimation of the type of installation that may be necessary to make the source usable. In addition, planners must have a good knowledge of the community that will use it, to judge whether it will be ultimately acceptable.

## *Technical Aspects of Extracting and Delivering Water*

- *Rain water*

Rain water can be collected off the roofs in receptacles placed under the drainpipes. In emergencies, plastic sheeting distributed for the construction of shelters can also be used to collect rain water.

**Technological input** is very minor.

- *Surface Water*

As noted previously, surface water must be considered as contaminated. Certain methods of exploiting it, can be used, however, to obviate the necessity of treating it. Such methods include, for example, sinking wells in the banks of a river, or

[18] S. Cairncross and R. Feachem, *Small Water Supplies*, Ross Bulletin 10 (Ross Institute, 1978), p. 6.

burying a filter box in the river bed. These methods are based on the principle of filtering water through soil, which will be studied later.

**Technological input** can be quite substantial, depending on the case.

- *Spring Water*

A spring is in fact ground water that rises to the surface at a certain point. The water has thus been naturally filtered by the geological strata and is usually potable. The trick is to draw the water immediately at the spot where it emerges (known as the "eye" of the spring). Spring water which has flowed above ground for too long becomes surface water, and is very likely to be polluted.

**Principal Steps for Using a Natural Spring as a Source of Water Supply**

- identify the eye of the spring (the point where the water emerges)
- develop a filtration system (natural or engineered)
- protect the area around the source from possible contamination
- set up a water-distribution system
- develop a drainage system for runoff
- set up a maintenance and surveillance system

**Technological input is considerable**. The filtration zone uphill from the point where the water emerges must be preserved and the filtration effect may have to be reinforced by the addition of new layers of sand or gravel. Uphill from the eye of the spring, a low retention wall is normally built, to which is adjoined a storage box. From it the water enters a distribution system (a simple pipe from which people help themselves directly to water, or a conduit to the village where distribution will take place).[19]

- *Ground Water*

Ground water is the water least immediately available. Consequently, the technological input necessary to gain access to it will be greater than for other sources. However, ground water has a naturally good microbiological quality that surface water, for example, does not. Surface water is easily accessible, but it must be treated before it can be consumed, whereas treatment is usually not necessary for ground water. In practice, the initial technological investment may seem large, but it later turns out to be in fact relatively minor. Thus, when potential water sources are being compared, the issue of technological input should be seen in perspective.

[19] Many manuals describing these techniques have been published, a notable example being the Ross Institute manual *Small Water Supplies* (1978), pp. 8-9.

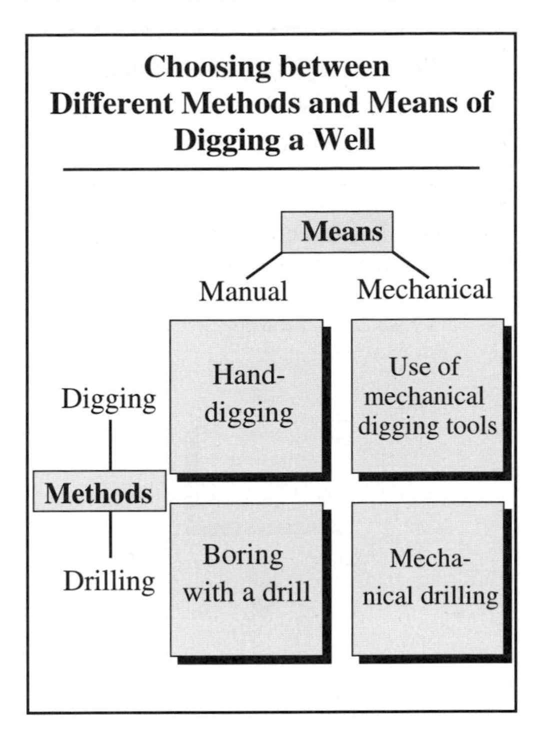


**Technological input** includes sinking a well and constructing its walls or lining.

There are four principal ways of sinking a well:

- manual digging
- mechanical digging
- manual drilling
- mechanical drilling[20]

The choice between these methods will depend on various factors, the importance of which varies from one situation to the next:

- urgency
- size of the population
- local availability of skilled labor
- alternatives (other sources of water)
- cost versus available funds

## 3.2 Technical Means for Extracting Water

### *Gravity*

Using gravity is the best way of drawing water, since it requires very little equipment. It can be used for some natural springs and for surface water (which can be diverted to a treatment unit).

### *Ancillary Means*

In developing countries, there are many local methods for drawing water from wells — for example, by means of a bucket attached to a rope and either thrown directly into the well or set on the end of a counterweighted pole. The major disadvantage of these systems is that the well usually remains uncovered.[21]

---

[20] Today, relatively compact drilling rigs are available which can be easily transported.

[21] The water in the well thereby becomes surface water and, accordingly, subject to contamination.

### *Pumps*

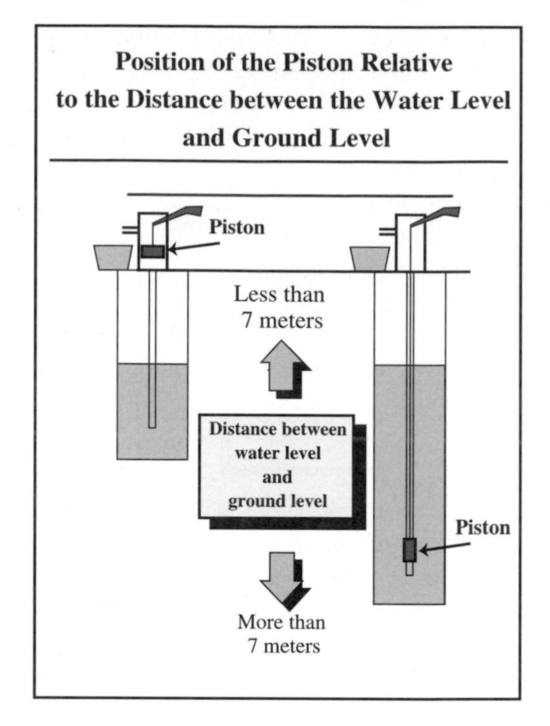


The use of pumps has the advantage of allowing the well to remain closed, and if measures for protecting the area around the well are correctly applied, the water is kept free of all contamination.

There are many types of pumps, which can be broadly classified as manual pumps or mechanical pumps. The technical specifications of each pump will not be described here; this section will focus instead on the criteria for choosing a particular type of pump in a given situation.

To avoid long lists,[22] decision-makers should focus on two main criteria and a few secondary ones.

- *The first criterion* is the operating mechanism of the pump, which may be one of two types:
  - the water is drawn up from above towards the outlet,
  - the water is pushed up from below, to the pump outlet.

In the first case, the operating cylinder is above the well; in the second, it is in the water. Although the first solution would appear to be simpler, it is limited by the laws of physics, since if the water level is more than eight meters down, the pump can no longer operate.[23]

The static level of the water table, then, will influence the choice of pump.

- *The second criterion* concerns the method of operating the pump:
  - manually (hand pump)
  - by an external energy source, such as wind, electricity, or sun.

The factors to be considered in this choice are as follows:

---

[22] See the chapter on rural water supply in Sandy Cairncross and Richard Feachem, *Environmental Health Engineering in the Tropics*, 2nd ed. (John Wiley and Sons, 1993), pp. 74-79.

[23] The pressure at the level of the piston/water interface becomes such that the water theoretically turns to vapor (triple point). The main idea here is that beyond a certain depth, the weight of the water column to be drawn up becomes too great.

- *Delivery capacity.* A hand pump can pump 750-900 liters an hour, and in theory could provide enough water for 1,000 people;[24] a motorized pump has a much greater output. For large populations, pumps operated by an external energy source are essential unless the number of water-supply points is increased.
- *The depth of the well.* If the well is more than 50-60 meters deep, a hand pump should not be used.
- *Long-term maintenance prospects.* Generally speaking, planners should try to "keep things simple."
- *Access to energy sources.* In conflict situations, where access to energy resources is limited and politically sensitive,[25] hand pumps are preferable. If an external energy source is used, it should be a non-strategic one such as wind or solar energy.
- *Cost.* Hand pumps are less expensive than the installation of systems dependent on an external source of energy.[26]
- *Capacity of the water source.* Since the consumption of water is linked to the volume of water provided,[27] the temptation is to install powerful technical means to provide maximum flow. If, however, water reserves (for example, the ground water) have been overestimated — or not been taken into account at all — they are apt to be quickly exhausted, with repercussions not only for the population's health status, but also for the environment.

## 3.3 Water Storage

Once the water has been drawn from its source, it can be put directly at the population's disposal or channeled into a storage unit from which it will be distributed.

### *Criteria Dictating the Use of a Storage Unit*

- *Water Quality*

If the water is of poor quality (for example, water pumped directly from a river), it must be treated. For proper treatment, whatever the technique (filtration, chemical treatment), the water must be stored. The storage area will depend on geography and the configuration of the distribution network that will be integrated with it. Ideally, distribution will be gravity-fed from the storage unit.

---

24 Ockwell, ed., *Assisting in Emergencies* (UNICEF), p. 337.

25 Diesel oil can fuel tanks as well as pumps.

26 It should be noted that solar-energy systems usually cost more to set up, but in the long run are more economical than diesel oil or gas.

27 And also to conditions of access, particularly the distance between the consumer's home and the distribution point.

• *Size of the Population*
Direct distribution at the source (a well equipped with a hand pump, for example) is satisfactory if the population is relatively small. But if the number of people depending on one source of water is high, there is a risk of "traffic jams!" The solution is to channel the water into a reservoir, whence it will flow into a network with a variable number of outlets, depending on the size of the population.

### *Technological Input*

The technical means required to construct storage units depends on several factors:

* available local materials
* local technical expertise
* the size of the storage unit
* the type of water treatment, if treatment is necessary

Treatment with sand filters may require the construction of several inter-connected storage reservoirs.

## 3.4 Treatment of the Water

Storage and treatment are closely linked. Water treatment procedures require that the water be stored, or at least held. Moreover, storage is in itself a form of water treatment.

### *Storage*

Storage plays a twofold role in water treatment. First, the sedimentation that occurs during storage reduces the amount of organic material in the water, so that less chlorine is required later, during chemical treatment. Second, storage helps eliminate certain pathogens — for example the cercariae that transmit schistosomiasis, and which die in the water after 48 hours. Moreover, holding the water in transparent reservoirs exposes it to ultraviolet rays from the sun, which eliminate most pathogens.[28]

*Technological input* varies considerably according to the circumstances. It may involve anything from building a family cistern to setting up reservoirs large enough to supply a whole city with drinking water.

### *Filtration*

This section will discuss only the technique known as the *slow sand filter,*[29] and not the rapid sand filter, nor filtration through special materials (ceramic

[28] "Exposure to sunlight in transparent vessels renders these solutions bacteriologically safe." A. Acra *et al.*, "Disinfection of Oral Rehydration Solutions by Sunlight," *The Lancet* (6 Dec. 1980): 1257.

[29] Speed of filtration is 0.2 m/hour.

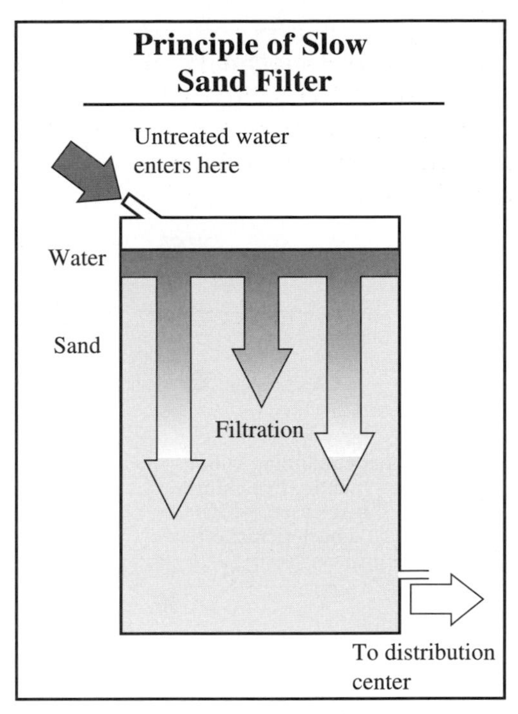


material, porous membranes, etc.). The sand filter is based on the principle of natural filtration through the soil. In this case, however, the soil is replaced by a layer of sand or alternate layers of sand, gravel, charcoal, etc., through which the untreated water passes.

Contrary to what might be supposed, the main mode of action is not the mechanical filtration process, which is related to the size of the space between the grains of sand,[30] but rather the biological action that takes place in the top centimeters of the filter.[31]

*Technological input* is not very substantial when the project is turning a barrel into a sand filter for use by a single household. It becomes rather more significant when prefabricated sand filters[32] have to be installed to provide clean water for a displaced-person camp, a hospital, or some other large institution.

*Chemical Treatment*

Chemical treatment has two uses. One use is to facilitate sedimentation during storage. Such treatment consists in adding aluminum salts, which accelerate the sedimentation of organic particles within the water by facilitating drainage. This does not kill the germs, but it reduces the quantity of organic matter in the water so that smaller quantities of chlorine can be used at the second, bactericidal stage of treatment.

---

30 This space is defined by granulometry; in general, a diameter of 0.5 mm is recommended.

31 "This biologically active zone, known as the 'schmutzdecke', is responsible for most of the water-quality improvement provided by a slow sand filter. In particular, the schmutzdecke retains or kills the great majority of viruses, bacteria, protozoal cysts, and helminth eggs and thus makes the slow sand filter a far more efficient pathogen-removing process than the rapid sand filter." Cairncross and Feachem, *Environmental Health Engineering in the Tropics*, p. 93.

32 The sand filters manufactured by Oxfam are the most widely used in emergency situations. They are composed of three reservoirs: the first receives the untreated water, the second contains the sand through which the water will be filtered, and the third holds the filtered water.

The other use of chemical treatment is to kill germs. This involves disinfecting the water. Although a number of different chemical products may be used for this purpose, they are all generally referred to as "chlorine." Two points are important here:

- Only free chlorine has a disinfectant action.
- Chlorine links with organic particles and is neutralized by the combination. Chlorine must therefore be added until all the organic particles in the water have been oxidized;[33] only then is free chlorine released in the water, allowing disinfection to begin.

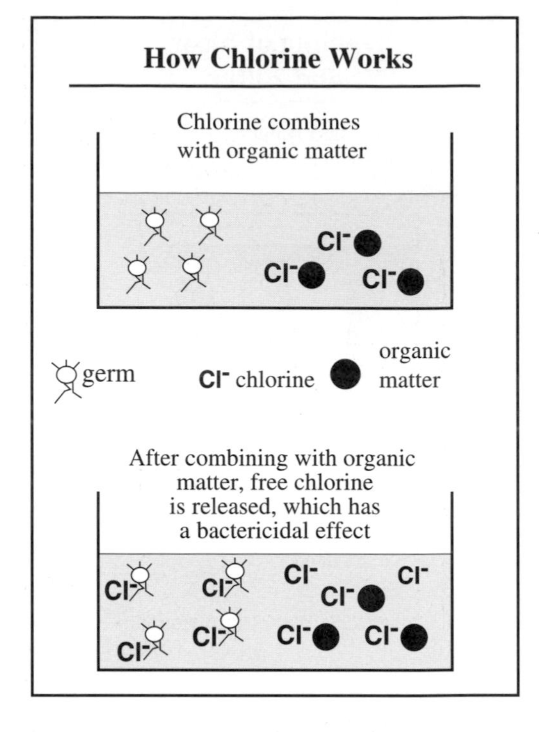


The effective dose of free chlorine is 0.5 mg/l, acting over a period of half an hour. There are numerous ways of measuring free chlorine in the water, colorimetric methods being the easiest and least expensive to use.

Chemical treatment may be implemented in different ways according to circumstances; it may consist in simply immersing a pot containing a product that releases chlorine, or it may involve specialized equipment.

*Technological input* consists of chemical products (basically chlorine and aluminum salts) and the equipment necessary to monitor the level of free chlorine in the water.

### *Boiling*

This method of treatment is seldom used in emergencies, since access to energy resources is usually difficult and uncertain.[34]

## *Decision Criteria*

The choice between the various treatment methods will be based on the following criteria:

---

33 Hence the importance of sedimentation, which reduces the quantity of organic matter.
34 Half a kilo of wood is needed to boil one liter of water.

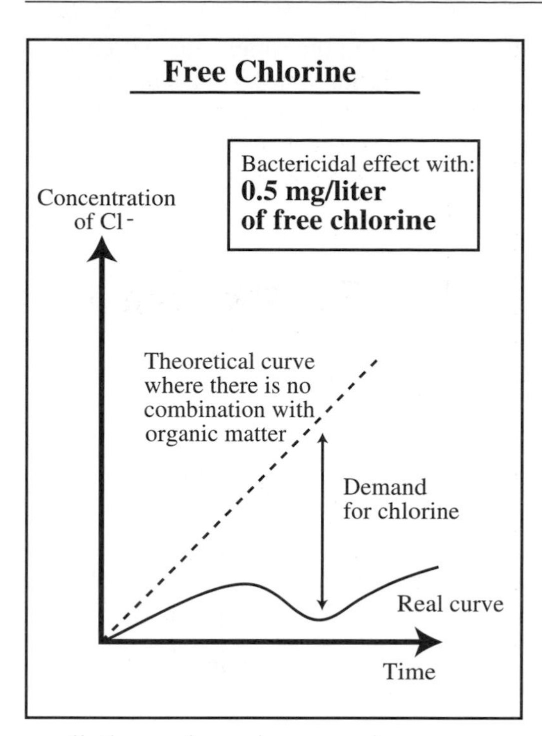


– *Cost*:
The use of chemical products requires a permanent capital investment, which some communities will not be able to afford without outside help. Sand filter systems, in contrast, once installed, can be operated without any major input of materials.

– *Simplicity*:
Chemical treatment is the most complex of all the methods. If it is misused — for example, where the optimum dose is exceeded[35] — it can lead to health problems.

– *Reliability*:
Correctly implemented chemical treatment will destroy all the pathogenic germs in the water, whereas slow filtration does not provide total safety.[36] A combination of methods can also be used, such as a sand filter followed by chemical treatment of the filtered water.

**Ways of Improving Water Quality**

1. Storage and sedimentation:
   - reduction of schistosomiasis
   - sedimentation of organic matter
2. Slow sand filter:
   - physical effect of filtration
   - bacteriological effect on germs
3. Chemical treatment:
   - flocculation with aluminum salts
   - disinfection with free chlorine
4. Boiling:
   - anti-germ action
5. Ultra-violet radiation:
   - anti-germ action

## 3.5 Distribution

The entire water-carrying network from the source or the storage unit to the user constitutes the distribution system. As

[35] An example is the episode of chlorine intoxication that occurred at the Khao-I-Dang camp in Thailand in 1980.

[36] "Slow sand filters improve the microbiological quality of water considerably, but if water completely free of pathogens is required, it is necessary to apply a chemical disinfectant." Cairncross and Feachem, *Environmental Health Engineering in the Tropics*, p. 94.

mentioned earlier, when the population is small and the water source is close to home, the user comes to fetch water directly from the source — a well equipped with a hand pump, for example, or a protected spring. In other circumstances, however, a distribution system will have to be set up.

### *Mobile Systems*

In emergency situations, tank trucks may be used to transport water from its source to the displaced-person camps. Instead of each person coming to the truck for water, the contents of the truck can be emptied into static tanks hooked up to a network providing simultaneous distribution to several users at a time.

### *Permanent Systems*

The classic water-distribution systems are permanent, and more or less ramified and complex depending on the circumstances. The options include:

- a simple connection between a protected source and one or more public taps;
- a public fountain equipped with several taps;
- a pipe network carrying the water into the houses;
- where the source is at a lower level, a distribution network equipped with pumps.

### *Selection Criteria*

In choosing the type of distribution system, the primary considerations should be simplicity and easy access. Several aspects must be taken into account:

- ***The distance between the distribution point and the user's home***
  This point is not as obvious as it might seem. Although in general reducing the distance leads to an increase in water consumption, this relation has not been demonstrated in all cases. Studies in Tanzania and Morocco, for example, have not established a correlation between the proximity of access to water and the quantity used per person.[37] The reasons are numerous, including cultural habits, traditions, and a rejection of new technologies.[38] In fact, within a certain distance (1.6 km), a substantial increase in water consumption

---

37 S.A. Esrey *et al.*, "Reviews/Analysis: Effects on Improved Water Supply and Sanitation on Ascaraisis, Diarrhoea, Dracunculiasis, Hookworm Infection, Schistosomiasis, and Trachoma," *Bulletin of the World Health Organization* 69, No. 5 (1991): 616.

38 "It was reported in East Africa that after providing water closer to the home, the use of increased amounts of water did not result if the traditional water source was less than 1 km from the home." Steven A. Esrey and Jean Pierre Habicht, "Epidemiological Evidence for Health Benefits from Improved Water and Sanitation in Developing Countries," *Epidemiologic Reviews* 8 (1986): 122.

occurs only if the water is piped into the home.[39] Thus, the impact on health will be maximal if water is piped into the home.

- ***The source's potential***
  If, in adherence to the first criterion, the plan is to set up a household distribution network, water consumption will increase 5-10 times over. It is therefore essential to confirm that the water source will be able to supply the potential demand.
- ***Urgency of the situation***
  In emergency situations, the population must be provided with water as quickly as possible. It is therefore advisable to settle for a simple system in which each distribution point serves part of the population. It must, however, be ramified enough to avoid long waiting lines at the distribution points.
- ***Local standards***
  Local standards should be respected. For example, installing a home water-supply system in a refugee camp is unwise if neighboring populations have to walk three kilometers to fetch water from a well.
- ***Cost***
  Transporting water by tank trucks may be acceptable at the very beginning of an emergency, but the cost of such a measure should lead relief organizers to seek an alternative solution quickly.

The "ideal" solution should take account of all these factors. The aim is to achieve the best possible compromise between the desired health benefits and the constraints of the situation.

## 3.6 Use

A number of factors influence the proper use of water.

### *Technical Characteristics of the System*

If the system functions badly (supply cuts), if it is badly planned (distribution points are too far away from users), or if it does not accord with local sociocultural habits, it will not be used.

[39] "When water is available within about 1 km or within half-an-hour's return journey of the home, water use does not significantly increase when the distance or time is reduced, unless it is less than 100 m. When the point is reached where a tap can be provided within each house, water use may increase dramatically from 10-30 l to 30-100 l/person." Cairncross and Feachem, *Environmental Health Engineering in the Tropics*, pp. 52-53.

### *Community Involvement*

The community must be involved at all stages of the project: choosing the source, deciding on the technical set-up (pumps, distribution system, etc.) and especially implementing the project. Systems that are supplied ready-made, without community involvement, are doomed to failure owing to lack of interest, insufficient motivation to insure maintenance, and, in the short term, lack of use.[40]

### *Level of Health Education*

The health-education factor is significant primarily at the family level. Strict water management implies preserving it from any contamination and using it advisedly (particularly during episodes of diarrheal diseases).

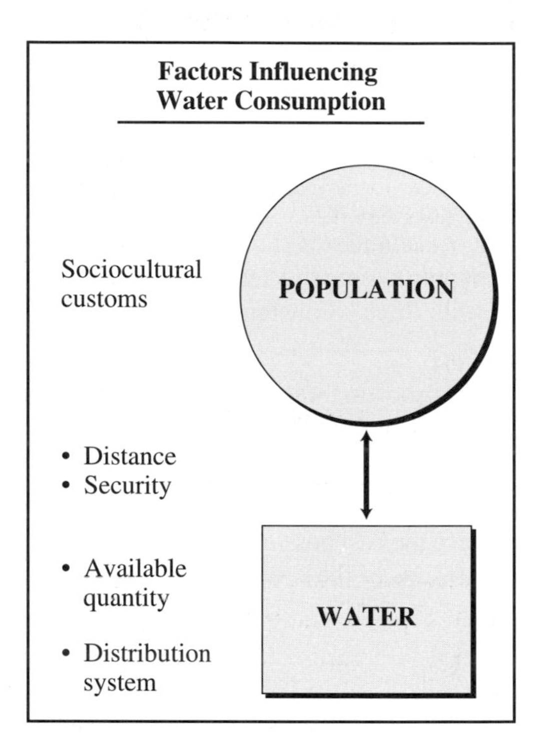


### *Cost*

Cost is generally not an issue in emergency situations where "everything is free."

*Water use represents the meeting point between technology and health.*

A water-supply system's performance is not judged solely by its capacity to provide water, but by the extent to which it is used by the beneficiaries and, consequently, by its impact on a population's health status.

---

40 "In water supply and sanitation programmes, planners have come to realize that community participation, among other things, is essential for projects to be successful. This represents a vast change from former projects in which the community was seen as a passive recipient of facilities planned and provided by the central government." Anne Whyte, *Guidelines for Planning Community Participation Activities in Water Supply and Sanitation Projects* (Geneva: WHO, 1986), p. 5.

# III. Environmental Sanitation

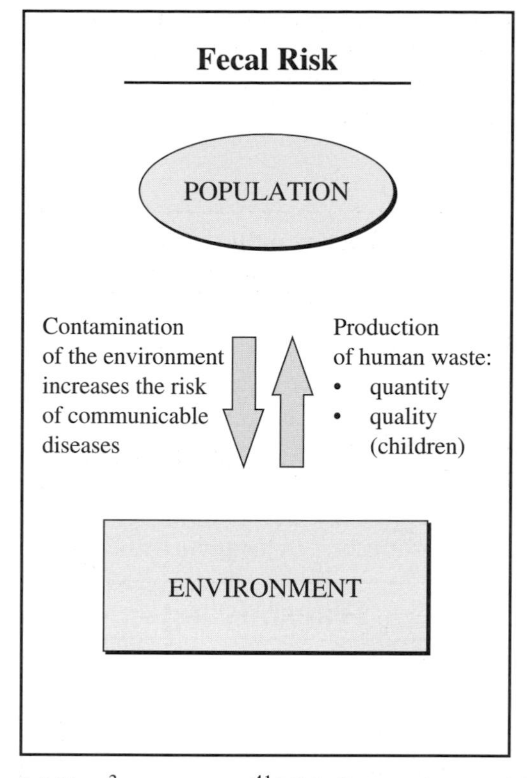


## 1. Human waste

Mention has already been made of the various diseases that can be transmitted to human beings through fecal contamination. Two basic ideas provide the starting point for a definition of the problem: production and transmission.

### 1.1 Nature of the Problem

*Production*

The **quantitative aspect** of human waste is considerable. On average, "production" of waste per person per day is estimated at 150-200 grams gross weight, and 60 grams dry weight. In terms of volume, this is the equivalent of 0.060 $m^3$ per person.[41] This figure gives an idea of the "volume" of the problem, but not necessarily of the size of the system required to dispose of the excreta, especially as other factors are involved — for example, cultural habits and the type of installation used (the main aspect of both these factors being whether or not water is used).

In any case, the volume in itself is not a problem; it is the **qualitative aspect** of waste production that will affect health — that is, the content of the stools. Stools may contain a whole range of pathogenic germs. The following is an approximate list of the contents of one gram of fecal matter:

- viruses: poliomyelitis $10^6$
  hepatitis A $10^6$
  rotavirus $10^6$

[41] Cairncross and Feachem, *Environmental Health Engineering in the Tropics*, p. 114.

- bacteria: *vibrio cholerae* $10^6$
  *salmonella* $10^6$
  *E. coli* $10^8$
  *shigella* $10^6$
- parasites: amoebas $15.10^4$
  *giardia* $10^5$
  ancylostomes 800 eggs
  ascarids 10,000 eggs
  schistosomes 40 eggs

Stools are variable. They do not all have the same pathogenic potential: children's stools are more infectious than those of adults, and sick people and healthy carriers excrete proportionately more of the germs related to their infection: cholera, typhoid, etc. Moreover, a stool's pathogenic potential changes with time; once the stool is excreted, the germs contained in it gradually disappear.

### *Transmission of Contamination*

Contamination may begin with the actual "producer." Inadequate hygiene after defecation may contaminate the hands, establishing fecal-oral transmission. This is the simplest route to infection, but contamination may occur through many other mechanisms of varying levels of complexity:

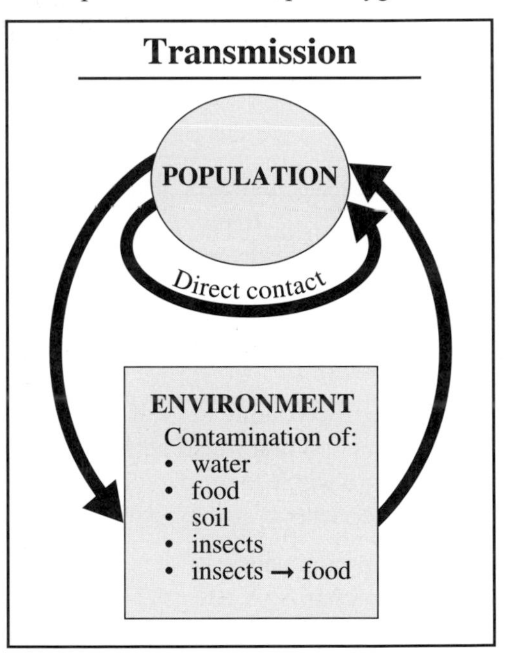


- transmission from person to person by dirty hands.
- fecal contamination of water, consumption of which will give rise mainly to diarrheal diseases, hepatitis, and typhoid fever. Such contamination can occur at all levels of the water chain: at the source, during storage, during distribution, or upon use. For example, water may be contaminated at its source by an adjacent latrine, or by the use of careless methods of drawing water.
- contamination of food, deficient personal hygiene (water can be contaminated by dirty hands), and/or the transmission of pathogens by insects such as mosquitoes which themselves are soiled with fecal matter.

## 1.2 Controlling the Problem

- **Control at the source:** The aim is not to try to reduce the quantity of fecal matter produced, but rather to control its content, by screening healthy carriers and implementing mass prophylactic chemical measures. These activities will be studied in more detail in Chapter 4 ("Communicable Diseases").
- **Proper disposal of human waste:** In many parts of the world, particularly in rural areas, there is no sanitary infrastructure.[42] This lack means that fecal matter is scattered in the vicinity of people's dwellings, thereby increasing the risk of disease transmission.

Numerous systems have been proposed for the proper disposal of human waste. For the sake of simplicity, they can be classified according to two basic principles:

- whether or not storage is at the site of production;
- whether storage is under dry or wet conditions.

The combination of these two factors, as shown in the table, will determine the choice of the system most appropriate to the situation.

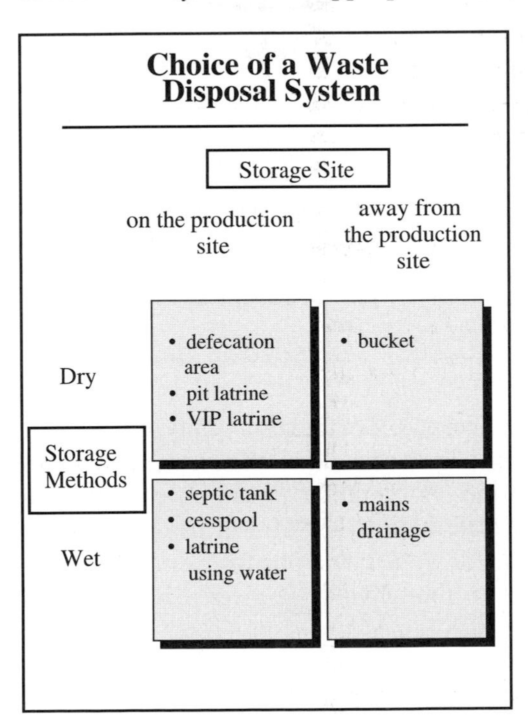


In this domain, however, technology comes into conflict with sociocultural habits, and the installation of sanitary facilities does not mean that they will be used. Obviously, the greater the community's involvement in the design and construction of such facilities, the more likely they are to be used.

Although the risk of disease transmission through fecal matter is reduced by the measures mentioned, it will nevertheless persist if health education is not provided, or if the quantity of water supplied is insufficient for adequate personal hygiene.[43]

---

[42] In 1985 it was estimated that only 18% of the rural population of the developing countries had access to sanitary facilities.

[43] In certain societies, water is culturally important for defecation.

## 1.3 Choosing a Method of Waste Disposal

In emergency situations, which usually involve a large concentration of people, preference should be given to systems that will be quickly effective:

- **Defecation area** – In the first days of the emergency, a defecation area can be designated, as a temporary measure until a more satisfactory system can be set up.
- **Dry pit latrines** – This is the ideal solution for displaced-person camps, for the following reasons:
  - They do not need water, an advantage in situations where water is scarce.
  - They can be quickly built, requiring little in the way of equipment.
  - They are simple to build.
  - They protect the privacy of the users.

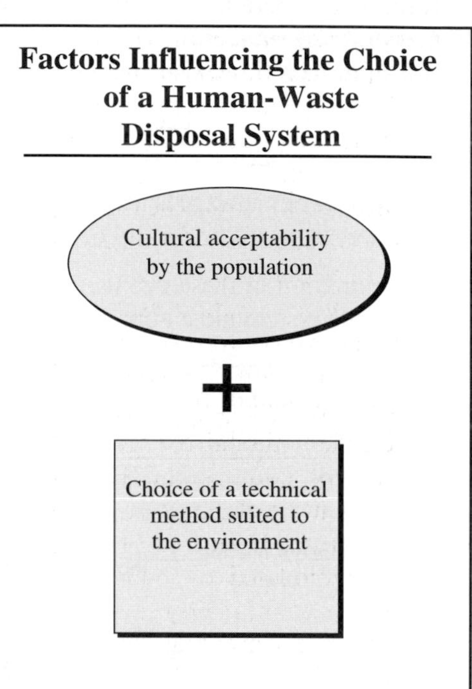


## 1.4 Building Dry Pit Latrines

Before embarking on a latrine-construction program, relief planners should examine certain parameters. As for all waste-disposal systems, three aspects must be considered:

- ***Social parameters***

  The most important requirement in a latrine is that it be socially acceptable to the community; otherwise it will not be used. In addition, more specific social factors must be taken into account, such as the use of latrines by children (meaning construction standards must be oriented towards safe and easy use). It will also be necessary to build two groups of latrines, one for women and one for men.

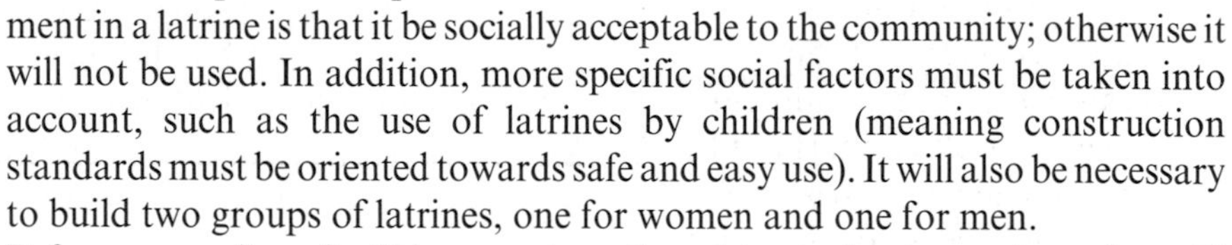

  Before any sanitary facilities are set up, thought must be given to how they will be maintained. Not only will badly maintained latrines not receive much use, but they themselves will increase the risk of communicable diseases.

  Among all these factors, one point in particular must be kept in mind:

  **Implementing a latrine-construction project requires community participation at all levels — choice of method, building, and maintenance.**

- ***What happens to the waste?***
  This may seem a hare-brained question to ask in an emergency situation. Nonetheless, "temporary" displaced-person or refugee camps sometimes remain in place for years, in which case the issue of using waste for agricultural programs arises. This will affect the choice of a technical solution, in order to limit the transmission of diseases as much as possible. The risk of disease is assessed on the basis of the life span of pathogenic agents in the soil. Normally, fecal matter is stored for a year before being used as fertilizer.

- ***Construction standards***
  The approach should be "tridimensional":
  - Depth — The main risk is that the waste from the latrines will contaminate the ground water. The bottom of the pit should be two meters above the water table.[44]
  - Distance — Two factors are essential. First, the latrines must be far away from water sources, especially wells, to prevent contamination.[45] Second, they must be quickly accessible — though the problem of odor should be taken into account as well. Both these factors can be accommodated by building the latrines fairly close to the users' dwellings, but downwind.
  - Conditions inside — A latrine should offer safety and comfort: its users, especially children, should feel secure;[46] and it should be sufficiently spacious and kept clean to encourage use.

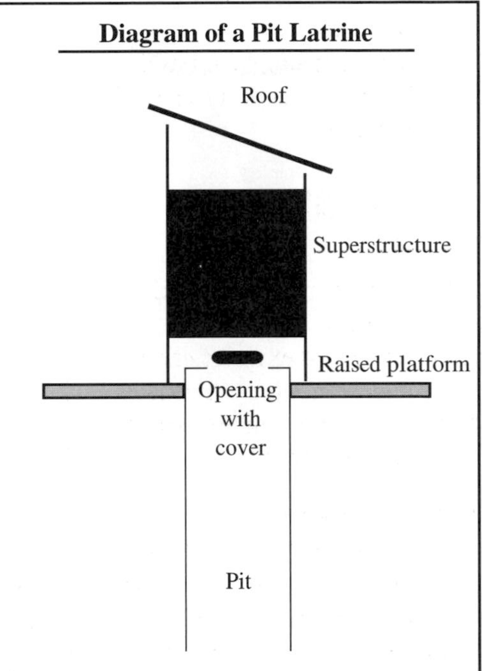


[44] This figure is based on the distance that bacteria are able to travel in soil. It may vary enormously, of course, depending on the type of soil.
[45] The recommended minimum distance between a latrine and a well is 15 meters.
[46] The type of materials used will depend on their local availability. Nevertheless, the aim must be to build latrines of good quality.

- *Types of Latrine*
  - *A pit latrine* consists of a pit three meters deep and one meter wide, a platform (of cement, if possible) and a superstructure built with local materials.
  - A *VIP* (*ventilated improved pit*) *latrine* has a ventilation system which prevents flies from gathering on the fecal matter in the pit[47] and, at the same time, reduces unpleasant odors inside the latrine. The principle and method of constructing this type of latrine are described in many sources.

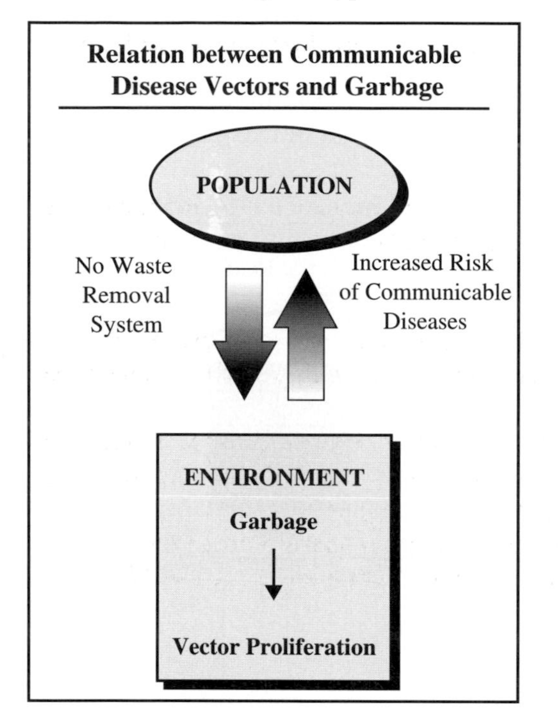


Fecal risk is reduced by the provision of facilities that are culturally acceptable to the population.

**The other modes of waste disposal (for example, septic tanks) will not be studied here, being too complex for use during emergency situations.**

## 2. Garbage

### 2.1 Nature of the Problem

The volume of garbage that a camp population can produce is difficult to quantify.[48] A number of factors must be taken into consideration, such as:

- the type of relief aid provided — there may be a substantial increase in the volume of rubbish if processed foods are provided, since they come in cans, packaging, etc.
- access to the local market, particularly for fresh food supplies (giving rise to food refuse).

Garbage constitutes an ideal breeding ground for communicable-disease vectors:

- insects:
  - mosquitoes develop in water contained in discarded empty cans and carry malaria, dengue, and yellow fever;

---

47 A pipe runs from the pit to the level of the latrine roof, where the end is closed off by fine mesh netting. The flies in the pit are attracted by the daylight, but are trapped by the netting.

48 Cairncross gives as an estimate for tropical countries 0.3-1 kilo per person per day. See *Environmental Health Engineering in the Tropics*, p. 173.

  - flies breed in garbage, alight on fecal matter, and contaminate food, eyes, etc.

- rats:
  - transmit leptospirosis and other diseases.

Particular care must be taken with rubbish from health facilities (field hospitals, for example), due to its specific nature: soiled bandages, syringes, and used needles.

The more general problem of chemical pollution caused by garbage will not be studied here.

### 2.2 Controlling the Problem

Control measures, to be effective, must obey the same rules as human-waste disposal — simplicity and respect for the cultural context are essential.

Four stages must be considered:

- garbage collection at the household level — this involves providing households with trash cans or containers and organizing a garbage collection service.
- transport to a dumping area — the dump must be away from the population and subject to strict hygiene measures to prevent the proliferation of communicable-disease vectors such as rats and flies.
- waste disposal — the disposal method will depend on whether the waste can be burned. In an emergency, the rule is simple: *Burn what you can and bury the rest.*
- reuse or recycling.

## 3. Control of Vectors

### 3.1 Nature of the Problem

Emergencies give rise to conditions (overcrowding, poor hygiene, etc.) that favor the proliferation of communicable-disease vectors. The main vectors that cause problems in emergency situations are the following:

- flies
- mosquitoes
- lice
- fleas
- rats

The modes of transmission have already been mentioned:

- flies → fecal matter → food → contamination through the mouth

- anopheles → stagnant water → eggs → larva → adult anopheles → infection by a parasite carrier → transmission of the infection

## 3.2 Controlling the Problem

The preceding pages show that vector control depends in large part on the measures taken to dispose of waste. In emergency situations, however, time is sometimes needed to explain to the beneficiaries the impact of these measures on vector proliferation. In this case, relief workers may have to resort to more specific methods of control. These should not, however, take the place of basic hygiene and become "the solution."

### *Physical Intervention*

Physical intervention may include:

- drainage of rain water and waste water
- prevention of overcrowding
- use of traps designed for a specific type of vector, such as flies or rats
- use of mosquito nets

### *Chemical Intervention*

Chemical intervention involves the use of chemical products, mainly insecticides and rat poisons. These products have only a temporary effect unless they are accompanied by the measures mentioned above. Moreover, their use may be detrimental:

- to the health of those who handle them;
- to the health of beneficiaries, if the rules concerning the concentration to be used, the mode of delivery, etc., are not respected;
- to long-term vector control, since in the long term improper use may lead to the development of resistant vector strains, as was the case with anopheles and DDT.

**Methods of Vector Control**

Vector-control methods are one of the forms of primary prevention of communicable diseases. They act on two levels:

- reduction of vector proliferation by:
  - drainage
  - insecticides
  - larvicides
  - vector traps
- reduction of opportunities for contact between vectors and healthy humans:
  - mosquito nets
  - repellents
  - long garments

### *Combined Modes of Intervention*

Vector control involves the implementation of various kinds of methods which can be combined in different ways:

- Type of measure
  - physical
  - chemical
- Mode of action
  - reduction of vector population
  - reduction of contact with humans

Thus, to control anopheles, the actions best suited to the situation would be chosen from among the following:

- drainage of stagnant water
- use of larvicides
- use of insecticides on inside walls
- use of insecticides outside dwellings
- use of mosquito nets
- use of insect repellents

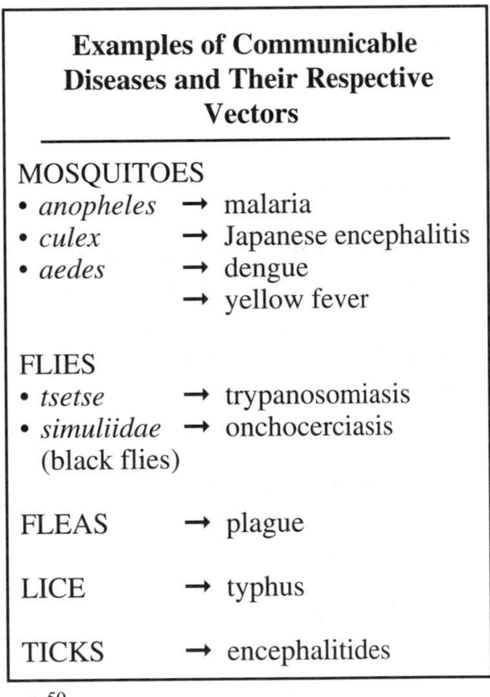

**Examples of Communicable Diseases and Their Respective Vectors**

|  | |  |
|---|---|---|
| MOSQUITOES | | |
| • *anopheles* | → | malaria |
| • *culex* | → | Japanese encephalitis |
| • *aedes* | → | dengue |
| | → | yellow fever |
| FLIES | | |
| • *tsetse* | → | trypanosomiasis |
| • *simuliidae* (black flies) | → | onchocerciasis |
| FLEAS | → | plague |
| LICE | → | typhus |
| TICKS | → | encephalitides |

In the battle against malaria, for example, the technical measures selected will depend on both the population's way of life and that of the mosquitoes in the area concerned.[49] These measures would be combined, as well, with public health activities (health education) and medical care (treatment of the sick).

One of the methods currently recommended is the use of mosquito nets soaked in insecticide (pyrethroids). Many studies have shown that this practice reduces transmission. As in every case where insecticides are used, the risk of resistant strains appearing must be continually assessed.[50]

---

[49] Certain kinds of anopheles live outdoors and others live indoors.

[50] The table on page 26 of the manual *The Use of Impregnated Bednets and Other Materials for Vector-Borne Disease Control* (WHO, Division of Vector Biology and Control, 1989) summarizes the impact of this technique.

*Specific Interventions*

In emergency situations which necessitate the storage of food reserves, sometimes for rather long periods, the control of rats and insects is essential.

# IV. Housing and Energy

Although the total or partial destruction of housing is characteristic of natural disasters (earthquakes, floods) and conflicts (bombings, pillaging), the problem of reconstruction will not be discussed here. This section will merely examine ways to provide adequate housing for displaced and refugee populations, taking into account energy and structural requirements. The other factors that help define a population's living conditions (water and sanitation) have already been studied in the previous sections.

The uninitiated are apt to assume that the relation between housing and health amounts to nothing more than protection against bad weather. Consequently, providing housing is sometimes considered as a measure to provide comfort, although the link between shelter and health is based on physiological and social needs.

## 1. Health Risks

The relation between nutritional needs and inadequate housing has been studied in particular by J. Rivers, who writes, "The fact that famine-affected populations often have reduced amounts of clothing and limited shelter can be very important because of its impact on energy requirements."[51]

In a situation where access to food is problematic, contending with the cold requires an additional caloric intake.[52] Thus, the absence of means of protection from the cold favors the development of malnutrition and increases mortality linked to hypothermia, which itself is fostered by malnutrition. Indirectly, then, "warming up" displaced populations by providing them with housing suited to the climate and, if necessary, sources of energy (wood, kerosene) as well makes it possible to reduce the quantity of food required for distribution.[53] The distribution of blankets is more economical than the distribution of a food supplement to cover energy needs generated by chill.

---

[51] J.P.W. Rivers, "The Nutritional Biology of Famine," in G. Ainsworth Harrison, ed., *Famine* (Oxford Science Publications, 1988), p. 87.

[52] "Thus at 15 degrees the total energy expenditure might be more than 750 kcal/day higher than at thermoneutrality unless the subject is able to reduce heat loss by, for example, putting on extra clothing." *Ibid.*, p. 88.

[53] "A blanket which reduced the heat loss by cold stress in an environment of 15 degrees C could save food equivalent to 1-2 kg of grain per adult per week." *Ibid.*, p. 90. If we multiply this by 100,000 people for a period of six months....

Unsuitable housing, such as, for example, the crowding of large numbers of people into collective habitations, causes an increase in certain communicable diseases, as well as psychological stress. An increase in maladies such as tuberculosis, measles, or scabies is directly linked to overcrowding. In addition, the absence of family privacy is a factor in psychological and social tension.

Access to energy sources is always a problem for displaced populations. First of all, most major population movements occur in disadvantaged countries, where energy supplies are traditionally unreliable. The arrival of masses of people exacerbates this problem.

## 2. Norms

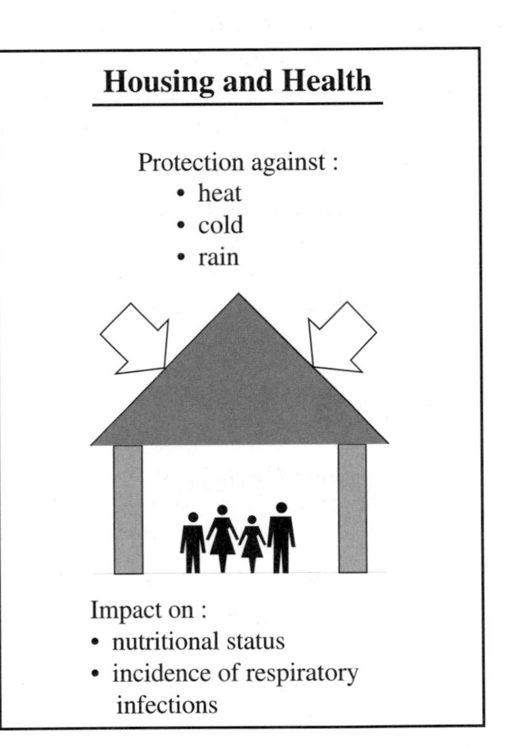


### 2.1 Habitable Surfaces

WHO recommends that a camp should provide 30 $m^2$ of space per person, 3.5 $m^2$ of that for housing.

### 2.2 Energy Needs

Camp residents need energy for cooking, warmth,[54] and light.

It is difficult to quantify energy norms. Climate, social habits, and available resources all influence the quantities consumed.

## 3. Solutions

### 3.1 Housing

In situations involving floods of displaced people, it is usually impossible to offer them at the outset housing that corresponds to the norms outlined above. At best, all that can be contemplated at first is ways to minimize the risks.

Temporary shelters can be used initially to give their occupants at least minimal protection from bad weather. Simple plastic sheets are enough to provide shelter from the rain and the sun. Makeshift shelters put together from materials found on the spot, as well as immediately available collective permanent shelters

[54] Depending on the climate.

(schools, hangars), must also be considered as merely provisional solutions, insofar as they do not permit respect for family or clan privacy.

Temporary housing should meet the following criteria:

*"Over and above their basic purpose of providing shelter against the elements and a focus for family life, human dwellings should afford protection against the hazards to health arising from the physical and social environments."*[55]

Other solutions are:

- tents
- dwellings modeled on those of the resident population
- reconstructions of the residents' original homes
- prefabricated dwellings

### 3.2 Energy Resources

Energy may be obtained from:

- wood
- charcoal
- electricity
- gas
- the sun (solar energy)

## 4. Selection Criteria

The criteria for choosing between these various solutions are given below.

For housing, the factors to be considered are:

- the speed with which the dwelling can be set up
- cost
- sociocultural habits
- climate

The use of prefabricated dwellings or imported tents should remain the exception, since they are more expensive and often are unsuited to both the climate and the population's social customs. The best solution is to use local materials to reconstitute simple dwellings acceptable to the population.

In the choice of energy supply, too, certain factors must be taken into account:

- *local availability*. The use of wood cannot be recommended in areas suffering from intensive deforestation.

[55] *Health Principles of Housing* (Geneva: WHO, 1989), p. V.

– *level of economic development*. The use of electricity cannot be recommended if the resident population does not have it.

– *social habits*. The use of gas cannot be recommended to populations who have never used it.

– *political context*. The use of kerosene cannot be recommended to civilian populations under strong military pressure, since kerosene has an obvious strategic value.

In short, there is no standard solution. In every situation, planners must analyze all these factors together to determine the most acceptable solution for the specific context.

The use of solar energy merits particular mention. The present state of technology does not allow this type of energy to be used on a large scale, for an entire population. It can be used, however, to supply the needs of facilities such as nutrition rehabilitation centers, dispensaries, and hospitals. Simple solar-energy systems can be built on the spot with local materials; if more complex systems are required, at least some of the necessary equipment has to be imported (solar pumps to equip wells, solar panels, storage batteries).

**Possible Housing Solutions**

Possible types of housing :

- emergency shelters (plastic sheeting)
- temporary dwellings:
  - tents
  - construction of shelters with local materials
  - prefabricated dwellings
- permanent dwellings in a program of reinsertion or rehabilitation

Factors to consider when choosing a solution:

- necessity of finding an immediate solution
- climatic conditions
- cost
- social customs
- probable evolution of the situation

Special efforts should be made to conserve energy — for example, in the selection of materials for building shelters, or by constructing energy-saving ovens. Such measures can be adapted to the needs of the population as a whole.[56]

# V. Site

It may seem paradoxical to wait until the end of the chapter to discuss the question of site, when site selection and organization depend largely on the factors that have already been discussed: the availability of water, energy sources, construction materials, and the possibility of removing solid and liquid waste. It

[56] Energy-saving ovens were built in Nicaraguan refugee camps in Honduras.

is true that, chronologically, selecting the site for a displaced-person or refugee camp comes first among the problems related to environmental hygiene; only after this choice has been made will measures involving water, waste, and housing be implemented. Nonetheless, to be capable of choosing the "right spot," planners must first achieve a technical mastery of the basic environmental principles studied previously. Thus, studying the principles involved in choosing a site constitutes a good revision of the entire unit.

# 1. Selecting a Site

As far as possible, populations in crisis should always be assisted in their homes, in order to avoid the major health risk entailed by population movements.[57] Nonetheless, many emergency situations do involve displaced populations,[58] in which case the problem of choosing a reception site may arise.

More often than not, however, humanitarian agencies have to deal with a *fait accompli.* Sometimes the victims themselves have already chosen their new location; more often, the local authorities have imposed a site on them. This *de facto* situation should not, however, prevent humanitarian agencies from standing back a little to consider whether the arbitrarily selected site meets the minimal requirements necessary to guarantee acceptable living conditions for the people who must live there.

## 1.1 Main Factors to Consider

The main factors that should be considered in assessing a site are:

- access to water
- sufficient space
- natural drainage
- physical and political security
- access to communication routes
- access to food
- access to energy sources
- possibility for inhabitants to return to their original homes
- ownership of the land
- potential for future expansion

Most of these factors have already been examined. Three of them, however, merit discussion here:

[57] Most of the major population migrations of the last ten years (Cambodia, Ethiopia, Sudan) were associated with a very high mortality rate.

[58] Such movements may be voluntary or otherwise, motivated by insecurity or organized for political reasons.

- ***Natural drainage***
  This factor is important for the removal of liquid waste. In displaced-person camps during emergencies, the systems recommended for waste disposal do not require water. But a system for removing liquid waste (the products of domestic use and personal hygiene) must be set up.

Methods of treating liquid waste, which involve installing settling tanks, will not be described here. This section will merely enumerate the general principles underlying emergency solutions to the most pressing problems. The main principle is to plan the camp on enough of a slope to permit waste water to drain naturally. This is plain common sense. More specific measures may be undertaken as well:
- drainage around water-supply points
- drainage ditches along the roads
- construction of a cesspool at the foot of the slope.

- ***Ownership of the land***
  Before setting up a camp, organizers must find out who the site belongs to and take all the necessary administrative steps with the proper authorities.

- ***Potential for expansion***
  The number of displaced people generally varies considerably over time. From a few thousand people to begin with, it may reach several tens of thousands. Although it is preferable to limit camp size and build several camps rather than a single, gigantic one, it is a good idea to allow for the possibility of expansion, "just in case." If the camp becomes a long-term fixture, organizers may consider initiating limited agricultural programs (vegetable gardens) or more ambitious projects (animal husbandry, farming). In this case, any camp extension must be made with the consent of the local authorities.

### 1.2 Selection Criteria

If a choice between two sites is possible, each factor must be analyzed in the light of the situation; at one site, security may be guaranteed, while at the other, the access to health services may be better. Or access to water resources may be convenient, but there is no possibility of expanding the camp. The decision to choose one site rather than another must be made with due consideration of all the factors weighed together.

## 2. Organization of a Site

The accepted space standard in a camp is an average area of 30 $m^2$ per person. This area comprises the actual dwelling space and the necessary space for community infrastructures (distribution areas, dispensaries, etc.). Usually the camp residents settle in by themselves before an administrative body can design a general plan for the camp. Whether organizers have the good fortune to be able to control the physical arrangement of the dwellings from the outset or whether they are obliged to restructure a haphazard settlement, the following general principles apply.

## 2.1 Organization of Housing

In a camp, the shelters are uniform, basic units lined up in rows; each family or group of families should have reasonably convenient access to latrines and water. The United Nations High Commissioner for Refugees (UNHCR) recommends, for example, that latrines be available within a radius of 50 meters, and water within about 100 meters.[59] If necessary, the camp can be divided into zones according to different ethnic groups.

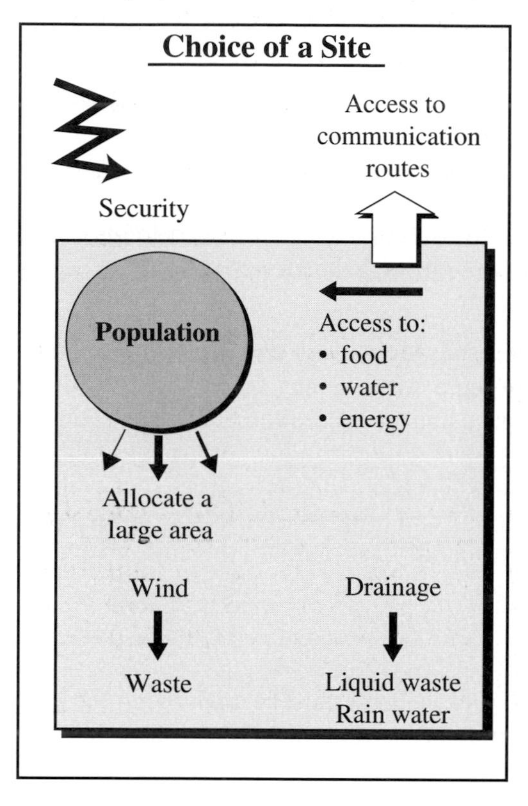


Around each dwelling, a drainage system should be constructed for waste water and rain water. Precautions should also be taken against fire.

## 2.2 Organization of the Infrastructure

The basic principle here is "think big."

- Access roads must be passable all year and navigable by relief trucks.
- Food distribution areas must be big enough to permit orderly distribution. Between distributions, they can be used as football fields!
- Locations must be reserved for infrastructural elements:
  - sanitary facilities: water storage, distribution network, latrines, and garbage dumps.
  - medical facilities: dispensaries or clinics, a hospital.
  - administrative facilities for the registration of new arrivals.

[59] UNHCR, *Handbook for Emergencies* (1982), p. 63.

# VI. Evaluation of Water and Sanitation Programs

First, the coverage of the programs set up must be evaluated. Coverage is reflected in such figures as the ratio between the number of people and the quantity of water available, and the ratio between the number of latrines and the total population.

Next comes an evaluation of the hygiene programs' impact on the beneficiaries' health, based on previously selected indicators. This is actually much more complex than it might at first seem. The evaluator must consider:

- the validity of the indicators chosen. For example, is the incidence of diarrheal diseases indicative of the impact of a sanitation program?
- the reliability of the information sources used. Not everyone may have the same definition of diarrhea..
- the incidence of all the variables — for instance, the importance of improved water, of latrine use, of education, etc., in reducing diarrheal diseases within a given population.

All these factors are routine elements of a surveillance program, which will be studied in Chapter 6 ("Epidemiology").

**Water is synonymous with survival. Environmental hygiene, too, is crucially important to a population's health, particularly in an emergency situation. From an evaluation of the water-supply situation to the elimination of communicable-disease vectors, measures concerning water and sanitation are now an integral part of medical care and humanitarian relief in general in cases of disaster or armed conflict.**

Chapter 4

# COMMUNICABLE DISEASES

***This work is not intended to cover all infectious pathologies. Numerous courses on tropical medicine and other subjects present the pathogenic, clinical, preventive, and therapeutic aspects of communicable diseases. This course, in contrast, will:***

1. ***Identify the main communicable diseases common in disaster situations.***
2. ***Discuss the risk factors associated with disasters, which help give communicable diseases a particular impact on public health.***
3. ***Describe the developmental cycle of infectious diseases, as well as potential levels of intervention.***
4. ***Examine the "tools" most often used in emergency situations.***
5. ***Identify the priorities in coping with communicable diseases.***
6. ***Survey the means used to control the most common communicable diseases in emergency situations.***

# I. General Overview

Disaster situations are often associated with the idea of communicable diseases; the media cannot speak of an earthquake without mentioning the risk of an epidemic or showing pictures of medical teams immunizing the victims. To put the issue into a proper perspective, it may be helpful to list the main communicable diseases and to examine the factors that make them potentially dangerous in a disaster.

## 1. The Main Communicable Diseases

Tropical-medicine textbooks tend to classify communicable diseases according to the pathogenic agents that cause them (virus, bacterium, or parasite). In emergency situations, however, these diseases are customarily classified according to the way they are transmitted — which may, in some cases, be complex, involving several different mechanisms.

### 1.1 Diseases Transmitted by Contact

- scabies
- trachoma
- conjunctivitis
- mycosis

## 1.2 Sexually Transmitted Diseases

- gonorrhea
- syphilis
- AIDS

## 1.3 Vector-Transmitted Diseases

- malaria
- recurrent fevers
- trypanosomiasis
- yellow fever
- onchocerciasis
- schistosomiasis

## 1.4 Diseases Transmitted through Fecal Matter

- non-specific diarrheal diseases
- cholera
- amebiasis and giardiasis
- bacillary dysentery
- hepatitis
- typhoid fever
- ascariasis
- ancylostomiasis (hookworm disease)

## 1.5 Diseases Transmitted through the Air

- acute respiratory infections
- tuberculosis
- measles
- meningitis
- whooping cough

Experience has shown that in emergencies, certain communicable diseases have a particularly great impact, as witness the mortality rates recorded among refugees in Thailand, Somalia, Sudan, and Malawi, where 50-95% of deaths were attributed to measles, diarrheal diseases, and acute respiratory infections.[1] Other important communicable diseases include meningitis (refugees from Sudan and Thailand), cholera (refugees from Somalia, Sudan, Malawi, etc.), and typhus (displaced populations in Ethiopia). Sometimes a refugee population contributes to an increased risk for a particular communicable disease in an environment

[1] M. Toole, "Causes of Deaths among Refugees," *Journal of the American Medical Association* 263, No. 24 (27 June 1990).

which was previously free from it. This was the case, for example, when Sudanese refugees arrived in northern Uganda, in an area where trypanosomiasis had been under control.

To define the kinds of intervention that can prevent such epidemics, it is essential to be familiar with the mechanisms that give these diseases a particular impact in emergency situations.

## 2. Factors Influencing the Impact of Communicable Diseases in Emergencies

The epidemics that develop in disaster situations are essentially a function of the large concentrations of displaced people or refugees living together in camps where living conditions are particularly hazardous. Natural disasters that do not entail mass population movements do not increase the risk of epidemics.[2]

The risk factors, listed below, are numerous, and the way they interact varies from case to case, so that they must be identified in every instance before the appropriate means of intervention can be determined.

### 2.1 Presence of a New Pathogenic Agent

Population migration may introduce new pathogenic agents into the host region. Usually it is not a new pathogenic agent in the strict sense, but rather a different strain from the one normally found in that particular environment. Thus, for example, the appearance along the border between Thailand and Cambodia of colonies of *Plasmodium falciparum* resistant to the major antimalarial drugs has been attributed in part to the intermixing of populations in that area.

The primary victims of this phenomenon are the displaced people themselves (although they may have a certain degree of immunity), but the local population may also be affected, being usually much more sensitive to a new pathogenic agent. Conversely, by changing environment, a displaced population may be confronted by a new pathogenic agent against which it has no immunity.[3]

### 2.2 Susceptibility of the Population

A population's susceptibility to disease is reflected at two levels: the population's immunity and the individual's immunity.

---

[2] C. de Ville de Goyet and M. Lechat, "Health Aspects in Natural Disasters," *Tropical Doctor* (Oct. 1976): 168-170.

[3] After several years in camps in Thailand, where antimalarial control is particularly strict, the Cambodians returning to Cambodia were exposed to *Plasmodium falciparum*, against which most of them had lost their natural immunity.

## *Immunity of the Population*

Every community possesses a certain degree of immunity: "There is nothing mysterious about the high resistance which certain groups of people have to particular diseases. It is a consequence of long continued exposure to a particular infection in any stable, relatively isolated community."[4] A population's resistance to a particular pathogenic agent depends on numerous factors, including the endemicity of the disease, and it is unequally distributed among the members of the population. In the case of malaria, for example, the mortality rate in endemic regions is very high during the first two years of life. In groups from non-endemic areas who move into endemic regions, all individuals run the risk of developing severe forms of malaria.

Besides the risks attributable to a new pathogenic agent, a certain number of other factors help modify the mosaic of a population's natural immunity. A change in the make-up of the population, such as a relative rise in the percentage of children,[5] proportionately increases the number of people sensitive to infectious agents.

## *Individual Immunity*

In developing countries, most people over the age of three or four are immune to measles, either because they have been vaccinated or because they have already had the disease. The group of individuals actually at risk, therefore, is restricted to children under the age of four or five. Similarly, in developing countries, most individuals over the age of five can be assumed to have been exposed to the tubercle bacillus, though it is impossible to say what percentage of them will actually develop tuberculosis. Another factor is malnutrition: malnourished children are particularly susceptible to infections. Thus, a study carried out in the Philippines in 1988 estimated that among children whose weight-for-age ratio was less than 60%, the risk of dying from an acute respiratory infection was 27 times higher than for children whose weight-for-height ration was over 90%; it was 11 times higher for children for whom this ratio was between 60% and 74%, and 4 times higher for 75%-89%.[6]

It is impossible to determine the immunity level of each individual in a population, but the groups at risk — those who are naturally most vulnerable to

---

[4] Derek Robinson, ed., *Epidemiology and the Community Control of Disease in Warm Climate Countries,* 2nd ed. (Churchill Livingstone), p. 24.

[5] Refugee or displaced populations generally contain a higher percentage of children than normal populations, because many adults remain behind in their original homes.

[6] T. Tupasi, M. Velmonte, *et al.*, "Determinants of Morbidity and Mortality Due to Acute Respiratory Infections: Implications for Interventions," *Journal of Infectious Diseases* 157 (1988): 615-623.

specific pathogenic agents — can be defined. The importance of this is evident when target populations must be identified for specific forms of intervention.

### 2.3 Increased Transmission

Several factors contribute to an increase in disease transmission, particularly:

- *overcrowding* — The concentration of a group of people in a restricted space presents an obvious risk of epidemics.
- *deterioration of hygienic conditions* — Lack of water for basic hygiene, accumulations of waste which encourage the proliferation of disease vectors, and the absence of sanitation measures are all factors that help increase the transmission of communicable diseases.

### 2.4 Deterioration of Health Services

The deterioration of health services affects disease transmission at all levels. For example, no vaccinations are given, vector-control programs deteriorate, and little or no care is provided for the sick.

Thus, not only do the risks increase in an emergency situation (fertile breeding ground for infections, increased transmission), but, in addition, the means of disease control are usually inadequate, if not nonexistent. All these factors contribute, in varying degrees, to an increased incidence of communicable diseases (sometimes to the point of actual epidemics), as well as to a greater severity of clinical manifestations, reflected in the mortality rates for specific infections.[7]

## II. Coping with Communicable Diseases in Emergencies

The difficulty in coping with communicable diseases lies in the diversity of diseases likely to pose problems in emergencies, as well as in the interaction of risk factors. A clear plan of action should be adopted, based on the natural cycle of communicable disease; that cycle will determine the different levels of intervention.

---

[7] In February, 1985, in the refugee camps in eastern Sudan, mortality rates for measles, diarrheal illnesses, and respiratory infections were 16/1000/month, 8/1000/month, and 2/1000/month, respectively. See M. Toole and R. Waldman, "An Analysis of Mortality Trends among Refugee Populations in Somalia, Sudan and Thailand," *Bulletin of the World Health Organization* 66 (1986).

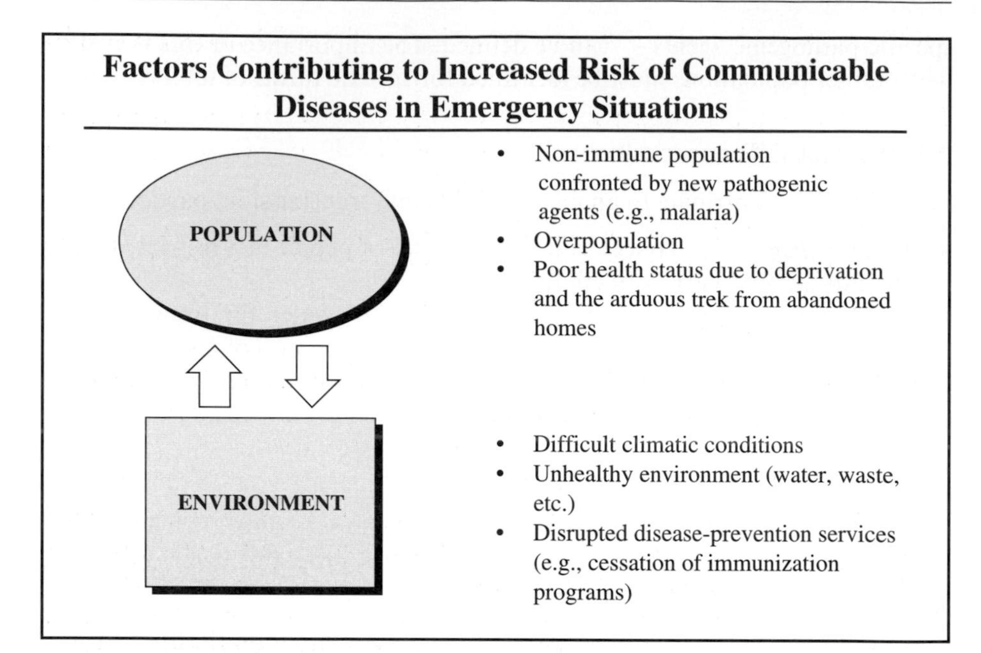


# 1. Natural Disease Cycle as Applied to Communicable Diseases

The classic model of the natural history of a disease comprises several stages:[8]

- risk/exposure factors
- population's susceptibility to the disease
- biological manifestations of the disease
- clinical manifestations of the disease
- progression of the disease
- return to a non-diseased state

This model can be reconstituted fairly easily, taking as its starting point the confrontation between a given population and the risk factors for communicable diseases (studied previously).

What provides the link between a population's susceptibility and an attack by pathogens? We have already seen that a population's susceptibility to a pathogen is not uniform, and varies from one pathogen to the next. The measles virus, for example, constitutes a problem for only a specific sector of the population. But the interaction between susceptibility and pathogenic agents is not always this simple. Although in the case of measles acquired immunity is permanent, this is

[8] Rougemont and Brunet-Jailly, eds., *Santé dans les pays tropicaux*, p. 8.

not true of other diseases — for example, malaria — for which immunity may be highly variable.

The degree of exposure must also be considered; for example, the development of clinical symptoms of tuberculosis in a healthy individual may depend on the extent and duration of contact with a contagious carrier.[9]

These are not purely academic considerations; on the contrary, they will have direct consequences concerning the type and method of intervention. The screening and treatment of contagious patients are sufficient to reduce transmission markedly.

If the pathogenic agent gains the upper hand, the subject will present biological and clinical manifestations. The biological form of the disease does not necessarily give rise to the clinical form. In regions characterized by endemic malaria, for example, individuals carrying the parasite are more often than not asymptomatic. By assessing the degree of imbalance between the subject's initial resistance and the magnitude of the pathogenic attack, we can anticipate the seriousness of the clinical manifestations, and take the necessary measures in time. The migration of a non-immune population to a region where the malarial agent *Plasmodium falciparum* is endemic should prompt fears of a considerable increase in cases of severe malaria.

A clinical case of disease may give rise to permanent damage (paralysis after poliomyelitis, for example, or keratomalacia after measles). Here again, consideration of both the immediate clinical aspects and the potential sequelae will help determine the measures to be taken.

A disease does not necessarily go through all the stages mentioned. Many infections go unnoticed. The fact that a disease produces only biological manifestations without any clinical symptoms is of course fortunate for the affected subject; but if that individual continues to carry the infectious agent, he or she may pose a danger to the community by contributing to the transmission and therefore the perpetuation of the disease.

## 2. Levels of Intervention

On the basis of these stages of the disease cycle, the main levels of intervention can be defined.

9 "As resistance acquired from the primary infection is not absolute, it follows that even immunologically competent individuals may eventually be overcome if the dose of mycobacteria is sufficiently high and persists for very long." Derek Robinson, ed., *Epidemiology and the Community Control of Disease in Warm Climate Countries*, p. 233.

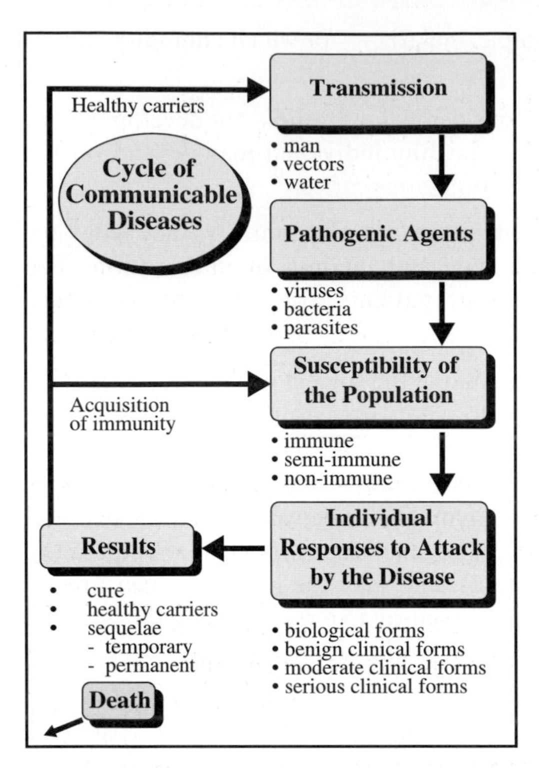


## 2.1 Intervention at the Source

Infectious agents can rarely be attacked directly in the environment; usually intervention must take the form of controlling transmission.[10] This kind of intervention may be:

– physical: mosquito nets to prevent contact between mosquitoes and humans
– hygienic: personal hygiene to reduce contact between fecal matter and humans
– chemical: water chlorination, insecticides against mosquitoes, etc.

## 2.2 Intervention to Modify Immune Status

The classic type of intervention here is immunization against pathogenic agents, if an effective vaccine exists. Together with direct intervention to improve immune status, many steps may be taken to help reinforce the body's natural defenses, such as maintaining a satisfactory nutritional status.[11]

## 2.3 Intervention at the Biological Stage

In an emergency, the possibilities of intervening at the biological stage are rather limited. Biological screening is of value only if it is followed by practical measures to control the disease it detects.

## 2.4 Intervention at the Clinical Stage

Intervention at the clinical stage is the level of intervention most familiar to medical personnel. However, when a communicable disease poses a problem for an entire community, certain adjustments in the treatment of individual clinical cases will be required.

[10] The "rule of the five F's": food, fingers, feet, flies, feces.

[11] "The most consistent changes in immunocompetence in PEM are in cell-mediated immunity, the bactericidal function of neutrophiles, the complement system, and the secretory IgA antibody response." R. Chandra, "Nutrition, Immunity, and Infection," *The Lancet* (26 March 1983): 689.

## 2.5 Intervention in the Aftermath of a Disease

Intervention in the aftermath of a disease means action to rehabilitate patients suffering the after-effects of a communicable disease — for example, treatment of paralysis, malnutrition, or other sequelae of a disease.

The levels of intervention can also be classified according to the type of prevention.

- *Primary Prevention*
  Primary prevention can be defined as the prevention of the biological and clinical manifestations of an infection. Immunization and sanitation measures fall into this category.

- *Secondary Prevention*
  Secondary prevention means preventing a harmless form of the disease from developing into a more serious form liable to cause death or complications. The use of oral rehydration salts (ORS) at the beginning of a diarrheal attack, for example, prevents the development of dehydration.

- *Tertiary Prevention*
  Tertiary prevention covers rehabilitation following the illness (social reintegration, nutritional rehabilitation after measles, etc.).

- *Curative Action*

*A priori*, the treatment of communicable diseases would seem to have nothing to do with prevention. It might even be argued that as far as the individual is concerned, the necessity for treatment represents a failure of primary and/or secondary prevention measures, which, after all, are intended to prevent the clinical forms of the disease. Nevertheless, to take

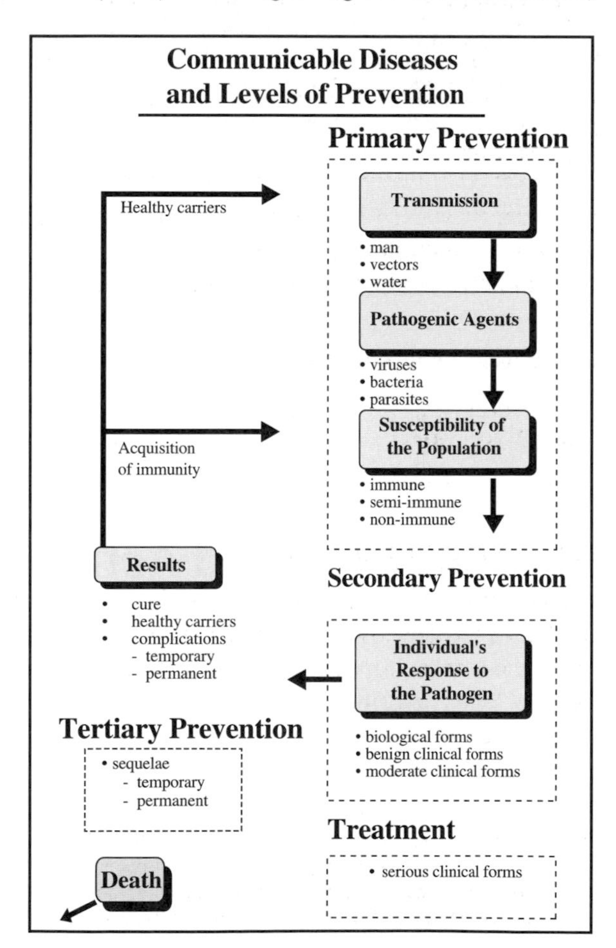

the example of tuberculosis, the identification and treatment of tubercular patients with positive sputum can be considered as a form of primary prevention from the community's point of view, insofar as this therapeutic activity reduces the source of contamination.

### 3. Intervention Strategies

The natural cycle described earlier can be considered as the framework of the system for controlling communicable diseases, which provides the foundation for the other intervention systems:

- environmental sanitation of the environment, in order to reduce sources of infection (primary prevention);
- feeding and nutrition, which contribute in some measure to maintaining immune status;
- therapeutic system to look after sick individuals requiring outpatient or hospital care.

The activities corresponding to these various strategies must be coordinated harmoniously in order to constitute an effective control program: treatment of diarrhea, provision of sufficient quantities of clean water, immunization against measles and the establishment of procedures for treating measles, etc.

The intervention strategy may be oriented in two different ways:

- *the vertical approach*: a health team takes charge of one particular communicable disease, to the exclusion of all others.
- *the horizontal approach*: a health team takes charge of a group of communicable diseases and, if necessary, the collateral interventions linked to them.

This subject will be discussed in detail in Chapter 7 ("The Health-Care System").

## III. Standard Activities: Tools

A certain number of activities related to the control of communicable diseases have already been mentioned in the context of environmental sanitation. This section will describe their role and integration in programs to control communicable diseases, but without reviewing the details of their practical implementation.

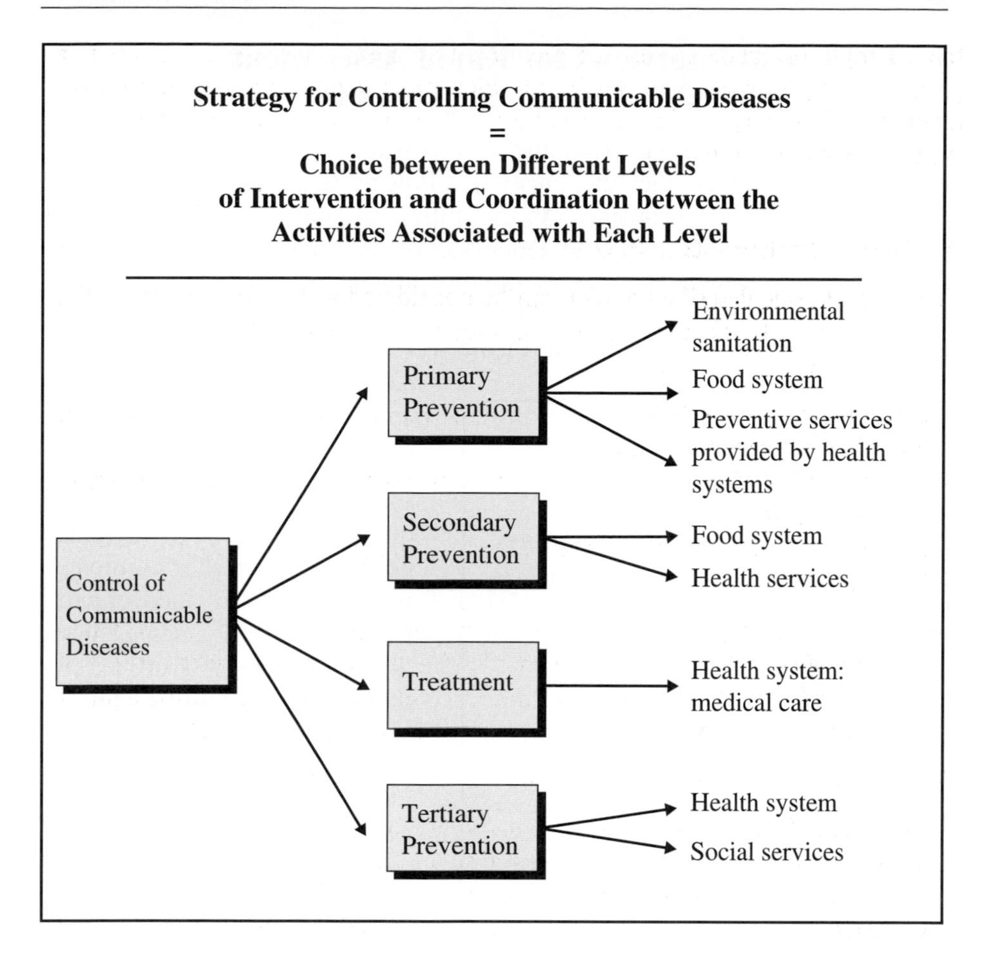


The following is a list of measures for communicable-disease control which have not been discussed in other chapters:[12]

- the use of interviews for rapid assessment of communicable diseases in emergencies
- immunization
- tests carried out in the field
- chemoprophylaxis
- therapeutic approaches
- health education

[12] Some of these measures are not specific to communicable diseases; health education and the use of interviews to evaluate communicable diseases are tools that are also used in other areas.

# 1. The Use of Interviews for Rapid Assessment of Communicable-Disease Problems in an Emergency

In emergencies, relief teams do not always have access to sources of information (dispensaries, hospitals, health ministries) allowing them to define the main communicable-disease problems. At the outset, the only available source of information is the population itself. Opportunities for direct investigation within a population are limited, and it is usually difficult to start off by running biological tests in order to diagnose the main communicable diseases. Initially, health workers will have to content themselves with the information they can collect through interviews with community members.

> **Rapid Assessment Procedures Applied to Causes of Death**
>
> 1. **Role :** to define quickly the main causes of mortality.
> 2. **Technique :** more or less structured interviews with the families and the representatives of a community.
> 3. **Limitations :**
>    - uneven description of the circumstances of death
>    - occasional difficulty in establishing the precise causes of death (linguistic problems)
>    - difficulty of determining the precise date of death
> 4. **Validation :** this technique should be validated by another method of investigation (for example, data furnished by the health services).

Depending on the data sought, such interviews may prove adequate to indicate which measures need to be taken. For example, a relatively simple questionnaire permits a rapid assessment of the main causes of death among the children of a displaced population. The procedure to follow can be summarized as follows:

- Draw up a list of syndromes which appear to be the main causcs of death. In the case of communicable diseases, these would consist primarily of measles, diarrheal diseases, malaria, and meningitis.
- Describe the symptoms used to identify the communicable diseases in question; the medical personnel and the individuals questioned may have markedly different interpretations of the same clinical manifestation. A minimal knowledge of local terminology is essential.[13]
- Verify the information. This is difficult in the case of mortality,[14] since the data received cannot be confirmed except by information from other sources — for example, the causes of death for hospitalized children.[15]

[13] "Clearly, a detailed understanding of local linguistics is needed before a VA [verbal autopsy] can be implemented." B. Snow and K. Marsh, "How Useful Are Verbal Autopsies to Estimate Childhood Causes of Death?" *Health Policy and Planning* 7, No. 1: 26.

[14] In the case of morbidity, confirmation by biological tests promotes greater exactitude.

[15] Keep in mind that the confirming source may also be inexact.

## 2. Immunization

This section will review the main elements of an immunization program, analyzing in succession:

- the indications for an immunization program
- the stages of implementing it
- the method for evaluating it

### 2.1 Indications for an Immunization Program

Some of the communicable diseases responsible for the high mortality rate found in displaced-persons' camps can be easily prevented by immunization. However, the situation must be analyzed to determine which diseases should take priority and what vaccinations are possible.

#### *Defining the Magnitude of the Problem*

The immediate impact of a disease is of less interest than its potential impact. Relief agencies should not wait until an epidemic of measles is declared to begin considering an immunization campaign (which by then would not be much use). This reasoning, however, does not apply to all the communicable diseases for which a vaccine exists. For example, there is no point in launching an immunization campaign against meningitis if no cases of the disease have been diagnosed in the population.

The approach, then, will vary according to the disease. It should be based essentially on the following criteria:

- ***Size of the group likely to develop the disease***
  The size of the group likely to develop the disease depends on several factors. One of them is the degree of immunity already conferred either by a case of the disease (regardless of immunization campaigns, practically all subjects over the age of five have had measles) or by a previous immunization campaign. The risk of contracting progressive tuberculosis does not depend on age. Although the entire population may be "at risk," some groups are nevertheless in greater danger than others: malnourished individuals, the family members of a tubercular subject with positive sputum, AIDS patients. The methods of quantifying each kind of problem will be discussed in greater detail in the sections devoted to specific diseases.
- ***Extent of morbidity or mortality***
  An immunization campaign puts a heavy demand on resources. In emergencies, therefore, immunization should be reserved for diseases with high morbidity and/or mortality rates. Many studies have proven that measles, neonatal tetanus, and meningitis cause high mortality in developing

countries, particularly in Africa. Poliomyelitis, too, is a major problem due to its potential sequelae.

### *Vaccine Effectiveness*

The effectiveness of a vaccine is judged by its ability to confer lasting immunity. After complete immunization, the seroconversion for measles, for example, is 90-95%, for polio 98-100%, for tetanus 100%, for whooping cough 70-95%, and for diphtheria 95-98%.

The duration of immunity is also an important factor. Immunization against measles provides indefinite immunity, while the immunity provided by the meningitis vaccine is limited to two or three years.

There is no interference between malnutrition and the post-vaccination immune response.[16] The vaccine against cholera is not very immunogenic and, moreover, the immunity it provides is of short duration.[17] Indications for an immunization program depend on a combination of both the importance of the diseases involved and the effectiveness of the available vaccines.

Accordingly, in its Expanded Program of Immunization (EPI) WHO has included immunization against measles, polio, tetanus, diphtheria, whooping cough, and tuberculosis, all of which are serious illnesses and against which effective vaccines exist. In emergencies involving large populations among whom non-immunized groups have been identified, the establishment of an EPI is absolutely essential.

## 2.2 Implementation of an Immunization Program

### *Determining the Target Population*

The WHO recommendations for an EPI[18] should be used as the basis for determining the target population.

- BCG at birth
- Polio at birth and, subsequently, with each DPT
- DPT at 6, 10, and 14 weeks
- Measles at 9 months

[16] B. Greenwood, H. Gilles, *et al.*, "The Immune Response to Vaccination in Undernourished and Well-Nourished Nigerian Children," *Annals of Tropical Medicine and Parasitology* 80, No. 5 (1986): 537-544.

[17] Major research has been carried out to improve the effectiveness of the cholera vaccine. The oral vaccine (B subunit/whole cell) provides 85% protection for six months. "New Cholera Vaccines," *Bulletin of the World Health Organization* 2 (1988).

[18] *Immunization Policy*, WHO/EPI/GEN/86/7, p. 3.

This schedule is applied in the framework of a routine program. In an emergency situation, the strategy used will be more along the lines of mass immunization campaigns, and the determination of target populations must be adapted accordingly. UNICEF recommends the immunization of all children under the age of five years.[19] In practical terms, the following schedule could be proposed:

- BCG for children under one year
- Measles for children aged six months to five years
- DPT for all children under five years
- Polio for all children under five years
- Tetanus for women of childbearing age

■ Immunization with BCG is limited to children under the age of one year. "There has been much controversy in the past about the efficacy of the BCG vaccine. It is now generally accepted that it provides a degree of protection, particularly in young children, against serious forms of the disease such as miliary TB and TB meningitis."[20]

■ The limits of the target group for immunization against measles should be reviewed in light of many recently published studies on the rate of measles incidence in children under nine months of age.[21] These findings should be weighed against the fact that the vaccine's effectiveness in children under nine months is inhibited by maternal antibodies. Therefore, the standard vaccine most commonly used (Schwartz strain) is recommended only from the age of nine months up. With the advent of a more immunogenic vaccine, the Edmonston-Zagreb (EZ) strain, the possibility of immunizing children from the age of six months has been suggested, which would reduce the number of measles cases.[22]

The duration of this vaccine's effectiveness, however, has yet to be proven. In October, 1991, a study carried out in Senegal showed that the risk of death in children who had received the EZ vaccine was 1.8 times higher than in children

---

[19] "Unless previous services are known to have had wide coverage, all children under 5 years may be vaccinated. First priority, however, is for children in the first year of life." Ockwell, ed., *Assisting in Emergencies* (UNICEF), p. 270.

[20] MSF, *Medical News* 4, No. 1 (April 1995): 21.

[21] Studies carried out in Africa, in countries where immunization programs are in progress, have indicated that the rate of measles in children under nine months is 20-45% of total cases of measles. Under these circumstances, it can be estimated that 5-10% of children under the age of nine months will contract the disease. See P. Aaby and C. Clements, "Measles Immunization Research: A Review," *Bulletin of the World Health Organization* 67, No. 4: 444.

[22] During the 1980s, the availability of the EZ strain, which, being more immunogenic, was better able to overcome the interference of maternal antibodies, made it possible to lower the age for measles immunization below the nine-month barrier. The minimum level has yet to be precisely defined, but it appears that children from the age of six months can be immunized. *Measles Control in the 1990s*, WHO/EPI/GEN (March 1992).

who had received the Schwartz vaccine.[23] Until the doubts have been resolved, the wisest course in emergency situations is to continue using the Schwartz vaccine.[24]

- Immunization against poliomyelitis can be started at birth.[25] The upper limit remains set at five years.
- Immunization against tetanus protects women of childbearing age and, in particular, reduces the incidence of neonatal tetanus.

These recommendations are applicable at the beginning of an emergency situation, when they should be carried out in the framework of a mass immunization campaign. Later on, when a routine program has been set up, the usual immunization procedures can be followed.

### *Contraindications*

Contraindications prompting a deferral of immunization are exceptional within the defined target groups. Under no circumstances should malnutrition[26] be considered a contraindication.[27] WHO has formulated this simple rule: "Routine vaccinations should be administered unless the child's condition makes hospitalization necessary." In fact, given the risk of hospital epidemics, immunization against measles is imperative for hospitalized children.

BCG is contraindicated for subjects presenting clinical signs of AIDS, but such patients can be given the other vaccines. "In general vaccination is avoided in cases of immune deficiency, but in developing countries the risk of measles and poliomyelitis is great in unvaccinated infants, whereas the risk entailed by immunization, even in the presence of a symptomatic HIV infection, appears minor."[28]

The uncertainty of being able to administer all the required doses for complete immunization within the recommended time limits should not rule out the

---

[23] "Child Mortality after High-Titer Vaccines: Prospective Study in Senegal," *The Lancet* 338 (12 Oct. 1991).

[24] "The standard Schwartz vaccine is recommended. The use of medium or high titer Edmonston-Zagreb (E-Z) vaccine is not yet recommended for refugee populations, since there are still concerns about its safety." *Morbidity and Mortality Weekly Report* (MMWR), CDC (24 July 1992), Vol. 41/N0.RR-13: 52.

[25] "Administration of TOPV at birth, in addition to establishing immunity against poliomyelitis at an earlier stage, produced a superior immune response to poliovirus type 3." L.Y. Weckx, B.J. Schmidt, A.A. Hermann, C.H. Miyasaki, and N.F. Novo, *Bulletin of the World Health Organization* 70, No. 1 (1992): 85.

[26] In nutritional rehabilitation centers, immunization against measles is imperative.

[27] "In fact, the presence of malnutrition is an additional reason to immunize." *Immunization Policy*, WHO/EPI/GEN (1986).

[28] WHO/EPI/GEN/86.7 Rev. 1, p. 6.

initiation of an immunization program. The interruption of vaccinations after the first or second dose does not mean the entire series has to be redone.

## *Objectives and Strategies*

The objective of immunization is simple: to immunize all the subjects (children and/or women) in previously defined age groups. Strategies to achieve this objective will depend on the relations between the health services and the population.

– ***Trust***
  - Is the population aware of the beneficial effects of immunization?
  - Are there any taboos relating to immunization?

  Some public relations work is necessary before an immunization program can be implemented. Usually this work will be carried out through the medium of the most representative members of the community.

– ***The proximity of health services to the population***

  In displaced-person or refugee camps, distances are not generally a problem. At the beginning of the campaign, mobile teams move from one place to another in the camp, following an itinerary jointly decided on with the representatives of the population. The campaign may be carried out either by mobile teams or through outpatient visits to medical facilities (dispensaries) set up in the meantime. These facilities are usually very close to where the camp residents live. This does not mean, however, that people will turn up in droves to be immunized. In camps, the simplest solution is to ask the local EPI to take charge of the immunization campaign; if that is not possible, all or some of the necessary equipment and personnel will have to be imported from abroad.

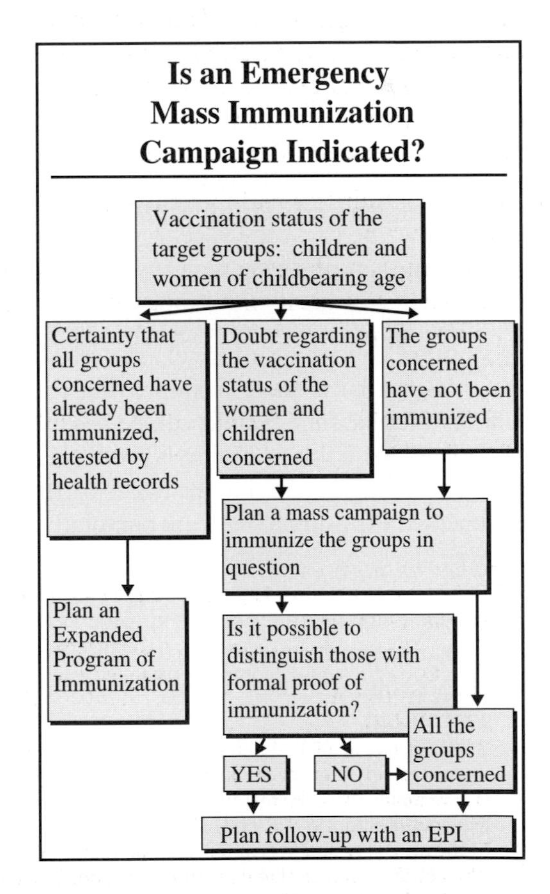

### Practical Organization

Once the general strategy has been defined, all the practical, organizational details must be arranged:

- Who will inform the population?
- What is the desired time-frame for the campaign? Different human resources will be required depending on whether immunization is to take place in a day, a week, or longer.
- How will the cold chain be organized?

Since practical organization depends on the circumstances of each situation, it is impossible to study all its aspects here.

### Material Resources

#### Vaccines

In calculating the number of doses necessary, health workers must take into account not only the total number of people to be immunized at the time of the campaign, but also:

- the coefficient of use[29]
- the necessity, after the mass campaign has ended, of immunizing new arrivals and children who were too young for inoculation at the time of the campaign.

#### Equipment

*Supplies for the cold chain:* WHO has published a number of technical brochures[30] describing all the characteristics of the components of a cold chain. Progress has been made in improving the thermostability of vaccines.[31] The tetanus vaccine, for example, can be used without refrigeration. However, these factors should not be a pretext for relaxing supervision of the cold chain. Each time a vaccine is exposed to the heat its effectiveness deteriorates, and the effects of repeated exposure to heat are cumulative.

*Supplies for injection*: WHO makes the following recommendations:[32]

- A sterile needle and a sterile syringe should be used for each injection.
- Reusable equipment must be sterilized by steam.
- Disposable equipment should be used only if its destruction after use can be guaranteed.

---

[29] The coefficients of vaccine use proposed by WHO are 50% for BCG and 75% for DPT, polio, and measles.
[30] "The Cold Chain," EPI Technical Series, Product Information Sheets. WHO/EPI.
[31] *Weekly Epidemiological Report* 30 (July 1990).
[32] *Immunization Policy*, WHO/EPI (1986).

- Since jet injectors (Ped-O-Jets) can theoretically transmit certain diseases, their use should be restricted to exceptional circumstances (mass campaigns).[33]

*Human Resources*

Organizing a mass immunization campaign means mobilizing substantial human resources, particularly if difficult techniques are to be used, such as immunization with BCG. These human resources include not only medical personnel, but also all the members of the population who will be directly involved in organizing the campaign. Each one must have a very clear idea of what he or she is supposed to do:

Who will register the subjects?
Who will take the vaccines out of the cold box?
Who will prepare the vaccine?
Who will prepare the syringes?
Who will inject the vaccine?
Who will sterilize the injection equipment?
Who will check the temperature control chart?
Who will decide on possible contraindications?

## 2.3 Evaluation of an Immunization Program

*Evaluation of Activities*

The measures taken should be evaluated. Note should be taken, for example, of the number of children immunized in a day, and the number of vaccine doses used; similarly, the temperature charts used throughout the cold chain must be monitored.

*Evaluation of Immunization Coverage*

Immunization coverage corresponds to the ratio between the number of subjects immunized and the number of subjects in the target group defined at the beginning of the immunization campaign.

*Evaluation of Vaccination Effectiveness*

It is difficult to measure the rate of seroconversion in an emergency situation. Instead, epidemiological evaluations should be made, based on the number of subjects immunized who develop the disease in relation to the number of non-immunized subjects who develop the disease.[34]

---

[33] The unreliability of these devices, however, makes using them at all inadvisable.

[34] VE = (RIN * RII/RIN) * 100
- VE = vaccination effectiveness
- RIN = rate of incidence in non-immunized subjects
- RII = rate of incidence in immunized subjects.

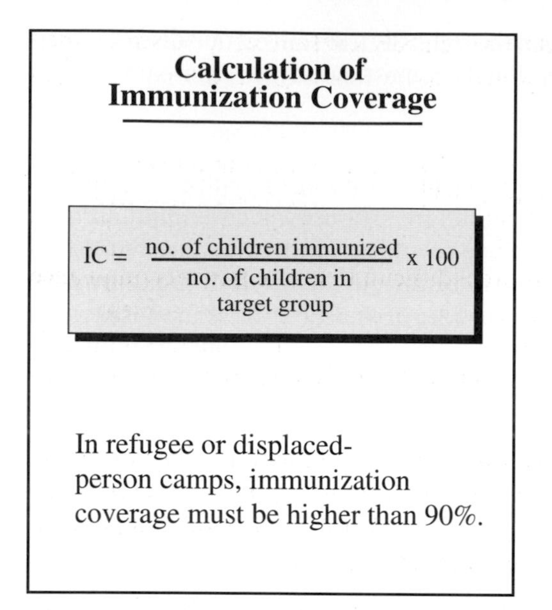

**Calculation of Immunization Coverage**

$$IC = \frac{\text{no. of children immunized}}{\text{no. of children in target group}} \times 100$$

In refugee or displaced-person camps, immunization coverage must be higher than 90%.

### *Evaluation of the Cost/Benefit Ratio*

The cost of resources is relatively low. In Ecuador, complete immunization costs $4.39 per person in a routine EPI and $8.60 in a mass campaign. The cost for each avoided death by measles is estimated at $1,900 in Ecuador, while in Gambia it is only $41. The difference stems basically from the low mortality rate for measles in Ecuador. Obviously, in an emergency situation, a very high measles mortality helps make the cost/benefit ratio much more significant. *The choice of intervention strategy will influence the cost of immunization.*

## 3. Chemoprophylaxis

Chemoprophylaxis comes under the heading of primary prevention. It prevents the appearance of clinical symptoms, but not the biological invasion.

The specific form of chemoprophylaxis appropriate to each disease will be discussed later in the context of comprehensive control programs. This section will deal only with the general problems posed by chemoprophylaxis.

The issue of chemoprophylaxis is frequently raised in emergency situations, usually by non-medical personnel and political officials. *A priori*, it would appear to be a simple, effective way of protecting groups of people liable to contract malaria, meningitis, cholera, tuberculosis, or intestinal parasitic infections; and, properly used, chemoprophylaxis can, of course, provide satisfactory protection against these diseases. However, several factors limit its appropriateness:

- **The right choice of drug** — The use of rifampin for protection against meningococcal meningitis is reliable in all latitudes. In contrast, chemoprophylaxis for malaria requires adjustments in the type of drug and its dosage depending on specific resistances in each region. A study on semi-immune subjects in Tanzania[35] indicated that chemoprophylaxis with chlorproguanil was effective at a dose of 20 mg twice weekly, whereas other studies have shown it to be ineffective.[36]

- **Length of use of the drug** — Chemoprophylaxis must be continued as long as there is a risk of developing the disease — for example, throughout an epidemic of cholera or meningitis, or as long as a risk of malaria persists.
- **The proper use of the drug** — It is often difficult to insure patient compliance with treatment regimens, and this is even more of a problem with chemoprophylaxis.[37] Certainly in the case of malaria, chemoprophylaxis has contributed considerably to extending the resistance of *P. falciparum* to the principal antimalarials.
- **The distribution of drugs** — When used for large populations, chemoprophylaxis demands a major logistic effort. The anticipated results must therefore be weighed against the fact that the operation will mobilize resources that might be more usefully employed in other kinds of activities.

Taking all these considerations into account, the conclusion is that chemoprophylaxis should not be rejected out of hand; but the decision to use it demands a case-by-case approach that weighs the risks involved and focuses on the selection of specific groups at risk (for example, the families of meningitis patients, or children under the age of five and pregnant women in a non-immune population exposed to endemic malaria).

# 4. Therapeutic Approaches

## 4.1 Mass Treatment

Mass treatment differs from chemoprophylaxis in that it is intended to treat within a very short time all the people susceptible to developing a given disease, the aim being to reduce propagation of the disease quickly.

In contrast, the search for and systematic treatment of individuals showing the symptoms of malaria or cavitary tuberculosis are intended more to reduce

[35] I. Rooth, "Proguanil or Chlorproguanil against Malaria in Tanzania," *The Journal of Tropical Medicine and Hygiene* 94, No. 1 (1991).

[36] M. Cosemans *et al.*, "Double-blind Study to Assess the Efficacy of Chlorproguanil Given Alone or in Combination with Chloroquine for Malaria Chemioprophylaxis in an Area with P. Falciparum Resistance to Chloroquine, Pyrimethamine and Cycloguanil," in *Transactions of the Royal Society of Tropical Medicine and Hygiene*, Vol. 81, pp. 151-156.

[37] Among the factors adduced to explain the failure of a chemoprophylactic campaign against malaria in Tanzania was the fact that the families involved did not believe the tablets would prevent the disease, and so saved them to use during acute attacks. *The Journal of Tropical Medicine and Hygiene* 86, No. 3 (1983).

mortality among these patients than to limit transmission of the disease in question. In such cases, therefore, mass treatments are not indicated.

The possibility of using mass treatment for ancylostomiasis (hookworm) has been suggested.[38] However, even in this particular case, a certain number of factors must be considered. Mass treatment does not take the place of environmental sanitation measures and personal hygiene. It is, rather, an auxiliary measure which, in the absence of a sanitation program, will have to be repeated every six months. In order to reduce budgetary and logistic costs, its use can be limited to the groups most affected by the disease (children under the age of 10).

## 4.2 Short Treatments versus Long Treatments

Patient compliance is a constant problem. In emergency situations, health-care personnel face the additional problem of following up patients from migrating populations. These two factors make short treatments particularly appropriate, for several reasons:

- *Better compliance with the treatment regimen*
  The health-care provider who administers single-dose treatments can rest assured that the patient has actually taken the medication. There are also fewer side-effects (one of the most common reasons for discontinuing treatment) — an important factor in tuberculosis, since treatment with isoniazid and thiacetazone for more than a year is badly tolerated.
- *Reduction of the work load*
  The reduction of the health services' work load is not a negligible factor, for in an emergency, particularly its initial stages, the number of patients requiring treatment is substantial.
- *Reduction of treatment cost*
  Treatment cost here is not the cost of the drugs used, but is calculated according to the number of patients cured in relation to those who would be cured by the conventional treatment. This analysis is particularly pertinent in the case of tuberculosis: in 1986, the cost of the short treatment was estimated at $158, while the cost of the long treatment was figured at $123. If figured on the basis of the cost per patient cured, however, this ratio was reversed (respectively, $314 versus $368).
  The availability on the market of generic drugs has made it possible to cut the cost of certain treatments considerably. It is worth keeping informed about

[38] "Mass anthelminthic therapy aims to treat all members of a community during a relatively short period of time without examining them individually and irrespective of whether or not they are infected. It may be used when infection is so prevalent and intensive that almost everyone may be assumed to be infected and to contribute significantly to the continued existence of parasites in the community." Z.S. Pawlowski, G.A. Schad, and G.J. Stott, *Hookworm Infection and Anaemia* (Geneva: WHO, 1991), p. 32.

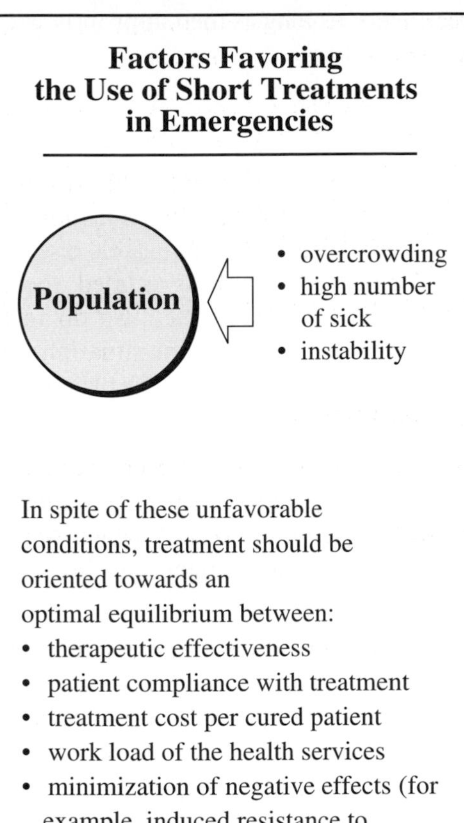


products which, although still marketed as patent medicines, will soon come into the public domain.

All these advantages, however, are of value only if the short treatment equals or surpasses the long treatment in effectiveness. Studies concerning tuberculosis are significant in this respect. Most of them agree that the rate of failure and relapse is 5-10% using the conventional treatments, whereas it is 0-2% for the short treatments. The rate of discontinued treatment is even more significant. According to an evaluation carried out in Peru, 41% of patients discontinued treatment (12 months). The rate of abandonment depends not only on the length of treatment, but also on economic factors (access to medicine) and sociocultural factors (whether the patient belongs to a nomadic or resident population).

Another aspect to be considered in tuberculosis is how quickly the treatment makes the patient's sputum negative. On average, after eight weeks of the short treatment the percentage of patients with negative sputum is 99%, while it is only 45-50% after eight weeks of traditional therapy. This is a key factor in a displaced-persons camp, where the reduction of transmission is a priority.

Single-dose treatments must nevertheless be prescribed with some care. It has been established, for example, that a single injection of chloramphenicol is an effective treatment for epidemic meningococcal meningitis;[39] but it is not suitable for other forms of meningitis.[40]

[39] "The efficacy of a single injection of an oily suspension of chloramphenicol in the treatment of patients of all ages with meningococcal meningitis has been demonstrated. This antibiotic is therefore the recommended form of treatment for the disease under epidemic conditions." *Weekly Epidemiological Record* 16 (20 April 1990).

[40] I. Friedland, "Failure of Chloramphenicol Therapy in Penicillin-Resistant Pneumococcal Meningitis," *The Lancet* 339 (15 Feb. 1992).

Most factors argue in favor of short treatments, as long as their appropriateness in a given context is assessed on a case-by-case basis.

## 5. Health Education

Health education is not limited to the problem of communicable diseases. However, communicable diseases are a useful lead-in for health education: the community must understand well the risks involved in communicable diseases, and participate in controlling them. Health education is related to the sociocultural milieu: "It is important to tell people what they can do to be healthy, but that is not enough. It must be realized that in many situations not only the individual must change. Other things influence behavior: the place where people live, the people around them, the work they do..."[41]

In emergency situations, relief workers rarely have much influence over the causes of the crisis. Unfortunately, they must settle for modifying or adapting the victims' behavior to conform to their new living conditions — which will be temporary, at best — without exercising any real impact on the social environment.

The problems that confront displaced populations are not new to them, but present themselves in a different form. Moreover, the urgency of certain situations necessitates immediate action, before the population has a chance to understand its purpose.

In its manual on managing refugee problems, the UNHCR notes: "The importance of health education is perhaps more widely recognized than are the difficulties in persuading those most at risk to change long-established habits. [...] At least in the emergency phase, priority topics should be those directly related to the immediate public health problems."[42]

A population confronted with an emergency finds itself obliged to change its behavior quickly. Such changes, however, cannot be dictated by outsiders; they must be formulated by the people concerned, and disseminated by them as well, in their own words.

On the basis of this principle, the following sequence might be proposed to begin the process of health education:

- *Have the community identify its problems* (in respect to communicable diseases, the examples are numerous: diarrheal diseases, fever, measles, etc.).

---

41 OMS, *L'éducation pour la santé* (1990), p. 1.
42 UNHCR, *Handbook for Emergencies* (1982), p. 84.

The technique of direct interviews with members of the population comes to the fore here.[43] The community may see its problems differently from the health professionals. They do not necessarily have the same priorities.

- *Study a population's behavior and customs when faced with the problems identified.* This includes factors such as:
  - care of sick children;
  - knowledge or ignorance of rehydration therapy for diarrheal disease;
  - propensity to seek help from health services or traditional doctors;
  - quality of personal hygiene.
- *Set objectives.* If the goal is to have mothers rehydrate their children during attacks of diarrhea, it will be necessary, for example, to:
  - make mothers aware of the risks of dehydration;
  - teach mothers to prepare a rehydration solution;
  - make mothers aware of the importance of continuing to breastfeed during a diarrheal episode.
- *Determine the appropriate measures.* Appropriate measures are:
  - culturally acceptable to the population;
  - effective in treating the health problem in question;
  - feasible in the context of the emergency.

Family members can administer oral rehydration only if they have access to potable water and to the ingredients necessary to prepare a rehydration solution. If these conditions are met, measures can logically be proposed that will change the way families deal with diarrheal attacks. The way these health messages are formulated should reflect the local cultural context: "A true health education necessitates the institution of a dialogue that takes into account the terminologies, the knowledge, the interpretations, and the local practices of the populations."[44] In other words, health messages can be formulated only by people who belong to the community or who are culturally very close to it.

- *Evaluate the impact of a health education program.* To do this, the evaluator must look back at the objectives set at the beginning of the program and assess the degree to which they have been attained. Oral rehydration therapy (ORT), for example, is promoted to reduce mortality caused by diarrheal diseases.

---

[43] "Listening to people talk about their health, expressing their needs as they experience them, and not only as the professionals see them. Individuals and communities must be allowed to express themselves: That is a fundamental element of health education." J.P. Deschamps, "La santé communautaire," in OMS, *L'éducation pour la santé,* p. 128.

[44] Y. Jaffré, "Elaborer un message sanitaire," *Santé et Développement.*

**Developing a Health Education Program**

- Identification of health problems by the community
- Study of behaviors adopted to cope with these problems: should they be modified?
- Determination of the objectives of a health education program
- Identification of practical measures, acceptable to the community, to modify these behaviors
- Implementation of the measures
- Evaluation of results

Improperly used, however, it may also result in complications. In Egypt, for example, when a campaign was launched to introduce ORT, a systematic surveillance program for dehydration cases seen in the dispensaries revealed a high rate of hypernatremia. A media-based education program corrected this misuse of ORT.[45]

Every program should be evaluated. Program organizers must not settle for the evidence of similar experiences in other contexts.

# IV. Setting Priorities

Every manual provides standard lists of priorities, but it is useful to make the intellectual effort necessary to understand the reasoning behind them. It may seem strange to discuss setting priorities after we have already reviewed the main measures applicable to the control of communicable diseases. Our purpose here is in fact to determine priorities in controlling communicable diseases, on the basis of two criteria:

- the importance of the disease, as reflected by morbidity, associated mortality, and the number of people apt to contract it.
- the feasibility of control measures, as reflected by their effectiveness in reducing disease, comparative costs of different measures, and duration of effect.

These two criteria, taken together, provide a basis for determining priorities for action.

[45] "Hypernatraemia Surveillance during Use of ORS, Egypt," *The Lancet* 339 (15 Feb. 1992).

# 1. Impact of Communicable Diseases

The impact of a communicable disease must be assessed at two levels: the impact on individuals and the impact on the population as a whole.

## 1.1 Impact on the Individual

It is known that diseases such as poliomyelitis, measles, and tuberculosis can cause infirmity, death, or incapacity. To the individual, each of them poses a major risk.

## 1.2 Impact on the Population

In emergency situations and in most developing countries, the concept of a disease's impact on the population is very important. In normal situations, the aim is to manage limited resources optimally, addressing the problems that have the most impact on the population as a whole. In an emergency situation, resource availability is still something to consider. However, it is most important to define as quickly as possible the crucial problems of the entire population, rather than focus on individuals first.

Diphtheria, for example, is a serious disease, but relatively rare, with limited contagiousness. Measles, on the other hand, is also a serious illness, more common than diphtheria, and highly contagious. It thus represents a definite risk for vulnerable groups. Intestinal parasites, in turn, may be a public health problem for a large proportion of a population; yet, except in rare instances, they are not life-threatening. The forms of tuberculosis with positive sputum are serious; without treatment, 50% of these patients can be expected to die within two years.[46] But tuberculosis's low contagiousness (compared with that of measles, for example) and its slow progression mean that some delay in implementing a control program is permissible.

## 1.3 Influence of the Seasons

The incidence of most of the communicable diseases is seasonal. For example, epidemic meningitis develops during the dry season; the incidence of malaria, diarrheal diseases, and respiratory infections increases in the rainy season; and measles epidemics spread more easily during the dry season.

It should be noted, however, that the different seasons sometimes correspond to occasions when large numbers of people are gathered together. In the case of

[46] Oxfam, *Guidelines for Tuberculosis Control Programmes in Developing Countries, An Oxfam Memorandum* (1985).

measles, for example, the concentration of a group of vulnerable subjects probably plays a more important role in the development of an epidemic than the season during which that gathering takes place.

# 2. Possibilities of Intervention

In emergency interventions, what is theoretically possible will be conditioned by practical constraints.

## 2.1 Theoretical Effectiveness of Technical Measures

The technical solutions appropriate for a particular problem can be determined at the outset. This, in fact, means deciding which of the tools studied above are the most effective for controlling a given communicable disease. It is known, for example, that immunization against measles and oral rehydration therapy are effective, and that immunization against cholera is not.

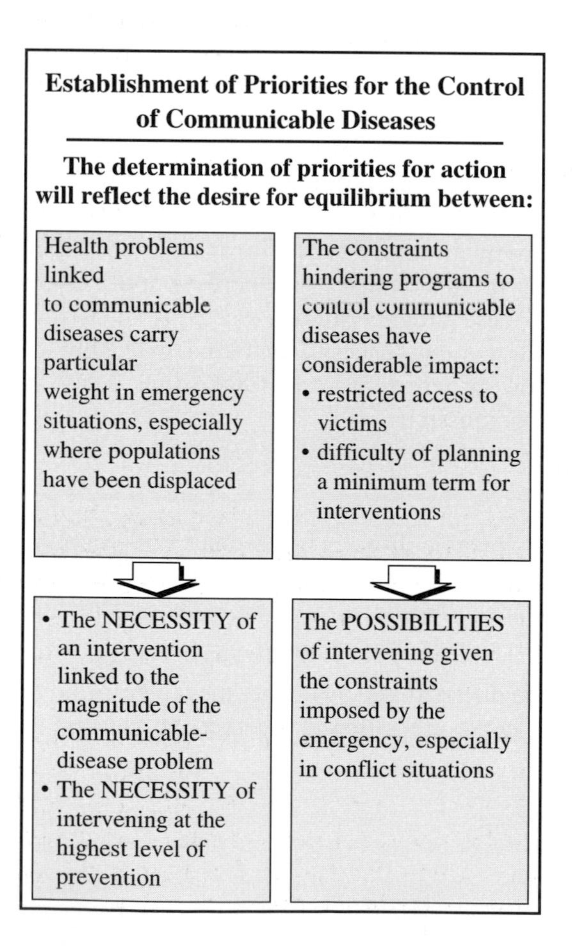


## 2.2 Duration of Effectiveness

Mass treatment of intestinal parasites will reduce the parasitic load of individuals considerably, but its effectiveness is temporary. Sanitation measures produce a slower but more lasting effect.

## 2.3 Limits Imposed by the Situation

The limits imposed by the situation may be budgetary, logistical, or political. Their importance and interaction vary from case to case; usually they impose a very down-to-earth approach to problems. The question is no longer knowing what ought to be done, but what can be done.

It is essentially in conflict situations that the implementation of technically feasible measures poses problems. The major constraint is lack of access to victims. Measures of control will achieve definite coverage and effectiveness only if they are implemented where the victims are living.

In addition, the theoretical technical effectiveness of control measures is often impaired. The reduction of mortality from *Plasmodium falciparum* malaria depends in part on the diagnosis and rapid treatment of cases. Yet how effectively can this be done in a migrating population for whom the quest for food, water, and safety takes priority?

# V. Examples of Programs to Control Communicable Diseases

Communicable diseases can be controlled by proper coordination of a series of measures implemented for that purpose. The combinations possible depend on both the diseases in question and the context in which they are found. The constraints of emergency situations — particularly conflicts — limit the possibility of taking all the steps which, together, would control the communicable diseases effectively.

The integrated, multidisciplinary approaches that can be instituted in an emergency, given the factors just mentioned, will be examined through the following examples:

- malaria
- measles
- diarrheal diseases (cholera)
- tuberculosis
- meningococcal meningitis
- intestinal parasitic infestation

These diseases do not necessarily constitute priorities as defined earlier, but as examples they serve as "puzzles" in which the different pieces vary in importance according to the disease. The intervention strategies for measles and poliomyelitis are fairly similar, in that they are based on the systematic immunization of groups at risk. In contrast, immunization does not have the same significance in the control of meningitis.

Most of the programs or activities coming under the heading of a general control program for one or another of these diseases have already been discussed in connection with communicable diseases, the environment, and food and nutrition. Thus, rather than trying to describe each activity in detail, this section will merely list them, assessing the relative importance of each with respect to the others in terms of its potential to influence the final outcome favorably.

To facilitate presentation, the recommended control regimens will be organized according to the natural cycle of the disease, as described at the beginning of this chapter. Measures will be categorized according to the level of intervention they represent — for example:

- immunizations -> primary prevention, modification of the immunological status of immunized individuals
- supply of potable water -> primary prevention, reduction of transmission
- chemoprophylaxis -> secondary prevention, prevention of clinical signs of disease

The "obligatory" interrelations between the different measures must be emphasized — for example:

Primary prevention of diarrheal diseases must include at the minimum:

  - a supply of clean water;
  - adequate personal hygiene;
  - correct disposal of excreta.

- To control malaria in emergency situations, the usual policy is merely to limit the mortality linked to this disease. From this perspective, coordinating effective clinical screening with quickly accessible medical treatment is essential.

There are more extended interventions. For example, immunization against measles, which prevents that disease, also helps prevent the concomitant diarrheal attacks. This impact on the global control of diarrheal diseases, however, is secondary.

# 1. Malaria

Dealing with malaria is complicated enough in ordinary situations; controlling it during crises depends on a combination of activities. In the framework of this course, a detailed analysis of highly specialized activities (for example, calculating vector capacity or using *in vitro* tests to determine the parasite's sensitivity to drugs), is less useful than an effort to link all these activities to the disease cycle, in order to establish a general framework for a disease-control program.

## 1.1 Impact of the Problem

The impact of the problem depends on a number of factors.

*Potential Seriousness*

The disease's potential to cause harm is based on several factors:

- *The nature of the parasite*: malaria caused by *Plasmodium falciparum* can be a major cause of death among displaced people, depending on the geographical region involved.
- *The presence of a vector capable of transmitting malaria.* This means establishing certain facts:
  - whether the vector is present in substantial numbers and close to human dwellings;
  - whether it exhibits tropism to man rather than animals;
  - whether its way of life involves eating and resting inside or outside of dwellings.
- *Factors favoring transmission*:
  - the population's way of life — specifically, the population's behavior with respect to the vector.
  - the season. During the rainy season, transmission is much greater due to the increased number of pools of stagnant water in which the vector can multiply.
  - environmental characteristics such as average temperature, vegetation, the presence of surface water at times other than the rainy season (irrigation water, for example).

The appropriate "parasite plus vector" combination is a key factor leading to the transmission of malarial infection within the population.

### *Susceptibility of the Population*

The susceptibility of the population depends on several factors:

- *the type of transmission*
  In areas where transmission is stable throughout the year (holoendemic and hyperendemic regions), the immunity that results is also stable, and although the number of people presenting parasitemia may be high, the number of people actually sick is relatively low. In contrast, in regions of unstable or low transmission, immunity fluctuates, and there may be a large increase in the number of malaria cases during periods of high transmission.
- *age*
  In regions of unstable transmission, all the members of the population are predisposed to attacks of malaria. In regions of stable transmission, certain age groups are more vulnerable than others. Essentially, children under the age of two years are most at risk.[47]

---

[47] "Clearly, [the study] cannot provide definitive rates for morbidity and mortality due to malaria in the community. Nevertheless, our finding that children have a 1 in 15 chance of being admitted to hospital with a severe, potentially life-threatening episode of malaria before their fifth birthday indicates the likely scale of the problem." R.W. Snow, J.R.M. Amstrong-Schellenberg, *et al.*, "Periodicity and Space-Time Clustering of Severe Childhood Malaria on the Coast of Kenya," *Transactions of the Royal Society of Tropical Medicine and Hygiene* 87 (1993): 388.

– *pregnancy*
  Mortality among pregnant women, especially primapara, is particularly high.[48]

Whether or not a certain immunity is present within the population is a key determinant for the development of "malaria disease."

*The Capacity of the Health Services*

In emergency situations, the disorganization generated by the disaster and lack of access to victims often prevent health workers from taking preventive measures such as controlling the vector's reproduction sites and combating the adult vector. In addition, the capacity to diagnose and treat malaria cases quickly is often too limited to cope with an epidemic.

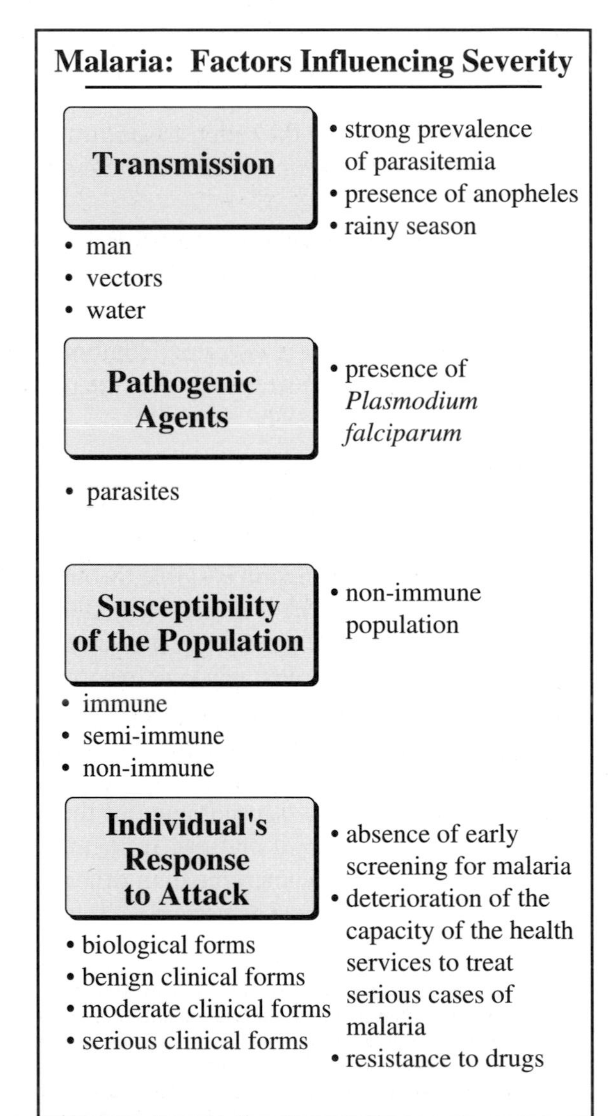


The combination of all these factors — presence of parasites and vectors, non-immune population, and lack of health services — will be reflected in a high incidence of malaria and, in the case of *P. falciparum* malaria, a large number of deaths.

*Qualitative Evaluation of the Problem*

In dealing with malaria, the first step is to seek

[48] "Pregnant women with malaria must be treated promptly, because the disease is more severe, is associated with high parasitemia, and is dangerous for mother and fetus." *Management of Severe and Complicated Malaria — A Practical Handbook* (Geneva: WHO, 1991), p. 34.

information from national and international institutions regarding the nature of the problem in the region in question. There are many possible sources of information, including the health ministry, institutions more specifically in charge of controlling malaria, WHO, and others. The data thus obtained usually provide answers to a certain number of questions:

- *What type of parasite is it?*
  Depending on whether the agent is *falciparum* or *vivax*, the consequences for the population will be very different.
- *What are the types and characteristics of vectors present in the region?*
  Ascertaining the vector's habits[49] makes it possible to avoid using insecticides indoors, since anopheles live principally outdoors.
- *Is the rhythm of transmission stable or unstable?*
- *Does the population concerned already possess a certain immunity?* In the case of a displaced population, information can be sought as to its previous exposure, stable or otherwise, to a given species of malaria parasite.
- *Is the parasite concerned susceptible to the standard drugs?*

*Quantitative Evaluation*

The numerous factors mentioned previously interact in a complex manner, and it is difficult to define the problem of malaria quantitatively. Attempts may, however, be made to quantify:

- *The prevalence of the parasitemia*
  Prevalence of the parasitemia can be measured directly from a sampling of the population. This measurement will indicate what percentage of the population presents *Plasmodium* in the blood.[50] The measurement of the prevalence of gametocytes in the blood indicates the percentage of infectious people.[51]
- *The vector's capacity to transmit malaria*
  The vector's capacity to transmit malaria depends on various factors, including the density of the vector in the human environment, the number of times it bites humans per day, its survival rate, and the period of incubation inside the vector. Estimating these factors is the job of an entomologist, who should be called in for the purpose.

---

[49] Endophilia, exophilia, endophagy, exophagy, anthropophilia, zoophilia, vector's life span, duration of sporogony (influenced by outside temperature).

[50] According to the classification system recommended by WHO, this measure can be expressed in various forms: plasmodic index, rate of parasitic density, rate of gametocyte infection, rate of infection by species.

[51] L. Molineaux *et al.*, "Malaria, Epidemiology and Its Measurements," in W.H. Wensdorfer and Sir I. McGregor, eds., *Malaria: Planning and Practices in Malariology* (1989), Vol. 2, p. 1045.

- *The degree of transmission*
  The degree of transmission can be measured by means of the splenic index in children from two to nine years old. Together with the plasmodic index (subjects carrying *Plasmodium*), it indicates the type of endemic involved.[52]

- *The population's degree of immunity*
  There are many tests to detect the presence of antibodies. These techniques are not very practical in an emergency situation, although large-scale studies have been made in remote regions.[53] The degree of immunity can also be estimated by indirect methods, such as measuring malaria-related morbidity and mortality.

- *The measurement of mortality must take account of age*
  A mortality rate associated primarily with children below the age of five years and pregnant women indicates that the overall population, with the exception of these vulnerable groups, has a certain immunity. A mortality which is distributed among all age sectors, on the other hand, is the earmark of a non-immune population confronted by a high level of contagiousness. This distinction makes it possible to quantify not the number of malaria cases that can be expected, but the size of the groups at risk: children under age five, pregnant women, or the entire population.

  Mortality figures can be obtained directly from the population (evaluation of mortality on the basis of symptoms) and from any existing health services.

## 1.2 Control Measures

Control programs are established on the basis of the disease cycle and with due consideration for the feasibility of the technical measures proposed. Later, any constraints limiting the use of these measures should be examined.[54]

---

52 Splenic index:
$<10\%$ = hypoendemic
11-50% = mesoendemic
$>50\%$ = hyperendemic
$>75\%$ = holoendemic

53 E.H. Benzerroug *et al.*, "Etude séroépidémiologique du paludisme au Sahara algérien," *Bulletin of the World Health Organization* 69, No. 6.

54 "However, it is not sufficient merely to identify the measures that could be used and that are known from experience to be technically feasible and to have a significant impact on the problem. It will also be essential to determinate the potentially useful measures which under the prevailing conditions would not be feasible from an operational, administrative or socio-economic point of view." P.F. Beales, S. Goriup, S. Litsios, L. Molineaux, E. Onori, and J.H. Pull, "The Planning of Malaria Control," in W.H. Wernsdorfer and Sir I. McGregor, eds., *Malaria: Principles and Practices in Malariology*, Vol. 2, p. 1299.

### *Treating the Parasite "Reservoir" (Gametocytes)*

Ideally, screening and treating all carriers of the sexual forms of the parasite would reduce transmission. Carriers of gametocytes are not necessarily symptomatic, however, and are therefore difficult to identify at clinics or other medical centers. Systematic screening within the population is unrealistic during the emergency phase.

### *Controlling the Vector's Reproduction Sites*

One of the main questions to ponder before deciding where to set up a displaced-person camp is whether the area in question contains many sites where anopheles can reproduce. It is simpler to choose a healthier site than to have to undertake sanitation measures. If it is not possible to choose the site, the following measures can be taken to limit the vectors' opportunities for reproduction:

- drainage
- pruning overgrown areas, which tend to develop into little swamps
- the use of anti-larval processes. There are numerous processes to develop predators of the larval forms of the parasite.[55] Another possibility is to spread a thin film of oily solution on the surface of local bodies of water.[56]

These measures require the participation of the population, and, therefore, a certain stability in the situation. Moreover, to implement methods of biological control, major investigations must be carried out first, something which is usually incompatible with an emergency situation.

### *Controlling the Adult Vector*

The use of insecticides against vectors[57] has been the basis of most programs of malaria control. This method has not eradicated malaria as was anticipated when it was introduced in the 1950s, but when properly applied it helps reduce malaria transmission significantly.

The feasibility of control depends on:

- previous knowledge of the type and characteristics of the vector, as well as its degree of resistance to insecticides;

---

55 In Colombia, introducing a nematode (*R. culicivorax*) into larval reproduction sites caused a rapid decline in the larval population and in the prevalence of malaria attacks in schoolchildren. W. Rojas, "Reduction of Malaria Prevalence after Introduction of R. Culicivorax in Larval Anopheles Habitats in Colombia," *Bulletin of the World Health Organization* 65, No. 3: 331.

56 This measure cuts off the larva's oxygen supply.

57 Two methods are possible, depending on the habits of the vector responsible for transmission: spraying inside dwellings, and spraying in the space around living areas. The use of mosquito nets soaked in insecticide is a method that combines a physical barrier to transmission between vectors and humans with the actual destruction of vectors.

- a reasonably stable population;
- the possibility of finding the necessary material means.

There are other ways of controlling adult vectors (chemical sterilization, genetic engineering), but they cannot be applied in emergency situations.

### *Controlling Transmission from Vector to Man*

Transmission from vector to man is controlled by means of simple measures designed to reduce the possibility of contact between the two. These measures include:

- *measures intended to repel the vector*. The use of insect repellent on the exposed parts of the body, clothing, and mosquito nets reduces the number of mosquito bites.
- *measures intended to prevent contact between vectors and humans*. The use of appropriate clothing (long sleeves) protects the skin and prevents bites.
- *the use of mosquito nets*. This has become an important means of control, especially since the use of mosquito nets soaked in insecticide was instituted. Studies on the use of mosquito nets impregnated with permethrin at a dose of 0.08 $g/m^2$ have shown a reduction in the number of mosquito bites,[58] as well as in the number of malaria attacks.[59]
- *measures to make housing mosquito-resistant*. This means mosquito screens on the windows, construction material that can be impregnated with insecticide, etc.
- *measures affecting the population's way of life*. This means staying inside during the times that the risk of being bitten is greatest.

Of all these methods, the use of mosquito nets is the only one directly applicable in emergency situations, provided that:

- the community's participation has been enlisted. Mosquito nets cannot be used on a large scale unless the population understands that this measure helps prevent malaria.
- the community's habits are compatible with the use of mosquito nets. The people at risk must be under the mosquito net at the time when the risk of bites is greatest; but unfortunately, that is often the time of greatest domestic activity.
- material means are available. It is possible to make permethrin-soaked mosquito nets locally.

---

[58] F. Darriet *et al.*, "Evaluation of the Efficacy of Permethrin-Impregnated Intact and Perforated Mosquito Nets against Vectors of Malaria," Burkina Faso, WHO document (1984).

[59] A study carried out in Gambia showed a decrease of 63% in clinical attacks of malaria. C.P. MacCormack, "Use of Insecticide-Impregnated Bed Nets in Gambian Primary Health Care: Economic Aspects," *Bulletin of the World Health Organization* 67, No. 2 (1989): 209-214.

## *Controlling Immune Status*

There is currently no vaccine against malaria, and there is very little choice in control measures in this respect. At most, the population's immune status can be taken into consideration. It had been thought that chemoprophylaxis inhibited the development of natural immunity, but in fact, several studies have shown that this is not the case for children under the age of five years. Chemoprophylaxis is never total, and the subject continues to receive enough exposure to the parasite to develop immunity, even if the immunoglobulin and antibody rates are lower in cases of chemoprophylaxis.

## *Controlling the Infection at the Biological Stage*

When the infected vector has managed to circumvent all obstacles and inject the parasite through the cutaneous barrier, chemoprophylaxis reduces the risk that malaria-disease will develop by neutralizing the pre-erythrocytic forms of the parasite. Although chemoprophylaxis does not prevent malaria absolutely — that could be done only by destroying the sporozoites the moment the vector injected them into the host — it can be used in emergencies. In that case, the relief team must:

- *define a prophylactic regimen*
  The appearance of drug resistance limits the choice of drugs that can be used for chemoprophylaxis. The use of certain drugs normally used for therapeutic ends is inadvisable, due to the risk of fostering resistance. Moreover, consideration must be given to the drug's side-effects which, in some cases, may be serious enough to contraindicate its systematic use in chemoprophylaxis. The choice is limited to chloroquine, proguanil, and chlorproguanil.[60] In each case, the medical team must assess the parasite's resistance, and choose the prophylactic regimen accordingly. There is no standard regime applicable to every situation.
- *define the groups needing protection*
  Pregnant women constitute one group at risk which requires protection. Chemoprophylaxis should also be contemplated for children under the age of five years, assuming that chemoprophylaxis does not prevent acquisition of natural immunity. Chemoprophylaxis for the entire population is not indicated.

The decision to use chemoprophylaxis will depend on the level of endemicity, the access to health services, and practical feasibility (cost and time compared with

---

[60] A study carried out in Tanzania on school-age children showed that taking chlorproguanil in doses of 20 mg twice weekly provided good protection. See I. Rooth, "Proguanil Daily or Chlorproguanil Twice Weekly Are Efficacious against Falciparum Malaria in a Holoendemic Area of Tanzania," *The Journal of Tropical Medicine and Hygiene* 94, No. 1 (1991): 45.

those for other measures). In the case of a non-immune population arriving in an area of strong endemicity, thought must be given to the feasibility of chemoprophylaxis for the two risk groups mentioned above.

### *Controlling Malaria in the Clinical Stage*

The purpose of treating the clinical forms of malaria is to reduce morbidity and especially mortality (caused by *P. falciparum*). The problem is not deciding whether or not to treat — that is imperative in every situation — but rather deciding which treatment to employ, taking into account drug resistances.

The information collected on the spot from the appropriate authorities usually indicates which therapeutic regimens are likely to be efficacious. Drug resistances are not uniformly distributed, however, and the right treatment for one area is not necessarily the right one for the area next to it. In an emergency, the relief team can begin treatment with a regimen based on the recommendations of local experts, while at the same time carrying out *in vivo* tests to determine the parasite's sensitivity to the drug(s) used.[61] *In vitro* tests clarify drug resistance, but they cannot take the place of *in vivo* tests.[62]

The strategy used to implement curative measures will depend on local capacities (available infrastructure) and the size and distribution of the population. If diagnostic means are unavailable and malaria appears (judging by endemicity and mortality) to be a major problem, then cases presenting clinical symptoms compatible with a diagnosis of malaria will be treated as such (presumptive treatment). If the necessary infrastructure for parasitological diagnosis is available, then confirmed malaria cases will be treated in the laboratory (radical treatment).

In the case of a mass influx of displaced people, many of whom are suspected to have malaria, presumptive treatment should be the first step, in order not to overload the laboratory (if there is one).[63] Establishing drug sensitivity is possible

---

[61] This process is based on parasitological observation of a sampling of patients who undergo certain tests (for example, a malaria smear) before treatment; every day for seven days the degree of resistance is assessed according to the WHO classification system:
- No parasites from day 6 and no new developments on day 7 — the parasite is amenable to treatment.
- The parasites disappear during treatment but reappear on day 7 — the parasite has an R I resistance.
- The parasites decline in number (to 25% of the initial level) but do not disappear at the end of 48 hours — the parasite presents an R II resistance.
- The rate of parasites remains unchanged or greater than 75% of the original rate — the parasite has an R III resistance.

[62] *Practical Chemotherapy, Report of a WHO Scientific Group* (1990), 91.

[63] The laboratory is best reserved for *in vivo* tests, which will make defining an effective treatment easier.

during an emergency, provided that enough of an infrastructure exists to permit tests to be read and patients to be kept under observation.

There is no standard program for controlling malaria. In a situation presenting specific epidemiological (vector, parasite, population immunity), logistical, and/or political (access to population) features, health-care personnel must analyze all factors and design a control program that treats malaria as a public health problem. For example, in the case of a non-immune population arriving in a region that is hyperendemic for *P. falciparum,* the risk of a malaria epidemic is great. The health team must therefore coordinate curative measures — to reduce morbidity and mortality quickly — with preventive measures, which will not be immediately effective but which will help reduce the disease's impact on the population.

**Modes of Intervention: Malaria**

**Primary Prevention**

| | |
|---|---|
| Transmission<br>• vectors<br>• water | • drainage of vector's breeding grounds<br>• the use of insecticides is difficult in emergency situations<br>• use of mosquito nets |
| Pathogenic Agents<br>• parasites | • determination of the parasite's sensitivity to antimalarials |
| Susceptibility of the Population<br>• immune<br>• semi-immune<br>• non-immune | • chemoprophylaxis for groups most at risk (children under five and pregnant women) is difficult to implement<br>• the vaccine is not yet operational |

**Secondary Prevention**

| | |
|---|---|
| • biological forms<br>• benign clinical forms<br>• moderate clinical forms | • early screening of cases |

**Treatment**

| | |
|---|---|
| • serious clinical forms | • effective treatment of cases |

***Reducing morbidity and mortality involves:***

- finding out what treatments the local authorities recommend on the basis of their experience;
- diagnosing and treating cases;
- monitoring the effectiveness of the treatments by *in vivo* tests.

***Preventing malaria involves:***

- mobilizing and educating the population. Most of the following measures depend on the population's ability to institute and continue preventive measures. Populations who have never used mosquito nets will not use them

now, unless they have received preliminary instruction on the subject (education program).
- controlling vectors with insecticides (selected according to the vector's habits and known resistances).
- controlling the vectors' breeding grounds.
- promoting the use of mosquito nets.
- using chemoprophylaxis for groups at risk.

This strategy must be regularly reviewed in order to determine whether the activities instituted at the beginning of the program are still valid (in the meantime, the problem may have been resolved, or the measures may have proved ineffective). This implies the existence of evaluation mechanisms.[64]

# 2. Measles

## 2.1 Impact of the Problem

All unvaccinated children between the ages of six months and five years[65] can be assumed to be liable to develop measles. In a displaced population, this age group represents 15-20% of the total population. Depending on the situation, the rate of complications can be very high. In a study carried out in Zimbabwe which followed 1,399 children hospitalized for measles, 804 (57%) of them developed complications.[66] The mortality rate varies considerably, depending on whether the sick children have access to health care or not. It may fluctuate from 1-3% up to 50%, the rate registered during epidemics in Sahelian villages. Measles also causes complications in the form of malnutrition and ocular lesions due to vitamin A deficiency.

Displaced-person and refugee camps must be considered by definition to present maximum risk, measles being unquestionably a high-priority problem. There is no point in trying to quantify the potential effects of a measles epidemic (number of possible cases, number of complications, and number of deaths). Any results that might be obtained will not change the control strategy in any respect.

---

64 The selection of indicators for a surveillance program is studied in Chapter 6 ("Epidemiology").

65 In general, in developing countries the presumption is that most children over the age of three have had measles. In an emergency situation, a wider margin is generally adopted.

66 The principal complications (for all ages together) were pneumonia (41%), tracheobronchitis (5%), diarrhea with dehydration (52%), and convulsions (2%). See R.A. Kambarami, "Measles Epidemics in Harare, Zimbabwe," *Bulletin of the World Health Organization* 69, No. 2 (1991): 213-219.

## 2.2 Control Measures

The recommended policy in emergency situations where immunization coverage against measles is limited is as follows:

UNICEF: "The immunization of all children 9 months–3 years old against measles will be a high priority in any temporary camps, crowded communities and areas where (seasonal) outbreaks are common."[67]

UNHCR: "The only immunization indicated in the early weeks of an emergency is of young children against measles."[68]

Immunization is the core of any control program; but it does not eliminate the need to plan other measures, such as standard procedures for treating declared cases.

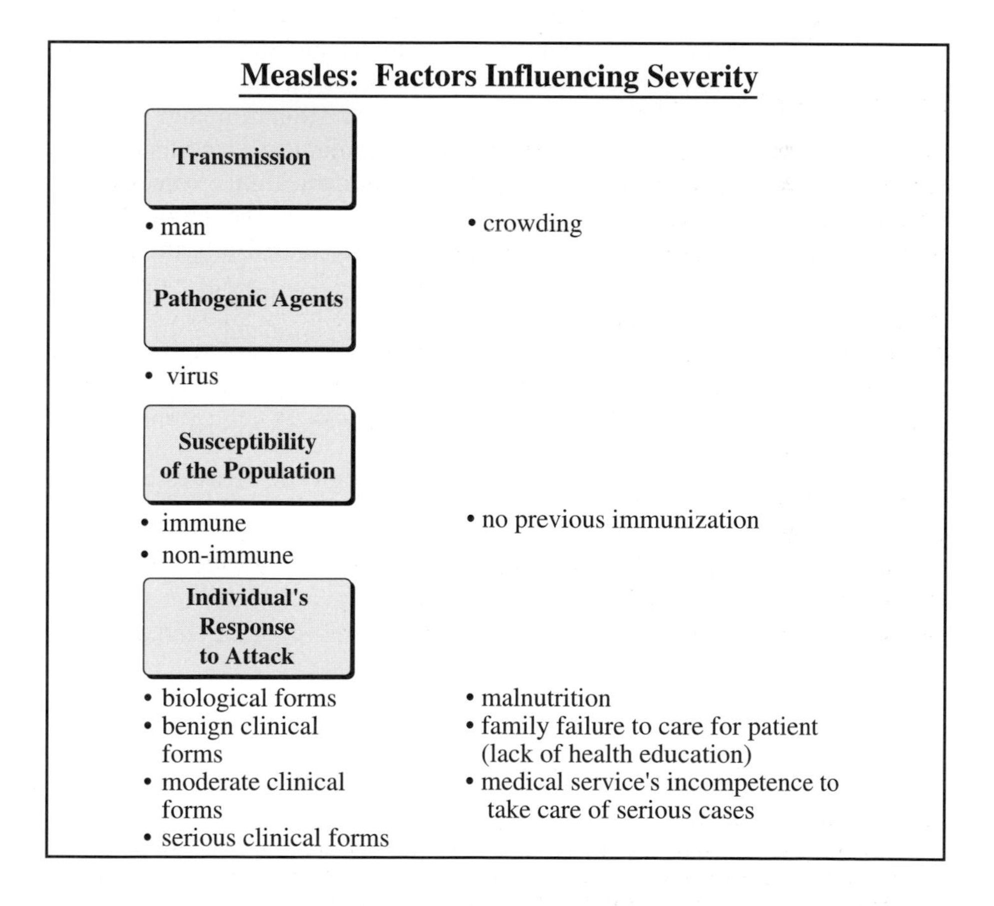


67 Ron Ockwell, ed., *Assisting in Emergencies* (UNICEF), p. 269.
68 UNHCR, *Handbook for Emergencies* (1982), p. 79.

### *Reducing Transmission*

Measures to reduce transmission of the disease have practically no effect. It is difficult to try to reduce overcrowding.

### *Reducing Vulnerability to the Disease*

Immunization against measles is a priority in situations where populations are gathered together temporarily. Where previous immunization is in doubt, all children between the ages of six months and five years must be immunized. For children under the age of nine months, a booster shot should be administered a few months later. A routine program should subsequently be instituted to immunize those children who were under the age of six months at the time of the mass campaign.

Despite these precautions, immunization coverage is never complete. Certain children outside the target group may not be immune, and develop the disease; others, although within the designated age group, miss the vaccination for one reason or another. Moreover, the fact that an immunization campaign has been carried out is no guarantee that a correct level of immunity has been achieved. Besides all the technical problems involved in the immunization campaign itself (effectiveness of the cold chain, vaccine efficacy, etc.), the percentage of seroconversion is in any case only some 90-95% in vaccinated subjects.

In camps, controlling measles is an imperative, and the aim must be to immunize more than 95% of the population if measles is to be eliminated.[69] In unstable populations, notably in the case of uncontrolled migration, it is unrealistic to try to eradicate measles; but this is no reason to postpone immunization. Under such circumstances, a strategy of mass immunization should be adopted.[70]

The overall effectiveness of an immunization campaign will be assessed on the basis of:[71]

- the percentage of susceptible subjects at the time of immunization;[72]
- the vaccine's rate of effectiveness (90-95%);
- immunization coverage (80%).

---

[69] F.T. Cutts, "Principles of Measles Immunization," *Bulletin of the World Health Organization* 69, No. 1: 2.

[70] "Days of tranquillity or 'corridors of peace' denote a cease-fire in areas or countries experiencing civil unrest or war that should be set aside for the purpose of immunizing all children in the conflict area, regardless of allegiance." *Weekly Epidemiological Record* [WHO, Geneva] 31 (August 1994): 5.

[71] N. Guerin and C. Fillastre, "Programmes de vaccination," in Rougemont and Brunet-Jailly, eds., *Santé dans les pays tropicaux*, p. 631.

[72] This depends on the percentage of children who will be immunized despite already having acquired immunity (from a case of measles or previous inoculation).

It should be noted that even when an immunization campaign has been properly implemented, groups of subjects susceptible to contracting the disease will still exist. As their numbers increase over the years, a major epidemic may be feared once they reach the critical threshold for transmission — that is, when a cohort of people at risk has developed.

### *Measures to Be Taken in Diagnosed Cases of Measles*

In emergency situations, no immunization campaign, however well implemented, can guarantee an outcome of 100% immunity. It is therefore necessary to consolidate the control program with supplementary measures, such as deciding on the procedures to be used in dealing with diagnosed cases of measles.

Certain steps are essential:

- antibiotic treatment;
- administration of vitamin A;[73]
- information on immunization history.

This last point merits particular attention, since it is the basis of the formula measuring vaccination effectiveness already mentioned: VE = (RIN — RII/RIN) * 100.

### *Integrating Identification of Measles Cases in the Epidemiological Surveillance Program*

The systematic collection of data on each case of measles diagnosed provides an indicator of the immunization's real effectiveness. If the rate of measles is high among immunized subjects, the effectiveness of the vaccine used must be questioned.

### *Monitoring Complications*

Surveillance of nutritional status and, if necessary, measures for nutritional rehabilitation are part of any program to control measles. Although such a program may focus mostly on immunization, many issues must be resolved, on a case-by-case basis:

- The selection of a target group: What age group should be immunized?
- Selection of the antigen to be used: Edmonston-Zagreb or Schwartz?
- Determination of intervention strategy: mass campaign or routine EPI?

---

[73] It was shown that the rate of mortality from measles was markedly decreased by the ingestion of vitamin A, and that complications were less severe. "Reduction of Mortality by Providing Vitamin A in Measles Complications," *The New England Journal of Medicine* 323, No. 3 (19 July 1990).

In addition, the importance of supplementary measures should not be underestimated.

**Modes of Intervention: Measles**

**Primary Prevention**

| | |
|---|---|
| Transmission<br>• man | • isolating patients is ineffective |
| Pathogenic Agents<br>• virus | • immunization of groups at risk. In emergency situations, particularly in refugee camps, the relief team should consider expanding the age bracket for the group at risk, and immunize children between the ages of six months and five years |
| Susceptibility of the Population<br>• non-immune | |

**Secondary Prevention**

| | |
|---|---|
| • benign clinical forms<br>• moderate clinical forms | • improve home care of moderate cases (health education, vitamin A, hydration, maintenance of breastfeeding, etc.)<br>• identify cases which must be referred to the hospital |

**Treatment**

| | |
|---|---|
| • serious clinical forms | • insure that serious cases are properly cared for<br>• administer vitamin A<br>• treat infectious complications with antibiotics |

**Tertiary Prevention**

| | |
|---|---|
| • sequelae<br>- temporary<br>- permanent | • prevent malnutrition<br>• treat the malnutrition associated with measles |

# 3. Diarrheal Diseases

## 3.1 Diarrheal Diseases in General

### *3.1.1 Impact of the Problem*

Diarrheal diseases may account for up to 39% of all medical consultations in a situation involving displaced people. It can be assumed that the etiology of an acute diarrheal disease in such a situation is identical to that found under normal circumstances. Studies[74] show that in ordinary times, the most frequent causes of diarrheal diseases in the children brought in for examination are:

[74] S. Huilan, "Etiology of Acute Diarrheal Disease among Children: A Multicentre Study in 5 Countries," *Bulletin of the World Health Organization* 69, No. 5 (1991): 549.

- rotavirus (20-40%)
- *E. coli* (16%)
- *shigella* (11%)

Interestingly, the distribution of pathogens changes with age. The age bracket in which children run the greatest risk of developing pathogenic germs is between 24 and 35 months. The risk of *shigella* is high for children in the first year of life, and in general it is estimated that 90% of deaths due to diarrheal disease (*shigella*) are children in the age group of 0-5 years. The rate of mortality caused by diarrheal diseases also varies according to the family's level of health education (use of ORT for diarrheal management) and its access to health-care services.

As a rule, then, it can be said that in the defective hygienic conditions that characterize displaced-person camps, the entire population risks developing diarrheal diseases (morbidity), and that the risk of death is particularly great for children under the age of five years. Such diseases are therefore a public health problem of primary importance.

### *3.1.2 Control Measures*

#### *Controlling Sources of Contamination*

The impact on health of measures to control contamination sources and their applicability in emergency situations have already been discussed in detail in Chapter 3 ("Water and Environmental Hygiene"). To review, the basic elements of controlling contamination are:

- a supply of clean water;
- waste disposal;
- personal hygiene (preventing the contamination of food and hands with fecal matter).

#### *Reinforcing Immunity*

Several vaccines are being developed[75] for diarrheal diseases caused by *shigella*, *E. coli*, and rotaviruses. However, they have not yet proved effective.

Every individual has a certain threshold of tolerance for pathogens, which depends on the immunity acquired against the particular germ and the infectious dose specific to each germ.[76] This is why a low level of contamination can be

---

[75] "Research Priorities for Diarrheal Disease Vaccines — WHO Memorandum," *Bulletin of the World Health Organization* 69, No. 6 (1991): 667.

[76] The infectious dose is the dose at which 50% of the people exposed to it will become sick. For bacterial agents this dose ranges from $10^3$ for *shigella* and $10^8$ for *vibrios*. S.A. Esrey, "Improving Water Supplies and Excreta Disposal for Control of Diarrheal Diseases," *Bulletin of the World Health Organization* 63, No. 4 (1985): 757.

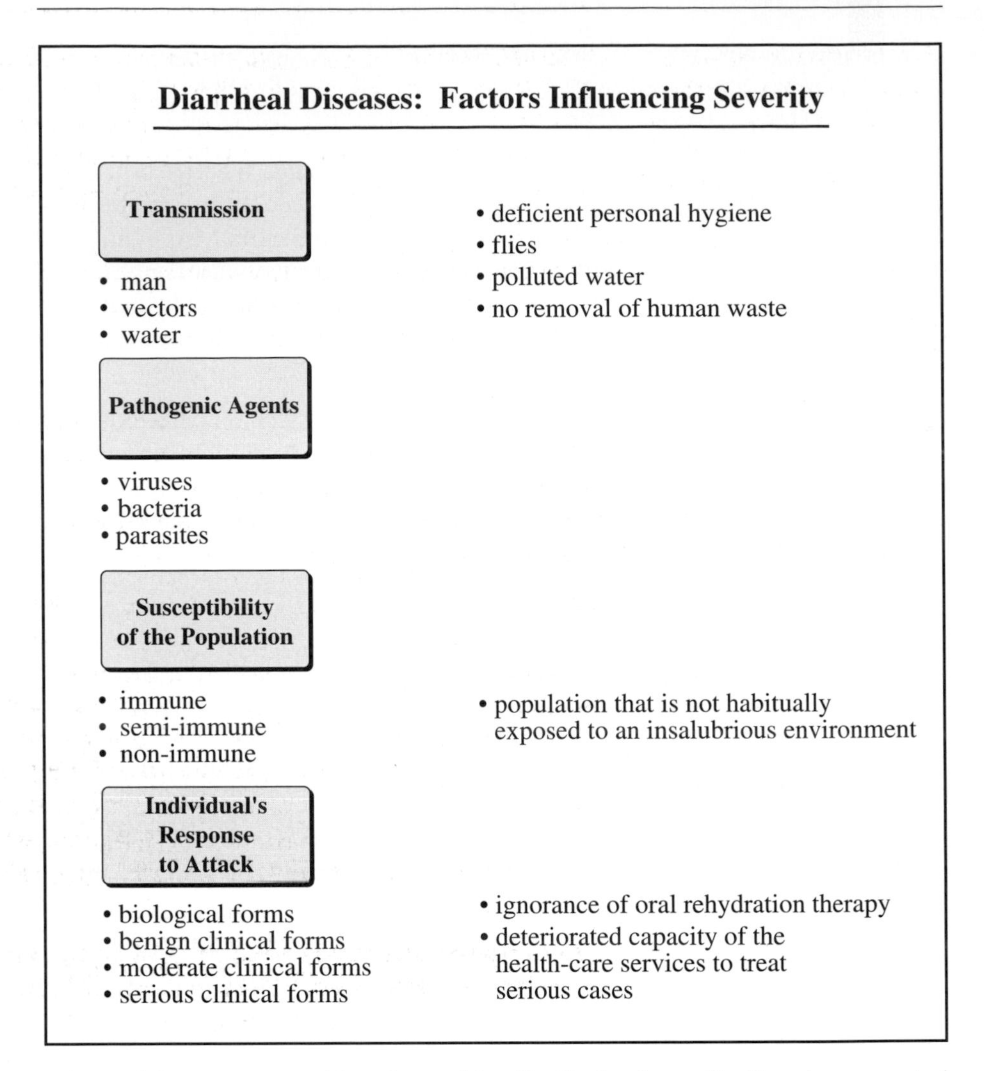


tolerated in water considered potable. Similarly, breastfeeding is promoted because mother's milk has been proved to contain protective antibodies against the main agents of diarrheal disease.

### *Treatment of Diarrheal Attacks*

- *Oral rehydration therapy*

  Every diarrheal episode, whatever the cause, is systematically treated with an oral rehydration solution. This treatment is universally recognized by health professionals. Its application by mothers is highly variable, depending on the mother's level of health education, traditional customs concerning diarrheal diseases, and the availability of the ingredients needed to prepare rehydration solutions.

Oral rehydration therapy (ORT) reduces mortality by preventing dehydration. A study carried out in Papua-New Guinea showed that the mortality rate fell from 3.3 per 1,000 to 1.3 per 1,000 after the institution of an oral rehydration program.[77] ORT is applicable in all emergency situations. In such situations, however, it is best to use solutions made from preprepared packets of rehydration salts,[78] rather than base a program on the constitution of solutions from ingredients found on the spot. Such packets should be widely distributed to all families. At the same time, an education program must be instituted to teach mothers how to use them properly.

- *Intravenous rehydration*
  Intravenous rehydration is reserved for cases of severe dehydration. Its feasibility depends on the existing infrastructure and, especially, on the availability of competent human resources.

- *Antibiotic treatmen*t
  Antibiotic treatment is indicated in some cases of diarrheal diseases with a specific etiology (for example, ampicillin for *shigella*), but other diarrheal diseases of bacterial origin do not require systematic antibiotic treatment.[79] To administer antibiotic treatment in emergency situations, the health team must be able to establish the etiology of the disease, or else treat cases on a presumptive basis. However, a study carried out in Ethiopia in a displaced-person camp has shown that the rate of resistance to antibiotics may be high, which makes the empirical approach very relative.[80]

### *Treatment of Sequelae*

Diarrheal diseases and malnutrition are associated. Ways of implementing nutritional rehabilitation are discussed in Chapter 2 ("Food and Nutrition").

---

[77] "ORT Combining Anthropological and Epidemiological Approaches," *The Journal of Tropical Medicine and Hygiene* 87, No. 3 (June 1984): 137.

[78] "Specifically, the standard WHO/UNICEF recommended formula consists of four constituents:
1. Sodium chloride 3.5 gr
2. Trisodium citrate, dihydrate 2.9 gr or sodium hydrogen carbonate 2.5 gr.
3. Potassium chloride 1.5 gr
4. Glucose 20.0 gr
to be dissolved in one litre of clean drinking water."
WHO/UNICEF, "The Management of Diarrhoea and Use of Oral Rehydration Therapy," a Joint WHO/UNICEF Statement, 2nd ed. (1985), p. 5.

[79] S. Gorbach, "Bacterial Diarrhoea and Its Treatment," *The Lancet* (12 Dec. 1987): 1378.

[80] J.C. Desenclos, "Clinical Microbiological and Antibiotic Susceptibility Patterns of Diarrheal Disease in Korem, Ethiopia," *The Journal of Tropical Medicine and Hygiene* 91 (1988): 296.

## 3.2 Cholera

Cholera is discussed in the context of investigating an epidemic, in Chapter 6 ("Epidemiology"). Accordingly, only the general principles of dealing with this disease will be addressed here.

Cholera is a distinctive diarrheal disease owing to its epidemiology and the severe dehydration it occasions. Fundamentally, however, it is treated in the same way as other diarrheal diseases.

### *3.2.1 Impact of the Problem*

Cholera is endemic in many parts of the world; under such circumstances, it is considered to be responsible for 5% of all cases of diarrheal disease. According to WHO, cholera incidence in epidemics reaches an average of 200/100,000. In refugee camps, a much higher incidence rate of 2.5% has been registered, with a mortality rate of 3.3% among those cases.[81] In camps in northwest Somalia, a mortality rate of 25% was recorded.[82] The explanations suggested for these mortality rates were poor hygienic conditions, which favored rapid transmission, and local personnel who were unqualified to manage a cholera epidemic.

Cholera is thus a potentially serious problem in displaced-person and refugee camps, and it affects adults as well as children.[83]

### *3.2.2 Control Measures*

#### *Preventing Transmission*

Prevention measures involving environmental sanitation and personal hygiene are similar to those used for other diarrheal diseases. They must, however, be reinforced, mainly by:

- sterilizing patients' stools with disinfectant solutions;
- following strict rules of hygiene when handling cadavers;
- promoting health education (concerning personal and food hygiene), a key factor in controlling cholera.

---

[81] A. Moren, "Field Epidemiology to Investigate a Cholera Outbreak in a Mozambican Refugee Camp in Malawi, 1988," *The Journal of Tropical Medicine and Hygiene* 94, No. 1 (1991): 113.

[82] "Mortality Related to Cholera in Various Refugee Camps," *Journal of the American Medical Association* 263, No. 24 (June 1990).

[83] This clinical fact can be evidence of a cholera epidemic.

### *Reinforcing Immunity*

Immunization with the current vaccine is not recommended[84] due to its ineffectiveness and the temporary nature of the immunity it provides (three to six months). Trials made with the oral vaccine WC/rBS (Whole Cell/recombinant B Subunit) look promising.[85] However, mass immunization against cholera during emergencies is inadvisable for several reasons:

- Confirmation of the effectiveness of the oral vaccine would have to be obtained.
- Such a campaign would involve considerable logistic problems, since two doses spaced two weeks apart would have to be administered to the entire population.
- There would be a danger of channeling the available resources (human and material) into the immunization campaign to the detriment of other essential measures, such as water management.
- Account must be taken of the advent of a new strain of the microorganism, "*Vibrio* 0139," which is not susceptible to the oral vaccine.

### *Treating Cholera Cases*

Treatment of cholera is essential to reduce mortality. Two factors should be considered:

- *The effectiveness of the treatment*
  Most cholera cases can be treated by oral rehydration. IV solutions are required only if initial oral treatment proves insufficient, or if the patient is in shock and unable to drink.[86] During an epidemic, 80-90% of cholera sufferers can be treated orally. In a study implemented during a cholera epidemic in a Malawi refugee camp, Epicentre calculated that:
  - the average quantity of rehydration solution per patient was 14 liters;
  - for IV patients, the average quantity per day of intravenous solution was 8 liters.

  WHO recommends a single dose of doxycycline for adults and trimethoprim-sulfamethoxazole for children.[87]

---

[84] *Guidelines for Cholera Control* (Geneva: WHO, 1993), p. 28.

[85] "Two doses of WC/rBS vaccine, given 1 to 2 weeks apart, provide rapid, short-term protection against symptomatic cholera in adult South Americans, who are predominantly of blood group O. Long-term efficacy studies in Peruvian adults and children are under way." José L. Sanchez, Bruno Vasquez, Rodolfo E. Begue, *et al.*, "Protective Efficacy of Oral Whole-Cell/Recombinant-B-Subunit Cholera Vaccine in Peruvian Military Recruit," *The Lancet* 344 (5 Nov. 1994): 1273.

[86] WHO, *Guidelines for Cholera Control*, p. 21.

[87] *Ibid.*, p. 23.

- *Access to health-care services*
  Treating patients before they reach a state of shock is essential if mortality is to be reduced. Diagnosis and the initiation of appropriate therapy will be facilitated if health-care services are directly accessible to the entire population.

  In emergency situations, the installation of facilities specifically designed to treat cholera cases may be considered if existing facilities are unable to cope with demand. The length of hospitalization is generally fairly short (about three to five days).

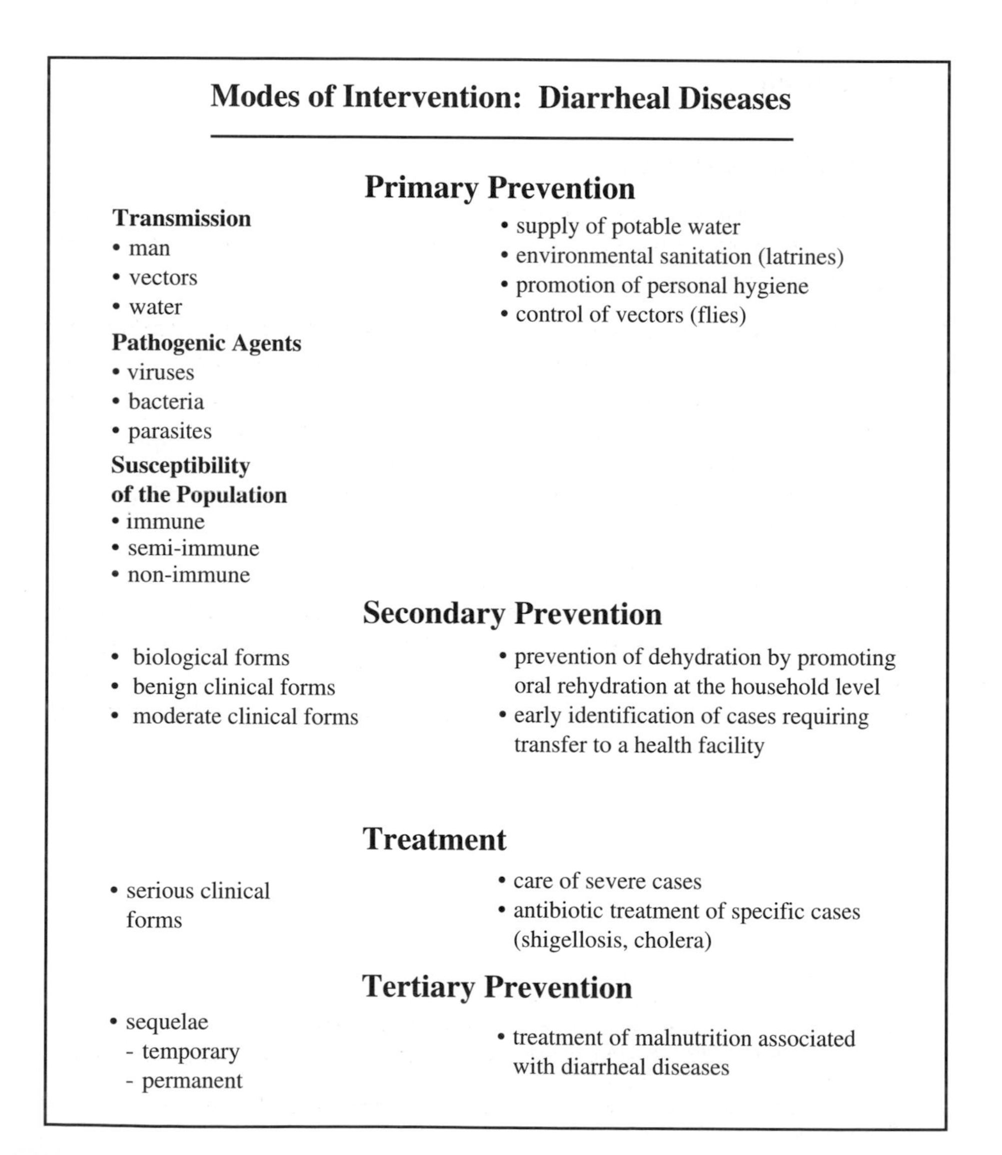

**Modes of Intervention: Diarrheal Diseases**

**Primary Prevention**

| | |
|---|---|
| **Transmission**<br>• man<br>• vectors<br>• water<br>**Pathogenic Agents**<br>• viruses<br>• bacteria<br>• parasites<br>**Susceptibility of the Population**<br>• immune<br>• semi-immune<br>• non-immune | • supply of potable water<br>• environmental sanitation (latrines)<br>• promotion of personal hygiene<br>• control of vectors (flies) |

**Secondary Prevention**

| | |
|---|---|
| • biological forms<br>• benign clinical forms<br>• moderate clinical forms | • prevention of dehydration by promoting oral rehydration at the household level<br>• early identification of cases requiring transfer to a health facility |

**Treatment**

| | |
|---|---|
| • serious clinical forms | • care of severe cases<br>• antibiotic treatment of specific cases (shigellosis, cholera) |

**Tertiary Prevention**

| | |
|---|---|
| • sequelae<br>- temporary<br>- permanent | • treatment of malnutrition associated with diarrheal diseases |

*Treating Healthy Carriers*

Treatment for healthy carriers is not recommended as a way of controlling a cholera epidemic.[88] Treating people who are in direct contact with a cholera patient is, however, an option to consider, depending on the rate of secondary cases.

*Other Measures*

Instituting a *cordon sanitaire* is ineffective, since it is difficult, if not impossible, to control population movements.

# 4. Tuberculosis

## 4.1 Impact of the Problem

Tuberculosis is not a disease involving an epidemic risk that necessitates immediate action. Nonetheless, it is a serious problem which must be dealt with, even during an emergency.

Where people are concentrated in large groups, priority is given to seeking out those tubercular subjects presenting positive sputum. Sputum containing tubercle bacilli ("Koch's bacillus") not only indicates the presence of a serious form of the disease,[89] but is in itself a certain means of transmitting the disease to groups at risk.[90] During an emergency situation, this pragmatic approach confines the problem, at least initially, to determining the number of cases presenting positive sputum.

Two methods are possible. The first method consists in determining the number of positive cases in the population, with the help of average prevalence statistics: Africa, 300-400 per 100,000; Asia, 110 per 100,000; Europe, 24 per 100,000, etc. Using an estimated prevalence as a basis, we can also estimate the rate of new cases per annum, which will correspond roughly to the prevalence figure divided by two.

---

[88] The reasons are:
- organizing mass chemoprophylaxis takes time, and the therapeutic effect lasts only a few days;
- the entire population must be treated at the same time;
- patient compliance is low. See WHO, *Guidelines for Cholera Control.*

[89] Without treatment, 50% of subjects with positive sputum will die within two years. Oxfam, *Guidelines for Tuberculosis Control.*

[90] A positive carrier may infect an average of 10 people (although not all will develop an active form of the disease).

A second, more sophisticated approach is to calculate the annual risk of infection,[91] which represents the percent of newly infected subjects in the course of a year. This percentage is linked to the number of sources of infection (subjects with positive sputum) in the population concerned. This rate is estimated to be 1-6%[92] in developing countries. On this basis, the presumption is that each time the annual rate of infection increases by 1%, incidence increases by 50/100,000 per year.[93] Thus, for a rate of 3%, incidence will be 150/100,000, and prevalence 300/100,000; for a rate of 6%, incidence will be 300/100,000 and prevalence 600/100,000; and so on.

The living conditions of displaced populations probably predispose them to an increased annual risk of infection, mainly because of poor nutritional status, overcrowding, and the many infectious sources (subjects positive for the disease who have had no access to health-care services for a long time).[94]

Using the calculations above, relief teams can:

- estimate the number of people who will die if no treatment program is initiated (one active case in two will die within two years);
- estimate the resources needed to implement a program to treat tuberculosis.

These elements provide a basis for deciding what approach to take.

## 4.2 Control Programs

Programs to control tuberculosis have long been controversial, due to the difficulty[95] and inherent risks[96] in implementing them. With the advent of

---

91 Proportion of the population infected with TB in the course of a year, determined by the rate of positive tuberculin skin tests in a population sample. The annual rate of infection is equal to the percentage of cases with positive reactions divided by the average age of the sample. For example, for a population sample with an average age of 30 years, the following values could be obtained:
- 36% -> 1.5%
- 60% -> 3%
- 80% -> 6%

The sample must consist of people who have not been vaccinated with BCG.

92 In exceptional circumstances, this rate may rise to 5%; moreover, the relation between AIDS and tuberculosis threatens to increase the rate in regions where AIDS is prevalent.

93 C. Murray, K. Styblo, and A. Rouillon, "La tuberculose dans les pays en voie de dveloppement: Importance, stratégie et coût," *Bulletin de l'Union internationale contre la tuberculose et les maladies respiratoires* 65, No. 1 (1990): 6-26.

94 R.G. Barr and R. Menzies, "The Effect of War on Tuberculosis: Result of a Tuberculin Survey among the Displaced Persons in El Salvador and a Review of the Literature," *Tubercle and Lung Disease* 75, No. 4 (1994): 251.

95 Essentially, the difficulty of implementing programs involving therapeutic regimens of 12-18 months.

96 Given the combination of long treatments (12-18 months) and unstable displaced or refugee populations, the main risk to public health is the development of resistance to antibiotics.

short treatments and a better epidemiological knowledge of the disease, the prospects for instituting a coherent program of tuberculosis control have improved. This section will deal only with programs specifically designed to control TB in emergency situations.

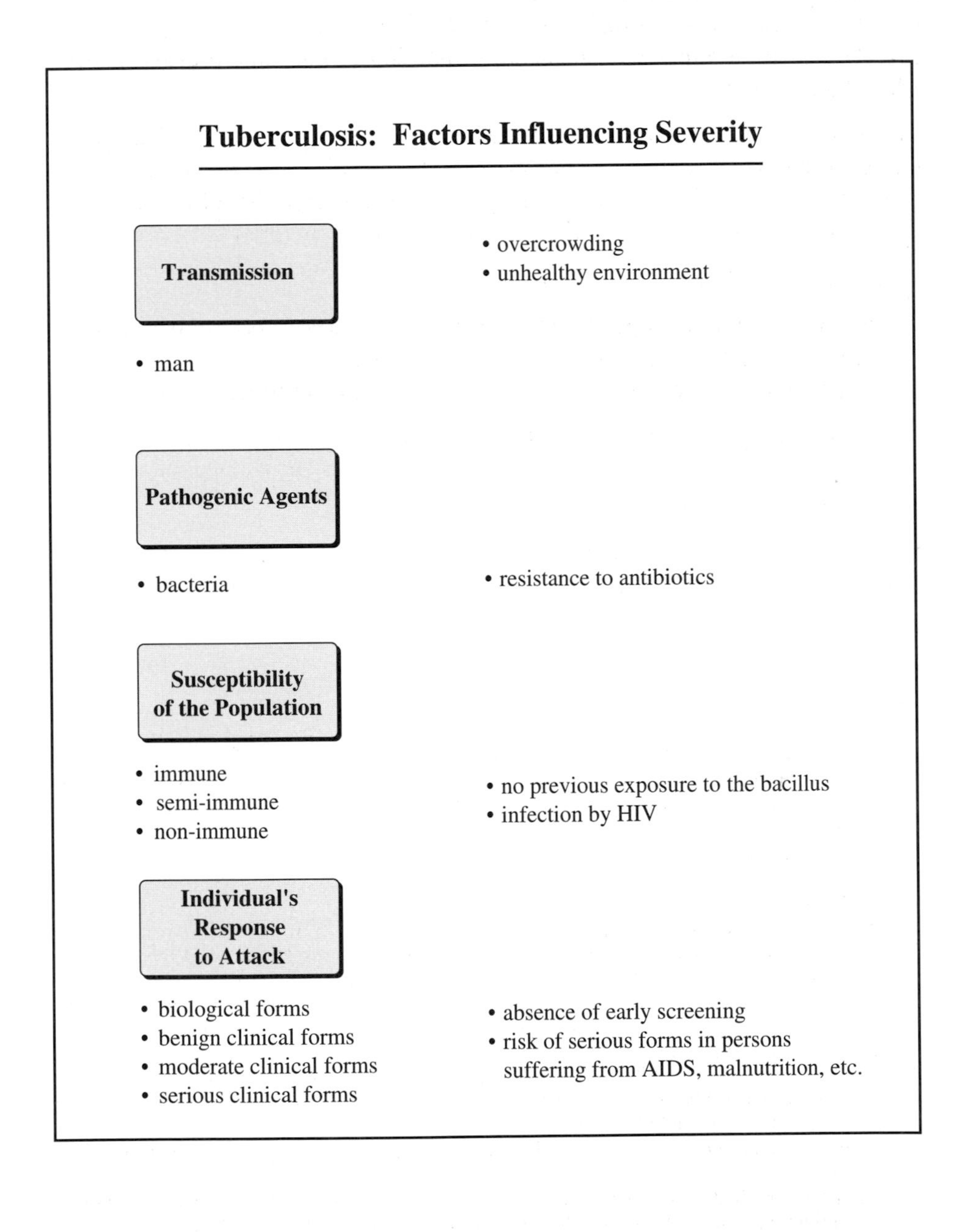

### *Reducing Transmission*

Improving living conditions (housing, hygiene) is a major factor in reducing the transmission of TB.[97] In emergency situations, it is recognized that seeking out and treating active cases of tuberculosis can reduce transmission. Primary chemoprophylaxis is used for subjects who have been in contact with active cases of TB and who are tuberculin-negative.[98] This type of intervention is not applicable in emergency situations, however.

### *Reinforcing Immunity*

The efficacy of immunization with BCG has not been clearly demonstrated except for children under the age of one year, and for the control of the miliary and meningeal[99] forms of the disease. In an emergency situation, then, immunization is recommended only for that age group.

### *Handling Cases Presenting a Biological Reaction*

Secondary chemoprophylaxis is used for all subjects who have recently become tuberculin-positive. Here again this does not apply to emergency situations, since there is no way of knowing when the change from tuberculin-negative to positive took place, and since this measure has little impact on transmission of the disease.[100]

### *Managing Active TB Cases*

Managing TB cases comprises four stages.[101]

#### *Defining the Disease*

In emergencies, a case of tuberculosis is defined as a patient presenting sputum that tests positive for TB bacilli. Diagnosis is a two-step process.

---

97 Tuberculosis is considered a disease of poverty. TB control in the developed countries began with improved living conditions, well before antibiotics were in use. Better housing conditions and a better diet were decisive factors.

98 In developing countries, most children have already been infected (tuberculin-positive). For example, a study carried out among Eskimos showed that 80% of children under the age of five years tested positive.

99 A. Lotte *et al.*, "Dimunition du risque de méningite tuberculeuse chez les enfants en France. Influence de la vaccination par le BCG," *Bulletin de l'Union internationale contre la tuberculose et les maladies respiratoires* 63, No. 4 (1988).

100 "Isoniazid preventive therapy for subclinical TB infection has no major role in TB control in temporary settlements." H. Rieder, "Considerations Prior to Initiating a TB Programme," *Tubercle* 70 (1989). See also C. Nolan *et al.*, "Active Tuberculosis after Isoniazid Chemoprophylaxis in South-East Asian Refugees," *American Review of Respiratory Diseases* 133 (1986); this study showed that the rate of active tuberculosis (subjects having a positive tuberculin reaction) after secondary chemoprophylaxis in 2,795 refugees was 2-3/1,000 per year.

101 H. Rieder, *op. cit.*

- *Clinical diagnosis* involves screening subjects who present some clinical symptom or combination of symptoms compatible with tuberculosis: cough for the last three weeks, weight loss, hemoptysis, thoracic pain, etc. Rather than trying to carry out active screening (door-to-door), health workers are advised to offer passive screening — that is, to wait until the patients come for consultation at a health-care facility.
- *Microscopic diagnosis* involves screening patients with clinical signs of tuberculosis for positive sputum. In an emergency situation, a laboratory must be found that is able to perform this test. At this stage, it is rarely possible to use cultures.

### *Treating Cases*

Long treatments (12-18 months) are no longer recommended.[102] Short treatments currently constitute the appropriate therapy. The patient's sputum becomes negative quickly (within two or three weeks), thereby also reducing the risk of transmission in the population. Under these circumstances, the treatment of patients with positive sputum can be considered as a form of primary prevention for the entire population.

The institution of a TB treatment program is subject to certain rules:

- Treatment is provided for subjects with positive sputum.
- The logistical arrangements must insure that patients are under care for the entire period required for their treatment.
- The quality of the bacteriological tests of sputum must be guaranteed.
- Patients' ingestion of medication must be stringently supervised.
- Cured patients must be followed up.
- Medical personnel and infrastructure must be available to meet all these requirements.

WHO[103] distinguishes between several categories of patients:

- Category I: New cases presenting positive sputum.
- Category II: Relapses and treatment failures.
- Category III: Patients with signs of pulmonary tuberculosis but without positive sputum, and patients with extrapulmonary forms of the disease.
- Category IV: Chronic cases — that is, patients who remain positive despite having correctly followed an appropriate treatment.

---

102 "The primary reason for the failure of the commonly used treatment regimen of 12-18 months of daily isoniazid and thiocetazone, supplemented by streptomycin during the first 2 months, is the delay in smear conversion from positive to negative." *Treatment of Tuberculosis — Guidelines for National Programmes* (Geneva: WHO, 1993), p. 1.

103 *Ibid.*

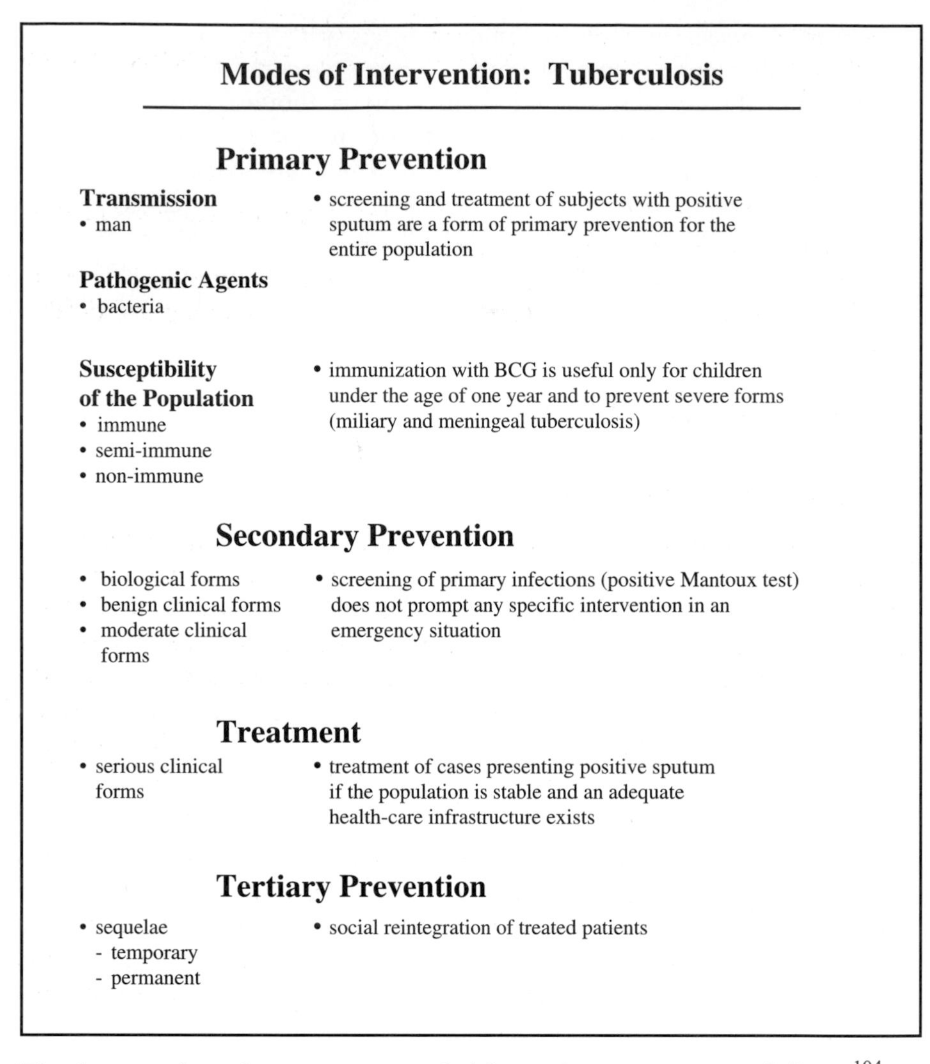

## Modes of Intervention: Tuberculosis

### Primary Prevention

| | |
|---|---|
| **Transmission**<br>• man | • screening and treatment of subjects with positive sputum are a form of primary prevention for the entire population |
| **Pathogenic Agents**<br>• bacteria | |
| **Susceptibility of the Population**<br>• immune<br>• semi-immune<br>• non-immune | • immunization with BCG is useful only for children under the age of one year and to prevent severe forms (miliary and meningeal tuberculosis) |

### Secondary Prevention

| | |
|---|---|
| • biological forms<br>• benign clinical forms<br>• moderate clinical forms | • screening of primary infections (positive Mantoux test) does not prompt any specific intervention in an emergency situation |

### Treatment

| | |
|---|---|
| • serious clinical forms | • treatment of cases presenting positive sputum if the population is stable and an adequate health-care infrastructure exists |

### Tertiary Prevention

| | |
|---|---|
| • sequelae<br>- temporary<br>- permanent | • social reintegration of treated patients |

The therapeutic regimens recommended for each category are as follows:[104]

- Category I: 2HRZS (E) + 4HR or 4H3R3
- Category II: 2HRZES/1HRZE + 5H3R3E3 or 5HRE

---

[104] H = isoniazid
R = rifampicin
Z = pyrazinamide
S = streptomycin
E = ethambutol
The first figure represents the number of months that the treatment with the drugs indicated will last (for example, 2HRZS), while the figure appearing after a particular drug indicates that treatment is intermittent, and corresponds to the number of times the drug is to be taken per week (for example, 4H3R3).

- Category III: 2HRZ or 2H3R3Z3 + 2HR or 2H3R3
- Category IV: According to resistances to antibiotics, but the chance of a cure is limited.

*Specific Points*

- Program effectiveness: It is generally accepted that a TB treatment program should aim to cure 85% of the patients.
- AIDS has increased the prevalence and incidence of tuberculosis — giving rise, in fact, to a veritable epidemic of TB, which will expand dramatically in the years to come.[105]

# 5. Meningococcal Meningitis

## 5.1 Impact of the Problem

The average incidence of meningococcal meningitis in endemic regions is estimated at 10/100,000. During epidemic years, this incidence may increase to 500/100,000 in disadvantaged urban areas (camps can be considered to fall into this category). Meningococcal meningitis is known to develop mostly in communal settings (cities, schools, etc.). The logical conclusion, then, is that displaced-person camps are favorable breeding grounds for meningococcal epidemics. The group most at risk to develop the disease is people between the ages of 1 and 25. A doubling of the usual number of cases per week[106] is considered to constitute an epidemic.[107]

It is difficult to quantify in advance the number of potential cases. The immune status of the population, the season (since it influences transmission), and the speed with which the health-care services detect the first cases must all be taken into account. The rate of attack is known to be high among infants up to the age of one year. Without intervention, the epidemic subsides by itself. An epidemic lasts 10 weeks on average, peaking at 4 weeks.

---

[105] "The human immunodeficiency virus is a nightmare-come-true for TB control workers and patients. Even though a third of the world's population is infected with TB, most people never become sick because their immune system keeps the TB germ in check. HIV destroys those cells that keep the TB germ in check. While TB/HIV co-infection currently produces just a small percentage of all TB deaths, it is one of the most rapidly growing factors in the TB epidemic. In 1990, TB/HIV co-infection was present in four percent of all TB cases. By the year 2000, co-infection will dramatically increase to nearly one in seven of all TB cases." *TB, A Global Emergency — WHO Report on the TB Epidemic* (WHO, 1994), p. 4.

[106] This implies that a surveillance system exists which insures that cases of meningococcal meningitis are regularly reported.

[107] P.S. Moore, M.J. Toole, P. Nieberg, R.J. Waldman, and C.V. Broome, "Surveillance and Control of Meningococcal Meningitis Epidemics in Refugee Populations," *Bulletin of the World Health Organization* 68, No. 5 (1990): 587.

The mortality rate for meningococcal meningitis depends on the time that elapses between the onset of the disease and the initiation of medical care, and on the quality of that care. Untreated, the disease has a mortality rate of 50%; with treatment, the rate is still 10%.[108]

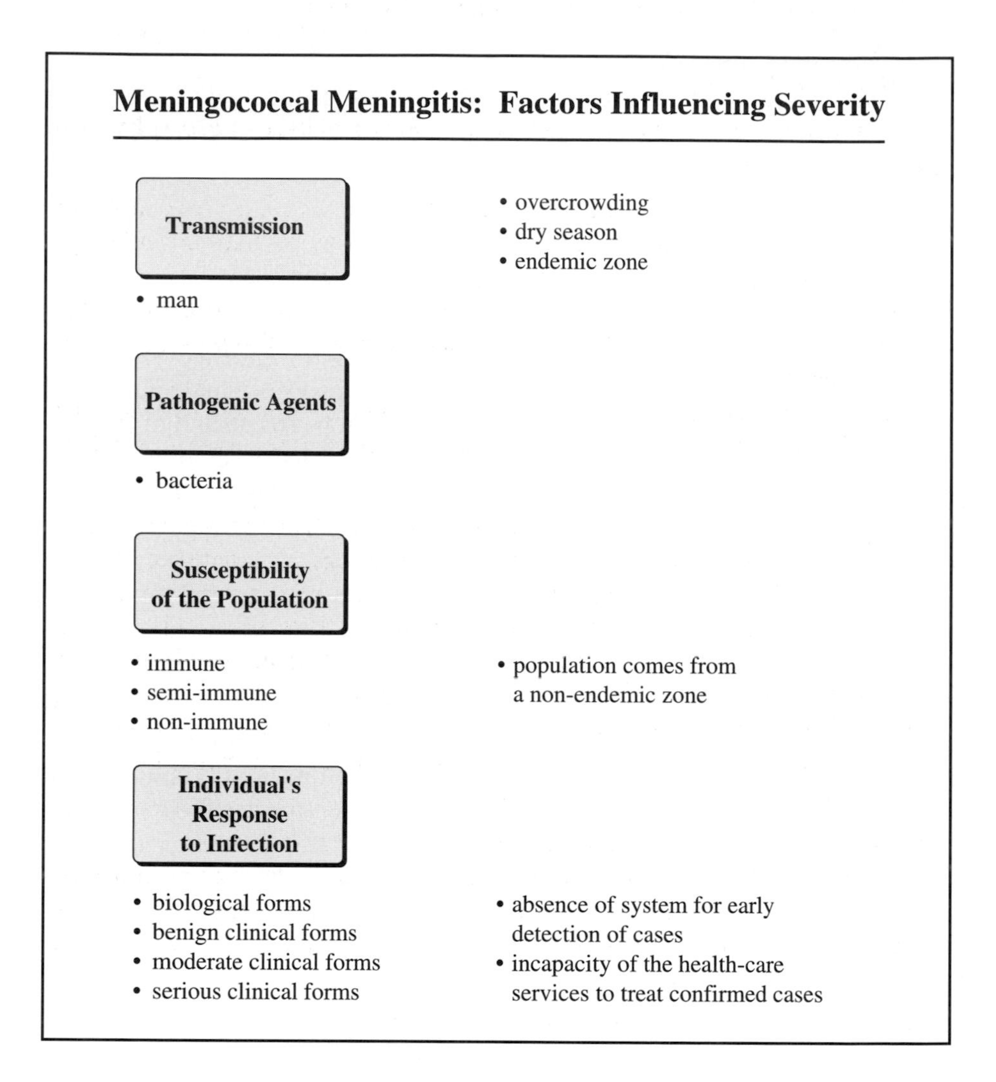


[108] P. Brès, *Public Health Action in Emergencies Caused by Epidemics* (WHO, 1986), p. 197.

## 5.2 Control Programs

### *Reducing Transmission*

The only possible preventive measure available for reducing the risk of transmitting the disease consists in limiting overcrowding.

### *Reinforcing Immunity*

Reinforcing immunity by means of immunization is a realistic measure, but two aspects warrant comment:

- Serogroups A, B, and C can cause epidemics, but no vaccine is available for serogroup B.[109] Immunization is relatively ineffective in children under age two (group C); group A requires two injections to produce a satisfactory rate of seroconversion. What is more, the immunity thus acquired is of limited duration. Immunization of children under the age of one year is not recommended.[110]
- Epidemics of the disease are naturally self-limiting, so that to be effective an immunization campaign must be implemented quickly (as soon as the first cases are diagnosed).

From these two observations it can be concluded, first, that routine immunization in the framework of an EPI, in the absence of any epidemic, is not recommended, due to the limited duration of immunity; and, second, that in an epidemic, immunization must be carried out immediately or not at all — hence the importance of a surveillance system able to spot the beginnings of contagion quickly. If resources permit, the entire population can be immunized; otherwise, immunization must be reserved for the groups most at risk. Alternatively, vaccination can be provided only for people coming directly in contact with the disease, to reduce the number of secondary cases.

To be effective, an immunization campaign must be carried out rapidly (at least before the peak of the epidemic, which occurs sometime during the first four weeks). A surveillance system is therefore fundamental, since it permits immediate detection of an epidemic. The determining threshold for an epidemic may be:

- a cumulative incidence higher than 100/100,000;
- a doubling of cases from one week to the next;
- a rate of attack higher than 15 cases per week for two weeks.

---

[109] "Four specific antigens related to serogroups A, C, Y and W135, are currently available. They are distributed in freeze-dried form, injectable by IM route, either as bivalent AC vaccine, or quadrivalent A, C, Y, W135 vaccine, containing 50 mg of each antigen." *Control of Epidemic Meningococcal Disease — WHO Practical Guidelines* (WHO, 1995), p. 28.

[110] P.S. Moore, M.J. Toole, *et al., op. cit.*

The procedure for organizing an immunization campaign need not be reviewed here, since the problems are similar for every disease.

### *Cases Presenting a Biological Reaction*

It is unrealistic to try to treat subjects showing meningococcus in a throat culture. There is thought to be no relation between the number of carriers and the imminence of an epidemic.[111]

## *Managing Cases of Meningococcal Meningitis*

### *Diagnosing Cases*

The clinical diagnosis of meningitis is based on a group of known symptoms, but differential diagnosis is complicated by a number of competing syndromes. If lumbar puncture produces purulent cerebrospinal fluid, meningitis of bacterial origin can be diagnosed; but clinical examination cannot confirm a diagnosis of meningococcal meningitis unless purpura is present.

In an emergency situation, health-care workers do not necessarily have access to a laboratory capable of identifying meningococcus in the cerebrospinal fluid. Agglutination techniques can be used to differentiate meningococcus from the germs responsible for other types of purulent meningitis.

The health-care team may need to aim for greater or lesser diagnostic exactitude depending on whether it is facing one or two isolated cases or an already confirmed epidemic. For isolated cases, an etiological diagnosis is essential in order to detect the beginning of an epidemic and to initiate not only the appropriate treatment for the patient, but preventive measures for the population. For cases in a confirmed epidemic, all patients presenting a meningeal syndrome can be assumed *a priori* to have meningococcal meningitis. Naturally, if all the facilities necessary for bacteriological tests are available, it is wise to seek confirmation for each case.

### *Treating Patients*

Treatment with an injection of an oily suspension of chloramphenicol is effective against meningococcal meningitis.[112] This is consequently the antibiotic of choice in an epidemic. A single injection is certainly preferable to ampicillin, which requires several injections a day and costs ten times more than treatment with chloramphenicol. On the other hand, chloramphenicol is not very effective against other forms of bacterial meningitis (*H. influenzae*, streptococcus,

---

111 Abram S. Benenson, ed., *Control of Communicable Diseases in Man* (1990), p. 282.
112 WHO, *Weekly Epidemiological Report* 16 (20 April 1990).

pneumococcus, etc.).[113] Before a treatment regimen can be decided, then, bacteriological confirmation of the germ's identity is necessary.

*Organization of Care*

Using the short-term treatment makes handling a large number of cases possible; but hospitalization is usually necessary.

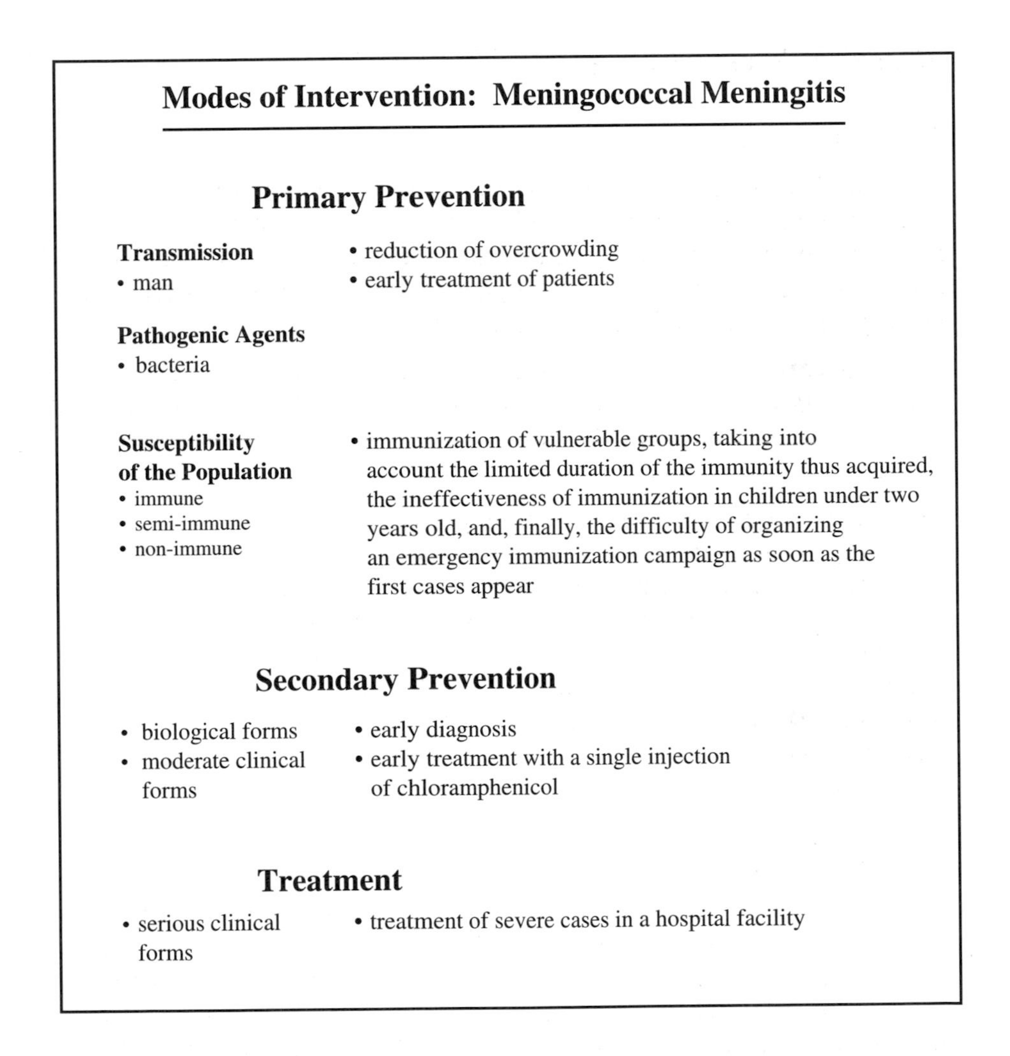

**Modes of Intervention: Meningococcal Meningitis**

**Primary Prevention**

| | |
|---|---|
| **Transmission**<br>• man | • reduction of overcrowding<br>• early treatment of patients |
| **Pathogenic Agents**<br>• bacteria | |
| **Susceptibility of the Population**<br>• immune<br>• semi-immune<br>• non-immune | • immunization of vulnerable groups, taking into account the limited duration of the immunity thus acquired, the ineffectiveness of immunization in children under two years old, and, finally, the difficulty of organizing an emergency immunization campaign as soon as the first cases appear |

**Secondary Prevention**

| | |
|---|---|
| • biological forms<br>• moderate clinical forms | • early diagnosis<br>• early treatment with a single injection of chloramphenicol |

**Treatment**

| | |
|---|---|
| • serious clinical forms | • treatment of severe cases in a hospital facility |

[113] See J. Friedland, "Failure of Chloramphenicol Therapy in Penicillin-Resistant Pneumococcal Meningitis," *The Lancet* 339 (15 Feb. 1992); and B. Pécoul *et al.*, "Long-acting Chloramphenicol Versus Intravenous Ampicillin for Treatment of Bacterial Meningitis," *The Lancet* 338 (5 Oct. 1991).

*Chemoprophylaxis for the Patient's Household*

Chemoprophylaxis for people who are in direct contact with a patient is not recommended.[114] If it is administered, however, rifampin should be used in a dose of 600 mg for adults and 10 mg/kg for children, twice a day for two days.

*Institution of a Surveillance System*

A surveillance system is most useful if it is set up before an epidemic appears, since it will allow the health team to detect the epidemic in time to take adequate preventive measures.

# 6. Intestinal Parasites

## 6.1 Impact of the Problem

Depending on the geographical and social environment, intestinal parasitic infestations may be very prevalent. They constitute, however, a less serious condition than the other diseases studied here.[115] Ankylostomiasis (hookworm) may be one of the main causes of anemia. Amebiasis and giardiasis cause diarrhea. Apart from the link between hookworm and anemia, intestinal parasites have not been proven to play a role in malnutrition.

No attempt will be made in this section to define the respective importance of each intestinal parasite, but it should be recognized that the complications these parasites occasion, particularly in pre-school-age children, can become a public health problem. Moreover, the relative importance of the measures designed to control parasitic infections differs from that of measures to control other communicable diseases (environmental hygiene, in particular).

## 6.2 Control Programs

The control of intestinal parasites can be limited to the control of the diseases caused by the parasites, or it can be expanded to include control of parasitic infection. The first case calls for an individual approach; in the second, the orientation is communal and focuses on environmental hygiene, the water supply, health education, essential drugs, food and nutrition, epidemiology, etc.

In emergency situations, when hygienic conditions are precarious and the rate of infestation is high, efforts must be made to reduce both the rate of infection and

[114] P. Moore and M. Toole, *op. cit.*

[115] A study comparing data from Asia, Africa, and Latin America ranked hookworm twelfth among infectious diseases in terms of mortality, amebiasis fourteenth, and ascariasis twentieth. J. Walsh *et al.*, "Selective Primary Health Care: An Interim Strategy for Disease Control in Developing Countries," *The New England Journal of Medicine* 301, No. 18 (1979).

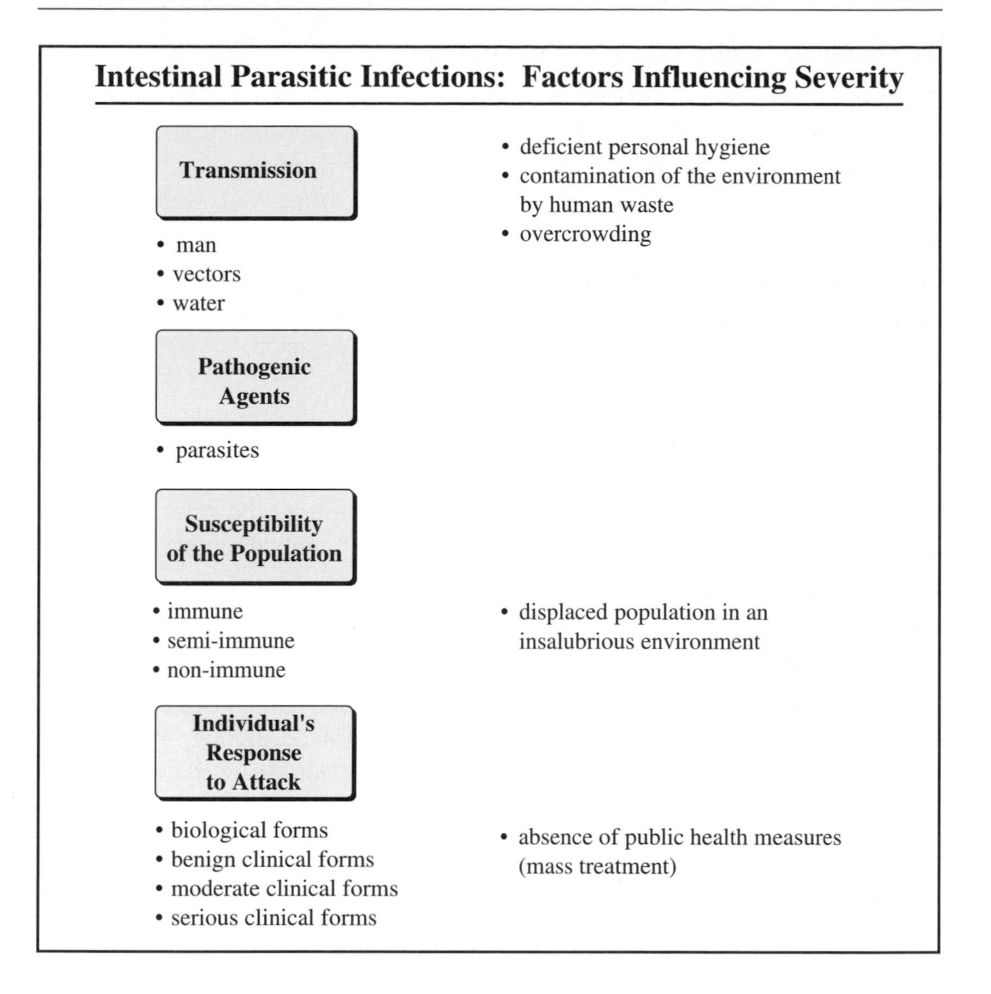


the rate of disease.[116] This approach is limited, however, by social disorganization and the channeling of resources towards more urgent problems.

---

[116] The measures that combine both approaches to amebiasis control can be listed as follows:
- Individual measures:
  - diagnosis and treatment of subjects with acute amebiasis;
  - supply of clean water;
  - food hygiene.
- Collective measures:
  - sanitation;
  - supply of clean water;
  - health education;
  - reinforcement of primary health care;
  - monitoring the hygiene of food products in the market.

See A. Martinez-Palomo, "Selective PHC: Strategies for Control of Disease in the Developing World: Amœbiasis," *Review of Infectious Diseases* 5, No. 6 (1983).

### *Reducing Transmission*

Transmission of most internal parasitic diseases reflects the local level of environmental hygiene and the conditions of water supply.[117] Reducing transmission depends on measures focusing on environmental hygiene (human-waste removal); health education; and an improved water supply, encouraging personal hygiene.

Depending on the parasitic infections to be controlled, potential measures will vary in importance. The following measures have been classified in order of their importance within the framework of a community approach:

- ascariasis: waste removal and personal hygiene
- ancylostomiasis: waste removal, personal hygiene, and the correction of anemia

In evaluating the relative importance of the different options, however, the health team should give thought to the cultural context and acceptability of the proposed measures.[118]

### *Managing Cases Presenting No Clinical Signs*

Cases presenting no clinical signs ascribable to intestinal parasitic infection (such as anemia, abdominal pain, or diarrhea) should not be treated, unless mass treatment is planned as part of a broader control program designed to reduce the parasite burden on the environment.

### *Managing Clinical Cases*

#### *Diagnosis*

The clinical symptoms of intestinal parasitic infections are not specific to them, and it is unrealistic to try to make an etiological diagnosis of every patient with presumptive symptoms who shows up for consultation. Treatment is often empirical.

#### *Treatment of Suspected or Confirmed Cases*

The advent of short treatments for most intestinal parasitic diseases has simplified the therapeutic approach to amebiasis (Fasigyne), and ascariasis and hookworm (Albendazole).

---

[117] WHO, *General Strategies for Prevention and Control of Intestinal Parasitic Infections within PHC* (1985).

[118] H. Gilles, "Selective Primary Health Care: Strategies for Control of Disease in the Developing World, Hookworm Infection and Anaemia," *Review of Infectious Diseases* 7, No. 1 (1985): 114.

*Mass Treatment*

According to WHO,[119] mass treatment can be undertaken in three ways:

- treatment of the entire population;
- treatment of all infected subjects, whether ill or not;
- treatment of the groups most susceptible to infection.

Mass treatment is justified if the prevalence of intestinal parasitic infections is very high — for example, 60-70% for ascariasis. It is only realistic, however, if the population affected is limited and lives in a restricted geographical area. Otherwise, intervention will have to be targeted to specific groups, such as children admitted to a nutrition rehabilitation center.

## Modes of Intervention: Intestinal Parasitic Infections

### Primary Prevention

| | |
|---|---|
| **Transmission**<br>• man<br>• vectors<br>• water<br>**Pathogenic Agents**<br>• parasites<br>**Susceptibility of the Population**<br>• immune<br>• semi-immune<br>• non-immune | • environmental sanitation<br>• provision of clean water<br>• promotion of personal hygiene<br>• health education |

### Secondary Prevention

| | |
|---|---|
| • biological forms<br>• benign clinical forms<br>• moderate clinical forms | • systematic screening is unrealistic in emergency situations<br>• mass treatment if the infection rate is very high<br>• systematic treatment of target groups (children) |

### Treatment

| | |
|---|---|
| • serious clinical forms | • treatment of serious forms of intestinal parasitic infections<br>• treatment of complications related to intestinal parasitic infections:<br>- anemia (hookworm)<br>- surgical complications of ascariasis |

119 WHO, *General Strategies for Prevention and Control of Intestinal Parasitic Infections within PHC*.

### *Managing Sequelae*

Managing sequelae may mean, for example, treating anemia caused by hookworm, or malnutrition (although intestinal parasites are not a determining factor).

The institution of a control program for intestinal parasitic infections must take into account the latent nature of each measure's specific effects. Environmental hygiene measures, for example, have an impact on health only in the long term. Mass treatments are more effective in the short term, but are soon followed by reinfestation unless steps are taken to improve hygiene.[120]

**This survey of communicable diseases has concentrated on the problems causing the highest mortality and morbidity rates in situations involving displaced people. The concept of therapeutic intervention introduced in this context will be studied in greater detail in the next chapter.**

[120] A study carried out in Peru showed that 98% of children treated for giardiasis were infected again six months after the treatment. R. Gilman *et al.*, "Rapid Reinfection by Giardia Lamblia after Treatment in a Hyperendemic Third World Community," *The Lancet* (13 Feb. 1988): 343.

# Chapter 5

# MEDICAL
# AND
# SURGICAL CARE

***This chapter covers medical and surgical care in emergency situations. Discussion is limited to the management of medical-surgical programs, without going into precise details regarding the diagnosis and treatment of each medical problem that may come up in this kind of situation. For greater clarity, a distinction is made between general care for displaced populations and surgical care for war-wounded.***

# I. Medical Care for Displaced Populations

## 1. Introduction

Medical care for displaced populations can be defined as the interaction between a patient with a health problem and a caregiver who must, if not find the solution to the problem, at least determine what should be done.

### 1.1 Nature of Medical Problems

The concept of health problems is part of a broader context which also includes the concepts of demand,[1] of needs assumed by the community, and of real needs.[2] This has implications beyond the realm of intellectual discussion. In fact, demand and real needs do not necessarily coincide, depending on the cultural context.[3] Clearly, in an emergency situation the presence of foreign health professionals compounds that dissociation between the conceptions of the community and those of the health professionals. There is no universal formula for itemizing these differences, which, moreover, are not limited to perceptions of disease, but encompass perceptions of health in general.

This chapter will study ways to approach classic medical problems, and will examine the tools essential for the institution of a coherent medical care program in an emergency situation.

---

[1] The expression of needs as defined by the patient himself.

[2] Needs as defined by health professionals.

[3] "There is a fundamental difference in perspective between health professionals and the community with which they work. If they are not careful, health professionals tend to formulate needs according to a medical interpretation of the situation, before communicating them to the population in the form of ideas, instructions, and recommendations. The population's responses to needs, in contrast, are not solely intellectual, but also entail behavioral changes. The behaviors in question are themselves part of the flow of daily habits and customs, linked to a way of life, rooted in history, and benefiting from the legitimacy conferred upon them by the family circle and the whole of society." J. Cook and D. Couet, *La santé communautaire: Concepts/Actions/Formation* (Paris: Centre International de l'Enfance, 1990), p. 111.

## *Types of Medical Problems*

Medical problems can be divided into three main categories.

- *Universal problems*
  This category includes, for example, non-specific diarrheal diseases, upper and lower respiratory infections, skin infections, scabies, intestinal parasitic infections, joint pain, cardiovascular ailments, etc. These pathologies are all found in both normal and emergency situations, but in emergencies they are much more prevalent and much more serious than they are normally.
- *Problems that are specific to:*
  - a region, such as malaria, kala-azar, and schistosomiasis;
  - a population group, such as sickle-cell diseases.
- *Psychological problems*
  Disasters give rise to psychological reactions during the event itself or after a variable lapse of time. These reactions include, for example, anxiety, depression, sleeping disorders, and alcoholism. Refugee or displaced populations are particularly vulnerable to psychosocial disorders, because of the social upheavals involved in the move itself, overcrowding, and, more generally, the reorganization of the social system, as well as the uncertainty of the future. Children are the most vulnerable, and this aspect of their health has become a major concern over the last few years: "Refugee children's psychological well-being is as important as their physical health. The term 'psychosocial well-being' is used to reflect the intimate relationship between psychological and social factors." [4]

In short, in emergency situations the types of medical problems are more or less the same as in normal situations; only their prevalence and seriousness change.

## *Prevalence and Seriousness of Medical Problems*

Several factors contribute to the increased prevalence and seriousness of medical problems in emergencies. Prevalence is usually a function of nutritional status, environment, and the deterioration of preventive services. One of the main reasons for the potentially greater number of serious problems in an emergency is that access to medical services is impaired, particularly in conflict situations. Owing to a lack of immediate care, such diseases as meningitis and cerebral malaria are likely to prove fatal.

The combination of prevalence and seriousness leads to high mortality. This idea can be formulated as follows:

---

[4] UNHCR, *Psychological Well-being in Refugee Children — Guidelines on Protection and Care* (1994), p. 37.

$$\frac{\text{Prevalence} \times \text{Seriousness}}{\text{Access to Medical Care}} = \text{Mortality}$$

Thus, the high prevalence of medical problems, the large number of serious cases, and the reduced access to health-care services all help explain the particularly high mortality rates found among displaced populations before an intervention takes effect. As an example, M. Toole has noted that in the refugee camps in Sudan, Ethiopia, and Thailand the mortality rate was 18 to 45 times greater than among the population of the host country. The establishment of health-care facilities is a priority in such situations.[5]

## 1.2 Care Providers

Care providers can be divided into two groups:

- providers of non-professional care;
- health-care professionals.

### *Providers of Non-Professional Care*

Certain activities related to medical care are directly performed by people within the household (mother, grandmother, neighbor, etc.).[6] The knowledge possessed by these caregivers may be empirical (based on what has always been done for a given medical problem) or technical (derived from health-education programs).

This category also includes traditional doctors and midwives, for they have received training — usually of an informal nature, of course, but which reflects the lore of generations. The social role played by this category of personnel varies from one culture to another, as does the nature of the problems they treat. This course will not examine traditional therapeutic methods in detail, but students should remember that traditional medicine is part of the organization of a health system, just as modern medicine is.

Community health workers (CHWs) fall into this category as well, although in some cases they may have had several months' training.

### *Health-Care Professionals*

Health-care professionals consist mainly in nursing personnel, doctors, specialists, and paramedical personnel such as pharmacists and laboratory assistants.

---

5 Curative and preventive measures will be discussed in Chapter 7 ("The Health-Care System").
6 Broadly speaking, this may be the clan, in which one person is recognized for his or her medical knowledge.

## 1.3 Level of Care[7]

There are three different levels of care.

### *Primary Level*

The primary level corresponds to the home and the health-care station where a sick person can expect initial contact with a non-professional. Oral rehydration and the treatment of fever and minor injuries are associated with this level. This type of care involves the family, community health workers, and traditional healers.

### *Secondary Level*

The simple facility where a sick person comes into contact with a health-care professional constitutes the second level. Depending on the country, this may be a dispensary or a health center. Usually, curative services are limited to ambulatory care, but some health centers are equipped with a few beds.

Depending on the competence of the personnel and the financial means available, the second level may offer the possibility of laboratory tests, though x-ray machines are rarely found in such facilities.

In a camp, the possibility of setting up a few beds for hospitalization may be considered if the number of patients does not justify setting up a hospital, or if the hospital serving the area is too far away or inaccessible (due to night curfews, for example).

It is essential to supply the facilities at this level with drugs in accordance with WHO norms.

### *Tertiary Level*

The tertiary level corresponds to the hospitals, both district and provincial. They represent the final link in the chain of care offered to patients. The level of care will depend on the competence of the personnel providing it and on the means available. Displaced people should have the benefit of hospital services (either local services or parallel services instituted especially for them).[8]

---

[7] The type of care offered at each level will be adapted to the complexity of the medical problems. It should be remembered that curative action is only one aspect of the activities carried out at each of these levels; preventive activities, for example, predominate (or ought to, anyway) at the primary level.

[8] The process of deciding between these two possibilities is examined in Chapter 7 ("The Health-Care System").

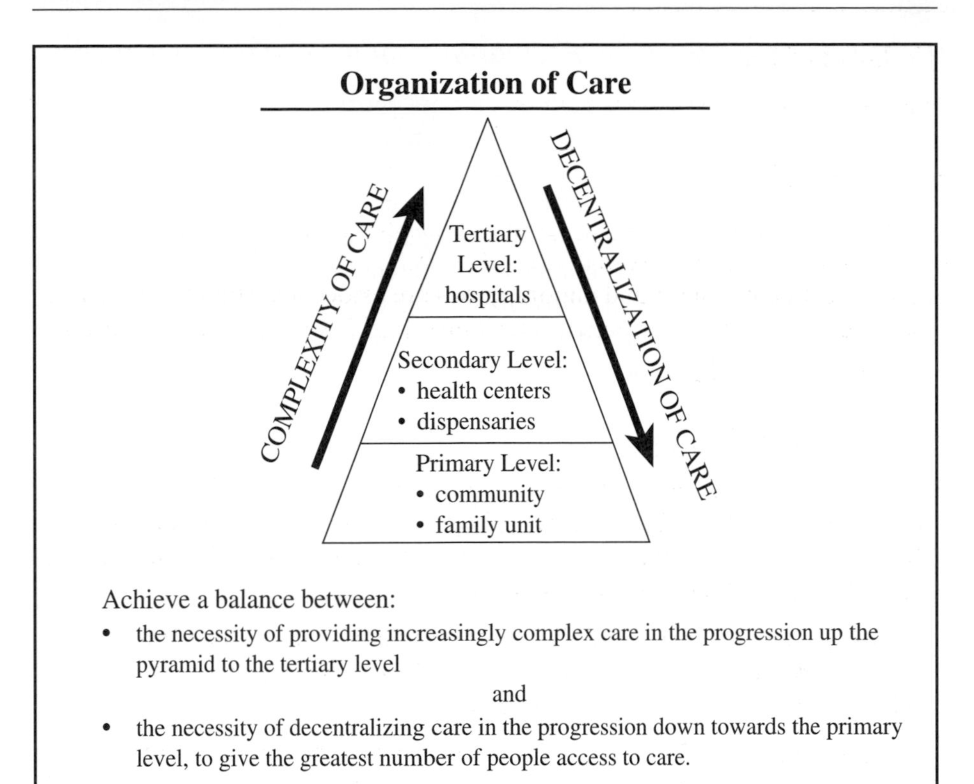


## 2. Principles of Managing Medical Care

The principles of managing medical care are based on the relation between the patients' medical problems and the ability of care providers to solve them. This concept has both a qualitative and a quantitative dimension.

### 2.1 Correspondence between Medical Problems and the Care Providers' Capacities

*Do the care givers respond to the real needs and demands of the victims?*

Certainly traditional healers respond more to the demands of the population than to medical needs expressed in terms of the technical criteria of Western medicine — although the two perspectives may intersect (in the case of setting broken bones, for example). Health professionals, in contrast, are more strongly oriented towards classic medical problems, a logical consequence of their training.

The key element to retain here is that the division of tasks should take into account the different capacities of each category of care providers.

*Do the care providers have the skills to treat the problems that arise?*

A case of meningitis treated with traditional medicines clearly exemplifies a problem of competence in the care provider. Conversely, bringing a gastro-enterologist in to treat simple cases of diarrhea raises the issue of a poor use of skills. A proper match between health-care personnel and the problems requiring treatment necessitates a definition of how the different tasks in a health-care system should be allocated among the different groups of caregivers. This allocation is not easy in displaced-person camps, due to the social intermixing which disrupts the activities of traditional healers, as well as the lack — or excess — of health professionals.[9]

## 2.2 Coverage of Medical Problems

Once the role of each type of care provider has been established, it remains to insure that each has the opportunity to respond to the maximum number of cases relating to the care provider's particular sphere of competence. Adjusting the number of qualified people to the mass of medical problems depends on several factors, in particular the distribution of the population. In a camp, this is a relatively minor problem, given the high population density[10] and the presence (sometimes stampede!) of health professionals. Most of the health problems are conventional ones, and a good number of them can be treated at the most peripheral level of care. An orientation based on primary health care is therefore indicated in displaced-person camps.

Decentralization is essential to avoid overloading facilities at the secondary and tertiary levels (dispensaries and hospitals, respectively). It is preferable to construct a care system in which 50% of the medical problems are treated by CHWs, rather than all cases being referred to health professionals. Otherwise the latter are likely to be completely swamped, and the quality of care becomes dubious.

A study on health-personnel needs in Papua New Guinea estimated that a CHW could treat a maximum of 30 cases per day, a nurse 50, and a doctor 40.[11] Another basis for comparison is the average consultation time. For example, in a study carried out in health centers in Ghana, R. Amonoo-Lartson[12] determined that the average length of a consultation was 7.1 minutes.[13] These, of course, are

---

[9] A flood of health professionals highly specialized in the latest medical techniques does not help solve everyday medical problems.

[10] Which gives rise to other problems, such as a heightened risk of communicable disease, lack of hygiene, etc.

[11] R. Kolehmainen-Aitken and P. Shipp, "Indicators of Staffing Need: Assessing Health Staffing and Equity in Papua New Guinea," *Health Policy and Planning* 5, No. 2: 167-176.

[12] *Soc. Sci. Med.* 15A (1981): 735-741.

[13] 8.6 minutes for a cough, 6.5 minutes for diarrhea, and 6.3 minutes for a fever.

theoretical figures which do not necessarily apply at the beginning of an emergency situation, when the volume of work imposes a reduction of consultation time.[14]

**WORKLOAD BY CATEGORY OF PERSONNEL**
***Factors to take into account***

1. AVERAGE LENGTH OF CONSULTATION:
   For example, 7 minutes for an acute respiratory infection
2. ESTIMATION OF AVERAGE NUMBER OF PATIENTS SEEN PER DAY:
   1 CHW -> 30 patients per day
   1 nurse -> 50 patients per day
   1 doctor -> 40 patients per day
3. OTHER TASKS:
   Supervision
   Preventive Activities
   Administration

In the case of a displaced population, relief workers should know how to use several management tools which all help insure a balanced division of tasks while affording all patients the opportunity to receive the care or instructions suited to their condition. These tools are:

- ranking medical problems in order of priority ("triage");
- approaching problems individually;
- standardizing methods, drugs, and supplies;
- training health-care personnel;
- planning medical facilities.

## 3. Aids Necessary for the Proper Management of Medical Care

### 3.1 Ranking Medical Problems in Order of Priority ("Triage")

When a displaced-person or refugee camp is first set up, it rarely has all the health personnel it needs at the outset. Even if it does, the health facilities, whether local or newly established for the occasion, will not be able to meet medical demand

[14] When consultations are conducted by foreign personnel, extra time must be reckoned for translation of the patient's complaint.

without a period of adjustment. Consequently, medical problems will have to be ranked in order of priority to optimize the use of personnel and material resources.

This policy must be clearly explained to the population, so that it does not see the procedure as a form of segregation for certain patients, but understands medical triage to be a normal technique of mass medicine.

Triage in this context involves first seeking out those severe cases for which an effective, short-term therapeutic solution exists — for example, pneumonia, severe dehydration, and malaria.[15] Moreover, certain pathologies (for example, epidemic meningitis) present a risk not only to the patient but also to the community if they are not diagnosed and treated quickly.

Conversely, care should *not* be provided for chronic cases in no immediate risk for which technical means — usually unavailable locally — would have to be mobilized. In these cases, the patient should be placated with palliative remedies (if necessary, pain killers), and an explanation of the necessity of postponing investigations until later. This category includes such ailments as degenerative joint diseases, cataracts, etc.

Serious cases requiring complex tests and/or treatments pose a completely different ethical problem. What should be done, for example, for a child with a congenital heart disease, or a patient with a very advanced form of cancer? It would be ethically questionable to try to draw up lists in advance of those complaints which should be treated and those which should not. On the other hand, it would be technically questionable to concentrate a substantial portion of available medical resources on these cases to the detriment of other cases which, although also serious, are simpler to treat. The decision must be made on a case-by-case basis, taking into account the patient's chances of survival and the local technical capacities.

This policy may seem to imply that simple medical problems of a non-serious nature require no attention. Yet many minor complaints have the potential to become major ones rapidly: diarrhea can lead to dehydration, for example, or fever may be linked to an attack of malaria. Consequently, the attention given these cases is not a function solely of the patient's condition at the time of consultation, but also of the potential risk of deterioration. The best way of resolving this problem is to develop quickly a network of community health workers to take charge of these kinds of ailments.

[15] Particularly in the areas where *P. falciparum* predominates, with its attendant risk of neurological complications.

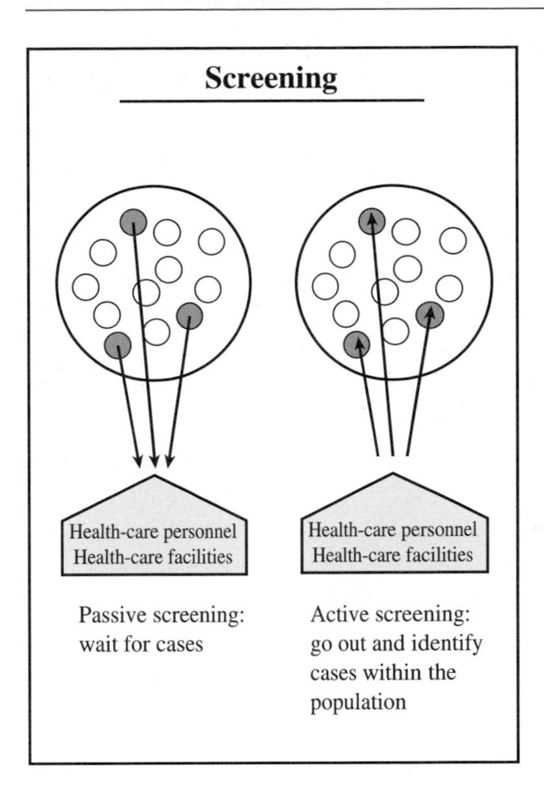


## 3.2 Screening

Screening is used for the systematic identification of high-priority medical problems within a population.[16] Thus, the health-care team may decide to screen for cases of severe malnutrition in order to refer them to nutrition rehabilitation centers. Other pathologies that may be screened for include tuberculosis, measles, malaria, and anemia.

The approach is both collective and individual, since the entire population may be examined or merely a specific sector of it (such as children, subjects with fever, etc.). The cases identified by the screening process will be treated, bringing about a short-term reduction in the frequency and incidence of the complaint screened for.

Screening differs from triage in that the problems looked for are identified in advance. Screening does not involve choosing from among a group of sick people those who will be given priority in treatment. It also differs from epidemiological investigation, the essential goal of which is to determine the frequency with which a particular medical or health problem appears, usually in a population sample. An epidemiological study may indicate the necessity of undertaking a systematic screening process.

## 3.3 Individual Approach to Health Care

Although mass medicine obliges health-care personnel to think in terms of groups, it should not be forgotten that the quality of individual care is equally important. So that this does not remain a subjective issue, the sequence and quality of the relations between a patient and a care provider must be analyzed.

[16] High-priority problems are those for which morbidity and mortality are high and for which an effective treatment exists.

The chronology of events is as follows:

- initial contact
- patient history
- clinical examination
- diagnosis
- decision on how to proceed:
  - advice
  - request for additional tests (x-rays, biological tests)
  - treatment
  - referral to a higher or lower level of care
- follow-up

### *Initial Contact*

A minimum of courtesy, if not consideration, is necessary. For example, should the patient be given time to sit down? This sort of question may seem trivial during an emergency situation, but relief workers should keep in mind that the warmth of the patient's reception will largely determine the quality of the relations between patients and health-care personnel.

### *Taking the Patient History*

An emergency often serves as an excuse to cut short the patient's recital of complaints. Lacking a complete patient history, however, the care provider risks misdiagnosing the problem. Moreover, when the health-care personnel (expatriates, for example) are working in an unfamiliar cultural context, the quality of the patient history is apt to suffer.

### *The Clinical Examination*

Traditionally, the clinical examination is an essential step in the care-giving process; in an emergency situation, its importance is all the greater because its quality must compensate for both the deficiencies of the patient history and the lack of the technical means for radiological and biological tests.

### *The Diagnosis*

A diagnosis falls into one of three categories:

- *"Symptomatic" diagnosis*
  Symptomatic diagnoses are made mostly at the peripheral level by non-professional personnel, on the basis of such symptoms as fever, cough, diarrhea, and abdominal pain.

- *"Clinical" diagnosis*
  Several symptoms are combined to arrive at a clinical diagnosis. Such diagnoses may be relatively precise, such as diagnoses of pneumonia or infected scabies, or may be merely presumptive (fever + chills + headache = malaria[17]).
- *Diagnosis confirmed by additional tests*
  Additional tests may support a diagnosis. For example, a diagnosis may be confirmed by:
  - laboratory tests (to detect malaria, or to determine the degree of anemia);
  - x-rays (pneumonia or bone fractures);
  - bacteriological cultures (to determine the bacterium involved in bacterial meningitis).

Analyzed in terms of the local context[18] and standard statistics on the main causes of morbidity or mortality in similar situations, the patient's symptoms in themselves are an adequate basis for proposing satisfactory therapeutic solutions. This approach, however, more empirical than scientific, poses the risk of numerous misdiagnoses (both false positives and false negatives). To limit this danger, diagnostic tests may be performed for a sample of controversial cases. The results obtained will help to define more clearly the way to proceed for all cases, obviating the need for systematic diagnostic testing for each.

### *How to Proceed*

Once a diagnosis has been made (within the limits described above), the care provider has several alternatives:

#### *Give advice but not treatment*

This approach must be clearly explained to patients, since they all expect to be given medicine when they go to see a health practitioner. If no satisfactory explanation is provided, not only will patients lose confidence in the care facility, but they will also be less than eager to undertake general preventive measures, for the same reason.

#### *Order additional tests*

At the beginning of the intervention, medical criteria can be used to rank the serious cases, most of which will not require additional investigation to determine

[17] These cursory diagnoses take into account the context of the illness. In a region where malaria is rife, such a combination of symptoms would logically arouse suspicions of malaria.
[18] Pathologies specific to the region.

treatment (respiratory infections, diarrheal illnesses, fever in a region of endemic malaria). Even later on, it is not always necessary to invest in sophisticated equipment. It is best, whenever possible, to refer "special" cases to specialized local services.[19]

### *Treatment*

"Effective treatment may be instituted by means of a single contact, or it may demand continued or repeated care; [...] or else treatment may be only a palliative, a placebo, or of dubious efficacy."[20]

In emergency situations, characterized by great population mobility, the aim should be to institute effective treatments that do not require repeated visits to the medical facilities. However, entrusting the patient with all the drugs he will need for a full course of treatment carries the usual risk of patient non-compliance (the drugs received may be sold, used for other members of the family, etc.).

For a certain number of pathologies, the care provider may choose between a conventional course of treatment (several daily doses administered over several days) and a single-dose treatment. Usually, they are equally effective. However, in view of the non-compliance so frequently observed in the longer course of treatment, the single-dose treatment often proves to be the more effective. In addition, it does not demand as much of the health-care personnel's time and energy. Its main disadvantages are that it is often more expensive, and that it does not correspond to local therapeutic practice.

In every situation, the pros and cons of the two approaches must be weighed. Conventional treatment proves more effective than single-dose treatment in diseases such as bacterial meningitis,[21] schistosomiasis, and amebiasis. The opposite is true for tuberculosis, owing to the difference in the cost/benefit ratio between the short and long treatments.

The use of placebos in emergency situations is controversial. Some believe that in the midst of all the urgent problems demanding concrete solutions, health-care workers should not "waste time" on insoluble problems. Others feel that the care provider should make some response to the patient's request, if necessary with a token therapeutic gesture. There are no precise rules in this domain. Every health

---

[19] If the local services are unable to perform this function, it is still wise to consider, before installing advanced equipment, the impact that such aid will have on local behavior. The resident population will see it as evidence of double-standard medicine, and the health professionals of the local services will be tempted by technical progress that they cannot afford.

[20] J. Brunet-Jailly, "L'évaluation économique des actions de santé," in Rougemont and Brunet-Jailly, eds., *La santé dans les pays tropicaux*, p. 431.

[21] P.S. Moore and M.J. Toole, "Surveillance of Meningococcal Meningitis Epidemics in Refugee Populations," *Bulletin of the World Health Organization* 68, No. 5 (1990): 587-596.

worker must develop his or her own philosophy in the field, in the context of the situation. The case is different with measures designed to make the patient more comfortable. A patient's suffering must be alleviated, even if lack of means precludes a satisfactory therapeutic response.

### *Means of Referral*

So that medical services are distributed with regard to the appropriate health-care level, provision must be made for mechanisms of transfer between the various levels. Thus, health-care personnel must be clearly informed of the services offered at each level of the health system, so that they can refer patients either to better-equipped medical units or to a lower level of care, confident that the medical attention received will be satisfactory.

In practically every situation, the caregiving personnel find themselves confronting the problem of particular medical cases requiring transfer to specialized units in the same country or in Western nations. Care providers must realize that they cannot deal with all the medical problems that arise, and that they must give priority to those for which an immediate solution exists.

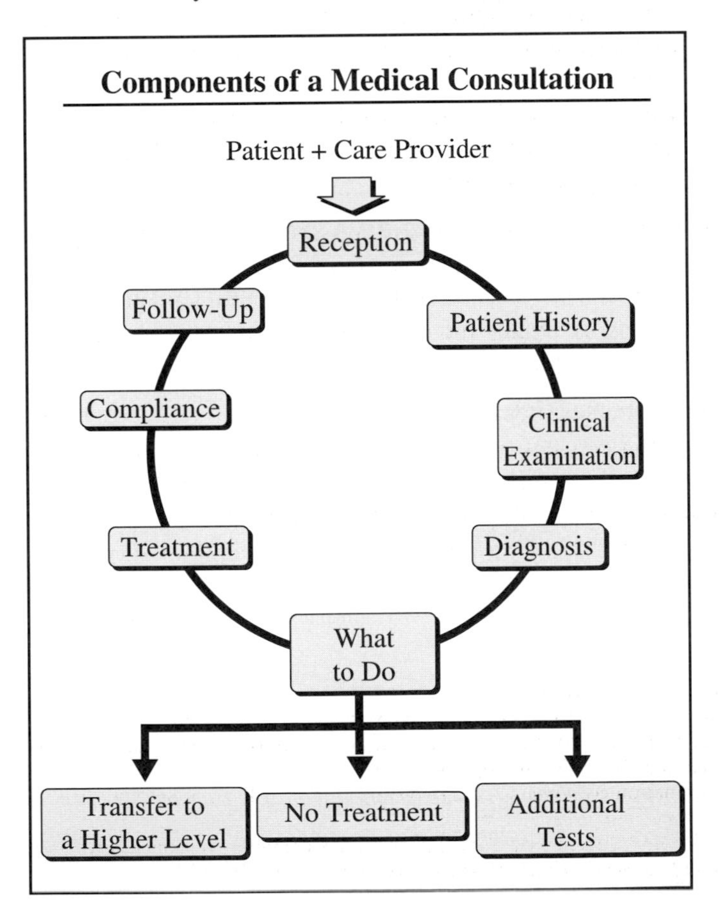


### *Follow-Up*

Once treatment is over, the attitude may be "out of sight, out of mind!" It is difficult to put together, at the very beginning of an action, a file system permitting proper patient follow-up. This is an administrative task which is often unpopular with the caregiving personnel, whose priorities lie elsewhere. Nonetheless, keeping files allows changing medical teams to follow up patients. It is, moreover, an essential element in the epidemiological monitoring of curative activities. Follow-up is also important when a patient moves from one level of care to another (for example, a patient referred from a dispensary to a hospital, or vice versa).

By definition, individual care depends on the interpretation of each care provider. This leaves the way open to numerous irregularities, unless certain measures are established to rationalize the approach — a rationalization which must still, of course, take account of the individual characteristics of the patients and those who treat them. The primary tool in this domain is standardization of the care chain.

## 3.4 Standardization Procedures

### *Diagnostic Standardization*

Many diagnostic procedures have already been laid down in the form of flowcharts. They can easily be adapted to the situation and to the type of personnel who will need to use them.

One good system involves using standardized cards for different symptoms: fever, diarrhea, abdominal pains, conjunctivitis, cough, lower-limb edema,

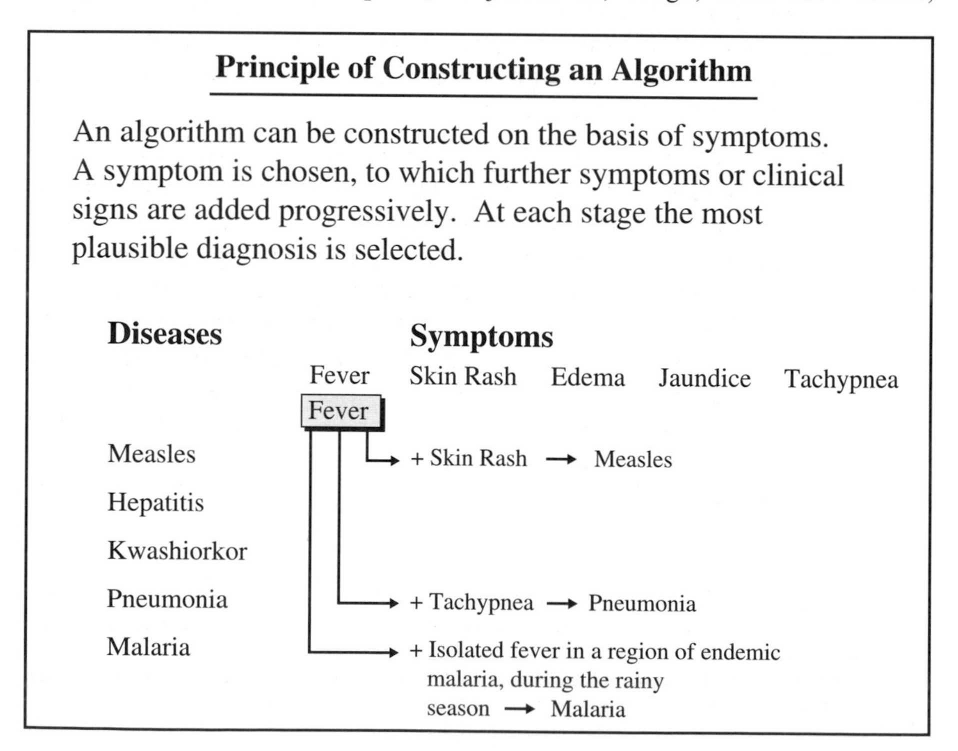

dyspnea, hepatomegaly, crepitation heard during auscultation of the lungs, etc. This is more useful than cards for etiologically defined problems such as pneumococcal pneumonia, amebic diarrhea, and left ventricular heart failure.[22] This standardization system can take the form of flow charts. Diagnostic standardization should reflect age (infants, children, adults) and sex.

### *Therapeutic Standardization*

According to A. Degrémont,

"The term therapeutic procedure means not only surgical action or the prescription of medicines, but also the decision to transfer the patient to another, more suitable health center, or else to abstain from intervention because it is useless or impossible."[23]

The standardization process is carried out on several levels.

#### *Standardization of Treatment*

In emergency situations, the use of biological tests and x-rays remains the exception. This restriction must be kept in mind when a course of treatment is planned.

Standardized treatment should be the rule at all levels of the medical hierarchy (CHWs, nursing personnel, doctors): "A vertical coordination must be achieved between the different standardization plans, to make sure they complement each other."[24] In this book, however, the emphasis is on the therapeutic tasks that the CHWs may need to carry out in a given context.

Standardization is particularly important in emergency situations. First, it should be remembered that in countries requiring relief assistance standard procedures usually already exist for treating the main pathologies, such as tuberculosis, malaria, and diarrheal diseases. Humanitarian agencies should try at the outset to standardize procedures, in order to harmonize their own emergency procedures with those employed by the health ministry. Occasionally, relief agencies may institute specific procedures which do not correspond to those advocated by the health ministry. A case in point is the introduction of short-term treatments for tuberculosis in refugee camps, when the host countries offer their own populations the conventional, long-term therapy. This problem must be negotiated with the local health authorities.

---

22 "Many decisions have to be made in the outpatient clinics. These include decisions about diagnosis, treatment, or the need for tests or referral and there is often less than five minutes to spend with each patient." B.J. Essex, *Diagnostic Pathways in Clinical Medicine* (Churchill Livingstone, 1980), p. 2.

23 A. Degrémont, "Organisation et gestion de la médecine curative," in Rougemont and Brunet-Jailly, eds., *La santé dans les pays tropicaux*, p. 431.

24 *Ibid.*

The standard treatment for the ailments listed below will indicate the level of care appropriate in each case. For diarrhea, fever, cough, abdominal pain, a rash, metrorrhagia, pruritis, weight loss, conjunctivitis, joint pain, etc., the course of action to be taken in each case will determine the care to be provided:

- at the household level;
- at the CHW level;
- at the dispensary level (nursing staff);
- at the district hospital level (doctors).

This means determining in advance what the people at each level should know how to do, and providing them with the wherewithal to do it.

Procedures are standardized at the hospital level as well, although here there are more therapeutic approaches specific to different doctors than at the primary or secondary levels.

*Standardization of Drugs*

Logically, the standardization of treatment regimens implies standardization of the drugs used. For many years now, efforts have been going on to rationalize drug use, and the principal humanitarian agencies accept WHO's recommendations.[25]

Lists of essential drugs, reflecting both the medical problems themselves and the different treatment levels, already exist:

- the WHO/UNHCR list of essential drugs;
- the ICRC list of essential drugs;
- the MSF (*Médecins sans Frontières*) list of essential drugs.

This rationalization must take into account four factors:

1. The population's health problems rather than the wishes of the medical teams.
2. The fact that the "essential" basic drugs will be used by personnel with varying levels of ability (the drug lists should therefore be adapted to the level of use). UNHCR, for example, suggests three lists:
   - the basic list for the CHWs who use the drugs at the most peripheral level;
   - a supplementary list for doctors and nursing personnel who use these drugs in dispensaries and general hospitals;
   - a specialized list for doctors and nursing personnel working in units where they encounter particular medical problems.
3. Cost (generic drugs).

[25] "After several years of study, field testing and modifications, standard lists of essential drugs and medical supplies for use in an emergency were developed. The aim was to encourage the standardization of drugs and medical supplies used in an emergency to permit a swift and effective response with supplies that meet priority health needs." *The New Emergency Kit* (Geneva: WHO, 1990), p. 1.

4. The policy of the local ministry of health on essential drugs.

**LIST OF STANDARD DRUGS**
**(for 10,000 people for approx. 3 months)**

| Drugs: | |
|---|---|
| Acetylsalicylic acid, 300 mg tablets | 3,000 |
| Benzyl benzoate, 25% lotion | 1 |
| Chlorhexidine (5%) | 1 |
| Chloroquine, 150 mg base tablets | 2,000 |
| Aluminum hydroxide, 500 mg tablets | 1,000 |
| Mebendazole, 100 mg tablets | 500 |
| Paracetamol, 100 mg tablets | 1,000 |
| ORS (oral rehydration salts), packet for 1 liter | 200 |
| Sulfamethoxazole + trimethoprim, 400 mg + 80 mg tablets | 2,000 |
| Ferrous sulfate + folic acid, 200 + 0.25 mg tablets | 2,000 |
| Tetracycline, 1% ophthalmic ointment | 50 |
| Gentian violet, powder | 4 |

Source: *New Emergency Health Kit* – WHO, 1992

This approach will also oblige the relief team, depending on the needs of the population, to:

1. coordinate action with the health ministry and the other agencies involved in a given emergency situation;
2. rationalize drug donations and prevent the dispatch of unsolicited drugs;
3. manage stocks more efficiently.

### *Standardization of Transfer Procedures*

The transfer of patients from one care level to another must obey precise rules so that the care given at one level of the health-care system will correspond to the skills of the health-care personnel associated with that level. Standardizing transfer procedures makes it possible to define what kinds of patients must be evacuated. This prevents complex cases from being treated at low-level facilities that do not have the capabilities for it, and, conversely, prevents simple cases from being too easily passed on to higher levels, where they would encumber operations.

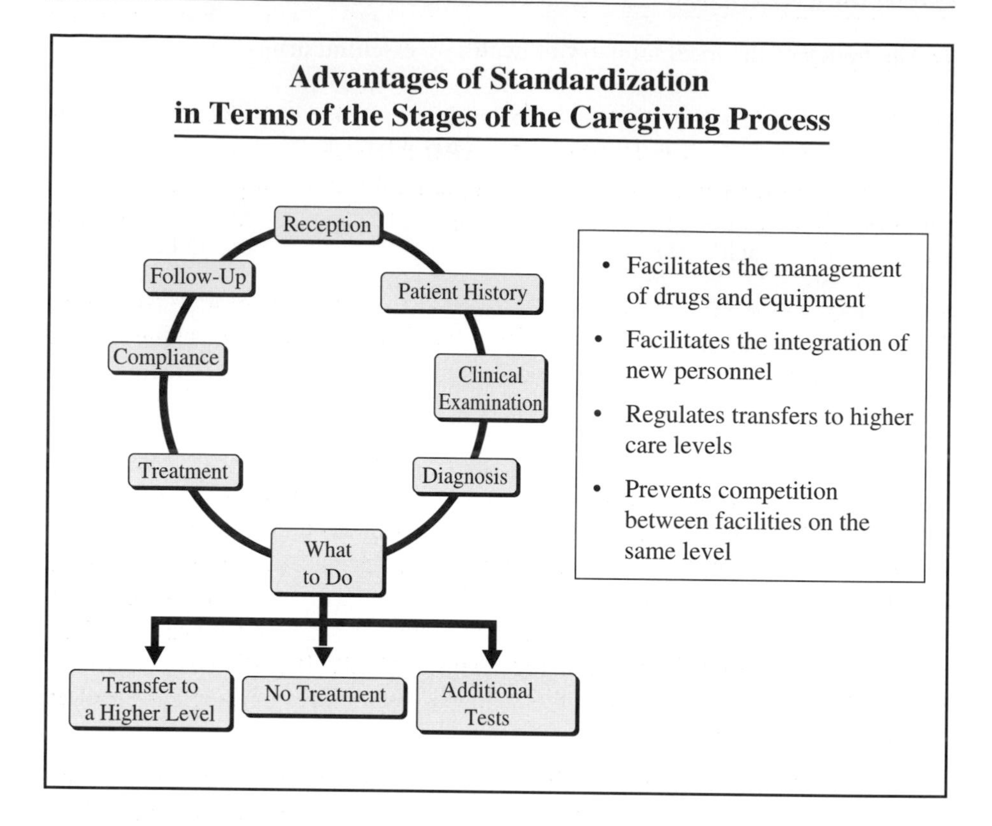


## 3.5 Training Health-Care Personnel[26]

The health professionals (nursing staff, doctors) working in emergency situations should already be trained. At most, additional instructions regarding specific problems may be given.

A certain number of medical tasks can be performed by non-professional personnel, as long as they have been properly trained to do them. Training programs have been instituted in most of the situations involving displaced or refugee populations. This type of training provides the basis for an effective teaching program for CHWs.[27]

---

[26] Training CHWs to perform a certain number of curative tasks will be the focus for a training program. This method of apprenticeship can be applied to all fields, not just healing activities.

[27] The information in this paragraph is taken from J.J. Guilbert, *Guide pédagogique pour les personnels de santé* (WHO, 1981).

## *Health Problems*

Every training program begins by defining the main problems of displaced populations. J.J. Guilbert proposes two basic principles:

"1. Training must focus on both groups and individuals, taking into account the health needs of the community in question: training is oriented towards the group.

2. Training must maintain the student in an active situation, gradually leading him to direct his own apprenticeship activities: training is centered on apprenticeship." [28]

## *Professional Tasks*

The approach described above is also appropriate for training CHWs in emergency situations. The preceding sections discussed the most urgent health problems and the necessity of defining and standardizing the professional tasks that have to be done. It was shown that CHWs may have to deal with patients suffering from fever, skin lesions, coughs, etc. Their training may permit them to identify these ailments. At the next stage, they must be able to diagnose the cause of the fever or other symptom — malaria, respiratory infections, etc. — and to treat it.

Choosing the level of skill that will be required of a health worker depends on the role the CHWs are expected to play in the health-care system. Should it be limited to screening cases of fever, or does it include the responsibility of making a diagnosis and providing treatment? This choice will determine which professional tasks CHWs should be able to perform. In an emergency situation, they must be quickly trained for specific tasks, such as taking anthropometric measurements, treating cases of scabies, and preparing rehydration solutions. In general, manpower is not limited, and CHWs can be speedily trained for a specific,[29] high-priority task. Later on, these tasks will be diversified so that they can be integrated into the more general framework of an activity.[30] The initial selection of priorities is therefore very important.

Controlling diarrheal diseases at the primary level, for example, encompasses a group of activities, such as:

- managing cases of diarrhea;
- controlling the water supply;

---

[28] *Ibid.*, pp. 1-19.

[29] "In general, simple tasks should be taught before complex ones. At the community level, complex health-care activities consist in the juxtaposition of several tasks." Rougemont and Brunet-Jailly, eds., *La santé dans les pays tropicaux*, p. 165.

[30] Breaking an activity down into tasks was discussed in Chapter 1 ("General Principles of Planning").

- controlling waste removal;
- promoting the rules of hygiene.

Each activity can be subdivided into several tasks. For example, managing cases of diarrhea breaks down into diagnosing cases of diarrhea, treating them, and identifying the cases that need to be referred to the dispensary or clinic.

## *Objectives of Apprenticeship*

The objectives of apprenticeship correspond to the tasks that the CHW will have to perform. To take the example of managing diarrhea cases again, the CHW must be able to:

- diagnose diarrheal diseases;
- explain to a mother the role of rehydration solutions;
- explain to a mother how to prepare a rehydration solution;
- explain the importance of continuing to feed the child normally;
- explain the importance of continuing to breastfeed;
- identify those diarrhea cases presenting severe dehydration;
- refer the most serious cases to the dispensary.

## *Training Content*

A distinction must be made between what the CHWs should *know* (knowledge) and what they should be able to *do*.

### *What a CHW should know*

Many training programs in emergency situations amount to a compilation of abstract facts, without any special connection to actual skills. Must the CHW be familiar with intestinal physiology to be able to treat a case of diarrhea? Should the CHW be familiar with the list of microorganisms responsible for diarrheal diseases? Or perhaps all he or she needs to know is that diarrheal diseases are characterized essentially by water loss; that the risk of death is linked to dehydration, and that rehydration salts are the basis for treating diarrheal diseases.

### *What a CHW should be able to do*

A CHW should be able to diagnose cases of diarrheal disease, treat them, and identify those cases that must be referred to a higher level.

Each of these tasks can be broken down into still simpler tasks. For example, to diagnose diarrheal diseases, the CHW must:

- determine — by means of the patient history or an interview with the mother — when the disease began, the number of stools per day, and for how many days.
- ask to see the stools.
- ask about the consistency of the stools.
- look for signs of dehydration: dry tongue, creased skin, tachycardia, sunken eyes, tachypnea.
- ask if the diarrhea has been accompanied by vomiting.
- ascertain whether the child has a fever.

## *Planning an Evaluation System*

A careful definition of what the CHW must be able to do also provides the basis for a system of skill evaluation. An observer can determine whether the CHW has:

- talked to the mother to find out when the illness began and verified the number of stools produced per day.
- asked to see the stools.
- looked for signs of dehydration during the clinical examination.

All these elements serve as reference points to evaluate whether the CHW is doing his or her work correctly and following exact instructions.[31] At this stage, the acceptable level of performance must be defined. For example, if the CHW has looked for creased skin and dry mucous membranes, but not the three other clinical signs of dehydration mentioned in the description of apprenticeship objectives, will his or her performance be considered acceptable? In such a case, the evaluator must weigh the relative importance of the signs sought.

Evaluation should cover the following aspects:

- *intellectual process* — The capacity to integrate the information derived from the patient history with that gained from the clinical examination in order to arrive at a diagnosis and make the appropriate decision.
- *attitude* — The CHW's manner while interviewing the mother and examining the child (kind or brusque, etc.)
- actions — Whether the CHW's actions conform to what has been taught.

Evaluation methods should be based on four essential criteria:[32]

- *validity*: whether the skills acquired do in fact conform to the educational objective.

---

[31] "Evaluation must begin with a clear and meaningful definition of educational objectives, derived from the most urgent health problems." Guilbert, *Guide pédagogique pour les personnels de santé*, p. 207.

[32] *Ibid.*, p. 235.

- *reliability*: measuring is consistent.
- *objectivity*: agreement between examiners.
- *simplicity* in the construction and use of the evaluation method.

The choice of a particular method of evaluation depends on the type of performance to be evaluated and the extent to which it meets the criteria above.

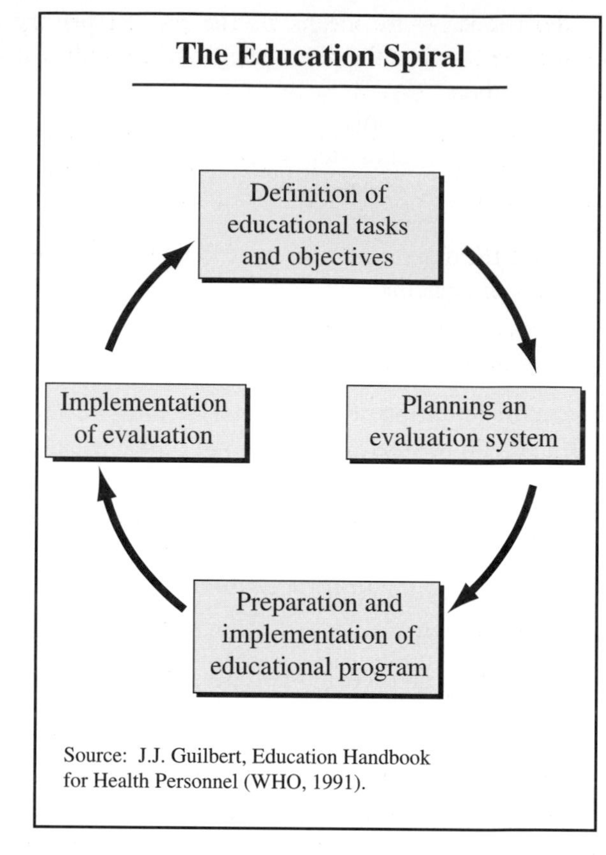

Source: J.J. Guilbert, Education Handbook for Health Personnel (WHO, 1991).

*Methods of Apprenticeship*

The methods of apprenticeship must be defined in terms of each objective. In an emergency situation, a CHW is generally expected to know how to approach people and to perform a few practical procedures. Learning is based on demonstrations, followed by a practical apprenticeship under direct supervision.

## 3.6 Architectural Design of Medical Facilities

Many plans for medical buildings are available; every book on health services presents a plan of its own.[33] Solving the facility problem consists in "importing" these plans, and making any changes necessary to adapt them to local conditions. Unfortunately, as alterations are added, the general appearance of the infrastructure no longer reflects a rational, comprehensive plan.

[33] See S. Simmonds, P. Vaughan and Sir W. Gunn, *Refugee Community Health Care*, p. 213 (Oxford Medical Publications, 1983) and M. King, *Medical Care in Developing Countries* (Nairobi: Oxford University Press, 1966), p. 1612.

Without discussing construction techniques per se, this section will attempt to define the health-care personnel's contribution to the architectural design of health-care infrastructure.[34]

By analyzing the activities and tasks that health-care personnel will be called upon to perform in a given facility, planners can determine how much space is needed and the best way to organize it.

A dispensary's activities, for example, could be broken down as follows:

- medical activities
  - registration of patients
  - consultations
  - bandaging
  - injections
  - distribution of drugs
- paramedical activities
  - laboratory services
- support activities
  - water provision
  - waste disposal
  - energy supply
  - cleaning

Each activity group can be further broken down into more precise elements, the end result being a definition of simple tasks. Consultation, for example, as defined in the section (3.3) on the individual approach to treatment, can be broken down like this:

- reception of the patient
- patient history
- clinical examination
- diagnosis
- treatment
- follow-up

The clinical examination can be further broken down:

- ask the patient to undress

[34] "In producing a schedule the medical planner has to take quasi-architectural decisions, e.g. the optimum size of the room. In this they are not adequately supported by medical advice. In interpreting a schedule the designers have to make quasi-medical assumptions, e.g. the optimum shape of the room. In this they are not adequately supported by medical advice." Jan Delrue, "Rationalization of Planning and Construction of Medical Care Facilities in Developing Countries," in B.M. Klezkowski and R. Pibouleau, eds., *Approaches to Planning and Design of Health Care Facilities in Developing Areas*, WHO Offset Publication No. 29 (1976), p. 63.

- ask the patient to lie down on the examination table
- examine the patient

Delrue suggests creating a list of all the tasks that need to be done, together with the material supplies required to carry them out. Subsidiary points should be added, such as provision for the CHW to wash hands after the clinical examination and lighting arrangements. All these data will provide the basis for determining how much space is needed and how it should be organized.[35]

**Basic Principles for Constructing a Dispensary**

1. Draw up a list of the activities that will be carried out in this dispensary:
   - consultations
   - immunizations
   - health education, etc.
   - ...
2. Draw up a list of the tasks involved in each activity:
   - consultations:
     - patient history
     - clinical examination
     - prescription
3. Determine the equipment and space necessary to perform each task.
4. Work out the dynamics of the dispensary by grouping together the tasks that will be done in sequence.
5. Design the layout of the dispensary, taking into account the space required for each task and the overall dynamics of the dispensary.

The architect's role, then, is to design a plan that will give the health-care personnel optimum ergonomic conditions. In emergency situations, of course, it is difficult to come up with satisfactory plans at the outset, particularly when the relief team is obliged to set up operations in non-medical buildings used as dispensaries or hospitals.

This approach can be used for all medical infrastructures.

**Community Health Station**

The community health station is the first concrete facility in the health system. Its organization will depend on the type of medical activities to be carried out there.

**Dispensary**

An estimation of a dispensary's work volume must take into consideration consultations, drug distribution, management of pharmaceutical stores, out-

[35] Jan Delrue, "Data Sheet, Consulting/Examining — General Purpose," in Klezkowski and Pibouleau, eds., *Approaches to Planning and Design of Health Care Facilities in Developing Areas*, p. 73.

patient care (bandaging), injections, etc. The layout of the dispensary must be designed rationally. The patients coming in should not bump into those going out, and the examination facilities should be set up in such a way that the privacy of the patients can be respected.

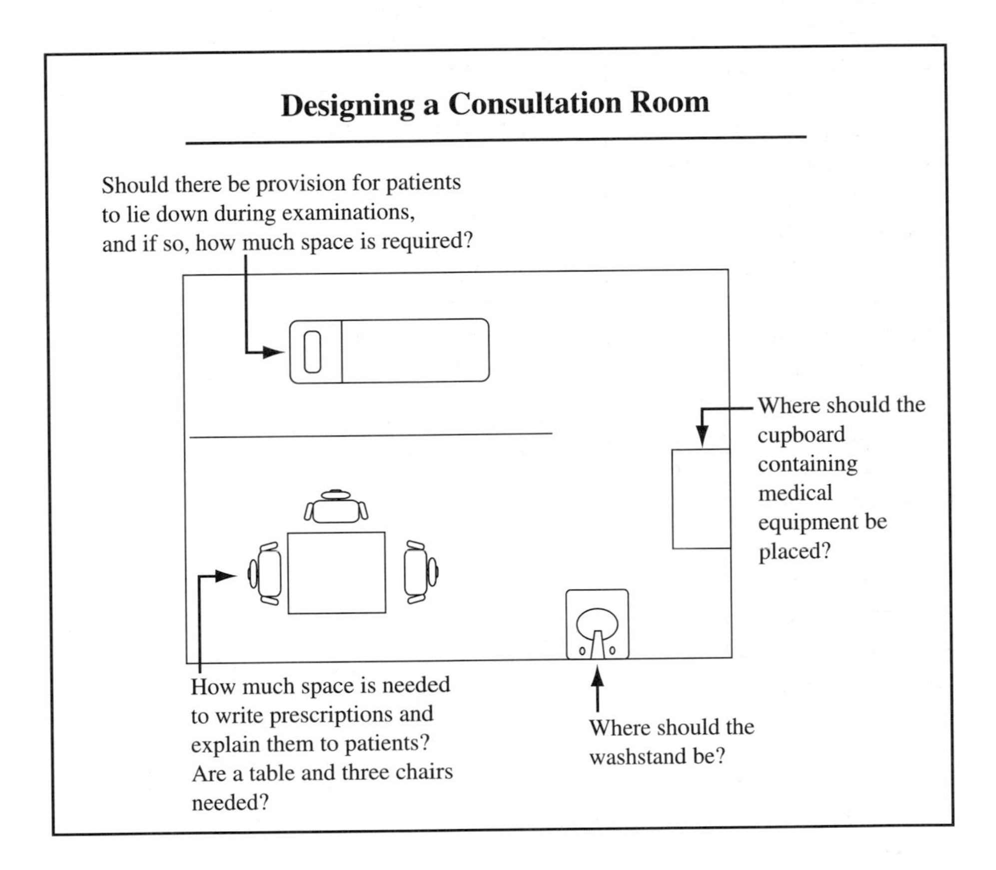


### Hospital

A hospital contains a greater diversity of activities than a small facility, and most of them are interconnected. This complexity makes it even more important to organize the place systematically by type of activity.

## 3.7 Evaluation of Health-Care Facilities

An evaluation of the activities carried out in a health-care facility is doubly useful. Before an intervention, it shows whether an existing facility has what it needs to cope with an emergency situation. In the course of an intervention, the evaluation process can be applied to a facility set up especially for the occasion; in this case, it falls into the more general framework of a surveillance program.

Most "check lists" for dispensaries or hospitals contain basically quantitative information; this chapter, however, will also discuss the qualitative aspect of health-facility structures. To decide whether an existing hospital will be able to meet the needs of a displaced population, several parameters must be evaluated.

## *Quantitative Evaluation*

*Patients*

- number of patients admitted per month
- average period of hospitalization
- number of deaths in the hospital
- number of consultations per month

*Health-Care Personnel*

- number of doctors (listed by specialty)
- number of nursing personnel
- number of paramedical personnel

*Equipment and Drugs*

- description of available equipment
- drug inventory

*Buildings*

- description of buildings
- description of support elements:
  - water supply
  - waste disposal
  - energy supply

*Organization*

- number of beds per ward
- rate of bed occupancy

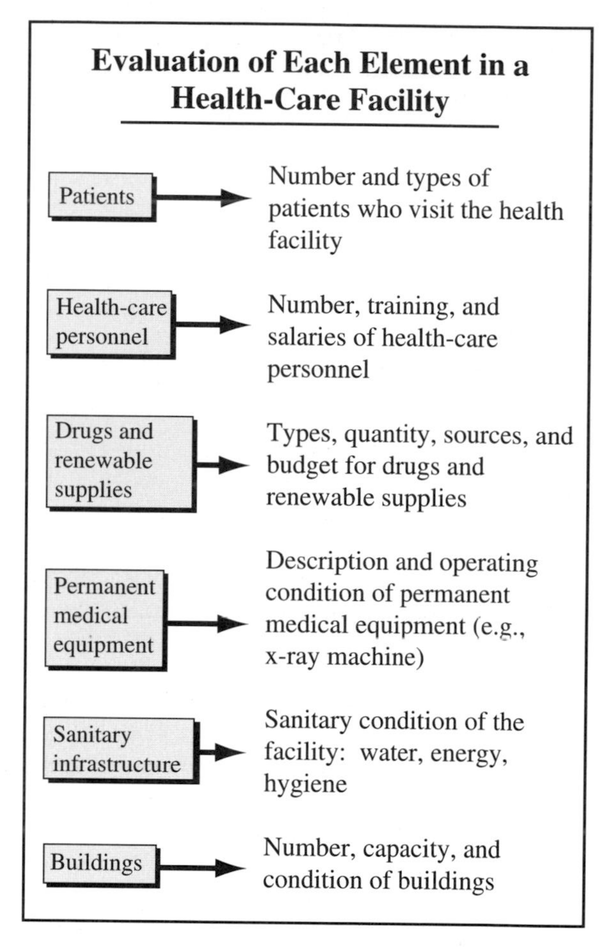

**Analysis of the Performances of Health-Care Personnel Conducting Medical Consultations**

Performances expected according to previously determined objective criteria

| List of activities | 5 | 4 | 3 | 2 |
|---|---|---|---|---|
| • Ability to communicate with patients | * | | | |
| • Pertinence of patient history | | | * | |
| • Validity of diagnosis | | * | | |
| • Appropriateness of treatment | | | * | |
| • Appropriateness of transfers to hospitals | | * | | |
| • Appropriateness of patient follow-up | | | * | |

Acceptable level of performance reveals points that need improvement

## *Qualitative Evaluation*

### *Patients*

- reasons for hospitalization
- causes of death in the hospital

### *Personnel*

It is always difficult to evaluate the performance of the health-care personnel objectively. The available means and the national context (medical standards in developing countries, disparities between rural and urban areas) must be taken into account. The standards normally considered acceptable must be adapted to emergency conditions. Although usually common sense is all that is needed to gauge the situation and to make such adjustments, some authors have suggested the use of grading systems based on the concept of "acceptable level of performance" mentioned in the section on training — in other words, performance profiles.[36]

This approach implies that acceptable levels of performance for the main activities conducted in a health facility have been defined in advance. For example, the following questions might be asked:

- Is the personnel's attitude towards the patients acceptable?
- Is the quality of treatment acceptable?
- Is the treatment of pneumonia in children acceptable (with respect to the choice of antibiotic, the length of treatment, etc.)?

The evaluator requires not only an adequate technical knowledge of generally accepted standards, but also solid field experience in order to judge technical performance in the context of the situation and to make a reliable pronouncement on the effectiveness of the care provided.

[36] F.M. Katz and R. Snow, *Assessing Health Workers' Performance*, Public Health Papers 72 (WHO, 1980), p. 34.

*Equipment and Drugs*

- Does the equipment function correctly?
- Are the stored vaccines always effective? Is the cold chain properly monitored?
- Have any drugs passed their expiry dates?

*Functioning of the Facility*

The combination of the quantitative and qualitative aspects of evaluation allows the relief team to assess the overall functioning of the health-care facility, and to determine whether it can absorb the extra workload occasioned by the arrival of a displaced or refugee population. If it cannot, the data collected will help pinpoint weaknesses and indicate solutions.[37]

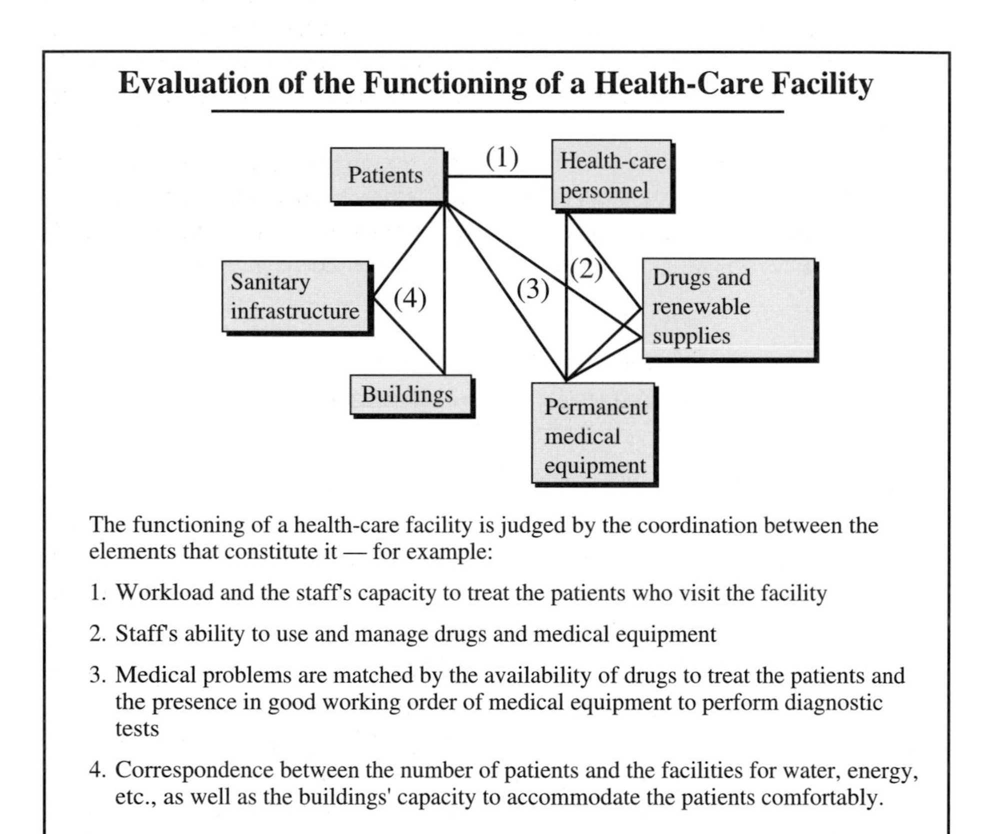


**Evaluation of the Functioning of a Health-Care Facility**

The functioning of a health-care facility is judged by the coordination between the elements that constitute it — for example:

1. Workload and the staff's capacity to treat the patients who visit the facility
2. Staff's ability to use and manage drugs and medical equipment
3. Medical problems are matched by the availability of drugs to treat the patients and the presence in good working order of medical equipment to perform diagnostic tests
4. Correspondence between the number of patients and the facilities for water, energy, etc., as well as the buildings' capacity to accommodate the patients comfortably.

[37] The role that local health-care facilities play in the options available to humanitarian organizations is discussed in greater detail in Chapter 7 ("The Health-Care System").

# 4. Planning Health-Care Facilities

## 4.1 Factors to Consider

In normal situations, planning the number and size of the health-care facilities for a given population is subject to the following considerations:

- *the concept of needs and demands* — The quantification of medical services depends on the volume of real needs that must be satisfied.
- *the availability of human resources* — The scarcity or surplus of health-care personnel will influence the profile of the curative services. If, for example, nurses are numerous, a network of relatively decentralized dispensaries can be set up.
- *the availability of financial resources* — The decision to establish health stations directed by CHWs depends largely on financial considerations. The cost/benefit ratio of a health station is particularly high, especially where the material (drugs) and human (CHWs) resources are the responsibility of the community itself.
- *the geographical factor* — It is necessary to estimate the size of the population these health units are supposed to cover. Thought must also be given to the distances that patients will have to travel to reach them. For this reason, no precise standard exists in this domain, merely indicative figures.

The general assumption is that:

- a health station (CHW) serves 500-3,000 people
- a dispensary or local clinic serves 5,000-10,000 people
- a district hospital serves 100,000-200,000 people

These considerations are completely different in emergency situations.

- Real needs are generally much greater in emergencies than in normal situations, due to the development of needs specific to the disaster (wounded) and to the particularly harsh environmental conditions to which the victims are subject (lack of food, cold, etc.).

- The geographical factor may be simplified, insofar as the refugee population is housed in a clearly delimited camp, so that the health-care facilities are immediately accessible. On the other hand, under the pressure of political events, refugee or displaced populations are extremely mobile. It is not unusual to plan health facilities which, after a few months of activity, stand empty because the population for whom they were established has moved on.

- The human resources mobilized for emergency situations are often completely out of proportion to the numbers that the health system of the country concerned can provide to its own population during normal times. There is a clear risk of fostering a double standard in health care, if no effort is made from the outset to match the level of care to that normally prevailing in the country. This, of course, applies to the cases where the local level is judged acceptable. If it is not, the whole problem arises of aiding not only the victims of a disaster, but also neighboring populations not directly affected by it.

- Financial resources usually correspond to the human resources. Certainly, the measures that have to be taken and, especially, the speed of the intervention impose a high cost. The relief team must know how to manage resources according to the victims' needs rather than the available funds.

These factors have a considerable impact on the "consumption" of medical services. Of course, the relation between the magnitude of real needs and the provision of appropriate medical services is clear — at least at the beginning of an intervention, when the preventive measures instituted together with the medical intervention have not yet had a measurable impact on the victims' health status. However, even if needs decline after a few weeks, the victims' demand for medical care is not necessarily less.

Physical access, free treatment, and the attraction of medical services that in many cases are based on Western standards are all factors favoring the consumption of medical services. Under these conditions, it is difficult to quantify with any precision the resources that must be mobilized to satisfy the medical needs of a population in an emergency situation.

## 4.2 Estimation of Necessary Resources

### *Ambulatory Care*

Average figures generated in normal times indicate that every individual comes into contact with the medical services twice a year.[38] A distinction should be made between preventive-care contacts (immunization, health education, etc.) and primary or secondary consultations.[39]

The number of medical consultations (at the dispensary level) can be empirically estimated at four to six consultations (primary and secondary) per year and per person in a refugee camp, at least during the first three months of the relief operation. This figure should normally fall to two or three per year and per person.[40]

This workload may be distributed differently depending on the degree to which ambulatory care (provided by CHW health stations, dispensaries, or local clinics)

---

[38] This is the average for an entire population. Some people may have five contacts, others none at all.

[39] A primary consultation is an individual's first visit for a given medical problem; secondary consultations are subsequent visits for the same medical problem.

[40] That is, if preventive measures are effective.

is decentralized. A study on refugee camps by the health ministry of Honduras showed that the average number of consultations per person and per year was 1.7 for refugees of Nicaraguan origin, 4.3 for refugees of Mosquito origin, and 3.9 for refugees of Salvadorian origin. The distribution of this workload between the community health workers and the health-care professionals (doctors and nurses) was respectively 18% for CHWs-Nicaragua, 51% for CHWs-Mosquito, and 53% for CHWs-Salvador.

These are not absolute values, applicable under all circumstances. The CHWs' volume of activity depends on their skill, their acceptance by the population, and, especially, their motivation. Although very uncertain, these figures give an indication of volume of work in a dispensary. At the beginning of an intervention, the number of consultations required to attend to the medical needs of 10,000 refugees will be 100-150 per day. This figure provides a basis for determining the number of medical staff and the quantity of drugs[41] necessary.

### *Hospital Care*

Similarly, it can be estimated that for a total population, 40-50 per 1,000 will need to be hospitalized.[42] Thus, for a population of 50,000 refugees, the relief team should reckon on 2,500 patients being hospitalized per year. If an average hospital stay is figured at seven days, this works out to 18,000 days of hospitalization. Accordingly, provision must be made for a hospitalization capacity of 50 beds.[43]

All these figures should be considered as very vague estimates which merely give an idea of the number of patients that can be expected in this type of situation. It is useful to know that for 50,000 people, a hospital with a maximum of 50-100 beds is needed, rather than a hospital with 500 beds.

**SUMMARY OF QUANTITATIVE NEEDS**

**Taking as a basis:**
**4 consultations/person/year**
**hospitalization rate of 40/1,000**
**average period of hospitalization = 7 days**

**It can be estimated that:**
**1% of the population will be seen by a medical worker each day**
**1% of those examined will have to be hospitalized**
**1 hospital bed will be needed for every 1,000 people**

[41] Lists established by WHO give the quantities of drugs and other supplies necessary to cover the needs of 10,000 refugees for three months.
[42] Excluding war-wounded, whose numbers cannot be predicted.
[43] This is the minimal capacity; in reality, an additional capacity of 10 beds is advisable to cover fluctuations in the number of admissions.

Certain constraints common to emergency situations should be kept in mind, however:

- Sometimes, at the beginning of an emergency situation, the need for beds is far in excess of the figures given above. This is no reason, however, to begin constructing large hospitals, since normally demand will soon be reined in by the preventive measures taken, to fall back within the margin of the estimates previously calculated.
- The total population can vary rapidly. It is not unusual for the number of refugees to rise in no time from 10,000 to 20,000. Plans for health-care facilities must take into account possible developments in the political situation, even though this usually involves considerable speculation.

## 4.3 Allocation of Responsibilities

### *The Family*

In a camp, at least at the beginning, it is difficult to organize family medicine cabinets; later on, the idea can be considered, but any drugs distributed in this way are very likely to be sold to offset the displaced people's lack of financial resources. Moreover, if secondary-level health facilities (dispensaries, health-care centers) are readily accessible, there is little sense in handing drugs over to the family.

### *The Community*

In a camp enjoying the services of trained CHWs, a framework should be created for them; where there are none, training CHWs is a priority in order to cover basic medical problems in a satisfactory manner. At the same time, facilities should be planned for them to work in.

### *The Dispensary*

If the number of displaced people is not too large, an effort should be made to find local facilities, if possible, that can meet the needs of the new population. The establishment of a network of dispensaries within large camps is essential.

### *The Hospital*

Building a hospital is justified only for large concentrations of people. In general, camp hospitals are flimsy structures able to accommodate only those cases that do not require very extended or complex hospital care. For those who do not fall into this category, a solution must be found in a local hospital.

### *Communication between Levels*

Setting up a communication system between the dispensaries and the hospital is usually not a problem (radio, ambulances). Maintaining regular communication between the primary level (CHWs) and the secondary level (dispensaries), however, is much more difficult, owing to the lack of personnel to supervise the CHWs and the absence of information on cases referred to the dispensary.

# II. Surgical Care

## 1. Nature of Surgical Problems

In disaster situations, particularly wars, surgical procedure is governed by very precise rules which derive from the necessity of adapting available means to demand. It differs both qualitatively and quantitatively from the requirements of normal situations.

### 1.1 Types of Problems

#### *Natural Disasters*

Among natural disasters, earthquakes are the greatest cause of injury. It is estimated that between 1967 and 1991, 741,420 people were injured worldwide as a result of earthquakes.[44] In a study on the 1988 earthquake in Armenia, E. Noji showed that of the total 500,000 people affected by the disaster, 130,000 were injured, 14,000 of them requiring hospitalization. Of the 1,500,000 people affected by the El Salvador earthquake in 1986, 10,000 were injured. Armenian injury figures were in a large part determined by poor construction and the pancake effect of the buildings collapsing.[45]

In certain villages, 85-90% of the people pulled out alive from the rubble of their homes were dug out by the neighboring civilian population. This fact, of course, has a direct implication for relief organization — basically, that emphasis must be placed on preparing populations living in vulnerable areas of disaster to provide the initial assistance, rather than on devising plans that give priority to international relief teams. Although the latter are certainly better equipped, they often arrive at the scene of the disaster too late.

---

[44] International Federation of the Red Cross and Red Crescent Societies, *World Disasters Report* (1993), p. 104.

[45] H. Armenian, E. Noji, and A. Oganessian, "Case Control Study of Injuries Due to the Earthquake in Soviet Armenia," *Bulletin of the World Health Organization* 70 (1992): 253.

### *Armed Conflicts*

Injuries caused by armed conflict can be classified as follows:

**a) Nature of the traumatizing agent**

- bullets
- mines
- bombing
- napalm, etc.

Each of these agents cause specific types of injuries:

- bullet wound
- foot injuries (mines)
- burns
- crush injuries

The lesions caused by a given agent may vary. For example, in bullet wounds, the extent of the lesion depends on the weight of the projectile, its stability,[46] the soundness of its construction,[47] its shape, and its velocity.[48] All these factors may combine to create particularly large lesions, due to the high transfer of energy.[49] Cavitation is produced, drawing debris and germs into the wound and causing additional lesions at some distance from the wound itself.

**b) Anatomical location of the injury**

- head
- upper limbs
- trunk
- lower limbs

Anti-personnel mine explosions cause localized injuries at foot and leg level; the location of bullet wounds is much more variable.

## 1.2 Extent of Needs

In disaster and conflict situations, it is impossible to predict the number of wounded who will require care.

---

[46] The bullet may go through various movements in the course of its trajectory: oscillations around its longitudinal axis, rotation, etc.

[47] Bullets that fragment on impact cause more extensive lesions than bullets that remain intact.

[48] A distinction is made between high-velocity bullets (800 m/s) and low-velocity bullets (150-200 m/s). The greater the velocity, the greater the amount of energy apt to be transferred into the body tissues.

[49] "The energy transfer determines the amount of tissue damaged." D. Dufour *et al.*, *Surgery for Victims of War* (ICRC, 1990), p. 14.

## *Disasters*

The number of wounded after an earthquake depends on:

- the intensity of the earthquake;[50]
- population density (whether its epicenter is located in the middle of a city or in a sparsely inhabited rural area);
- the degree of earthquake protection in the affected area. Constructing buildings to earthquake standards reduces seismic damage considerably.[51]

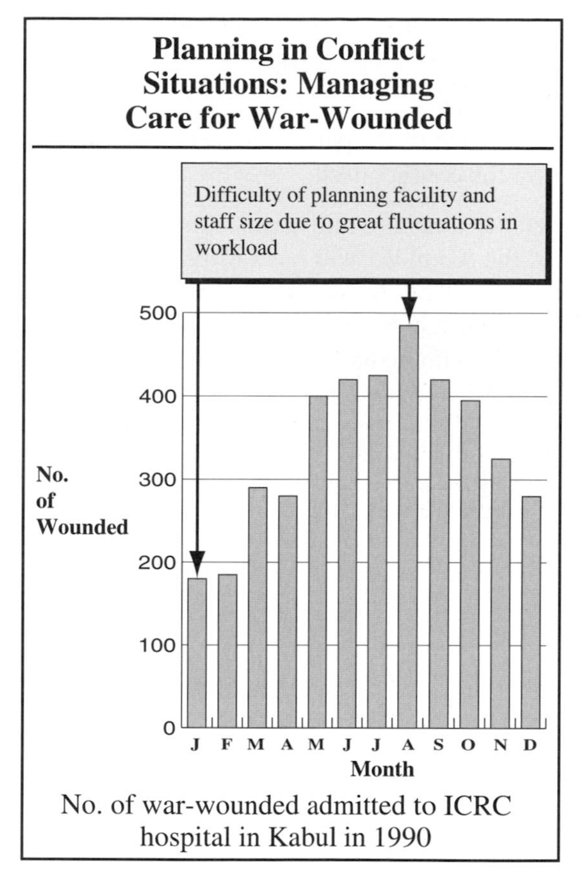


No. of war-wounded admitted to ICRC hospital in Kabul in 1990

## *War Situations*

It may seem obvious that the more intensive a combat is, the greater the number of people involved in it will be[52] and the greater the number of wounded. However, many other factors play a part as well: the degree to which combatants respect (or do not respect) the civilian population,[53] and the type of weapons used. Weapons now have greater blast effect and may cause delayed internal injury.

The interplay of these factors prevents a quantitative approach. Usually there is a tremendous flood of wounded for a few days, followed by variable periods of respite. The impossibility of anticipating the magnitude of needs influences the organization of surgical services, which must be prepared to work in spurts.

---

[50] Measured on the Richter scale.

[51] The degree of protection depends directly on the level of economic development. This subject will be discussed in Chapter 8 ("Disasters and Development").

[52] This means all persons involved in the conflict, whether directly (soldiers) or indirectly (civilian populations).

[53] Indiscriminate bombing of cities is an example of failure to respect the civilian population.

## 2. Handling the Wounded after Disasters or Wars

This section examines the specific problems of war surgery and managing the wounded (the techniques of war surgery are a specialized field).

### 2.1 First Aid

Conflict situations make speedy evacuation of wounded people difficult, owing mostly to:

- the geographical location of the conflict;
- the level of medical development of each of the parties to the conflict;
- security constraints deriving from the conflict itself.

If the fighting is in geographically remote areas and the parties to the conflict have only very minimal medical means, the wounded will have to be evacuated to hospitals behind the lines, often quite far from the combat zone. The increased time required for evacuation affects the condition of the wounded. For this reason, the quality of the first aid provided immediately or soon after the injury is essential to the patient's chances of survival.

Certain simple measures can be taken which in some cases will save lives, or limit further deterioration of injuries. Initially, rescuers must examine the wounded quickly to ascertain whether any of them are suffering from:

- an obstruction of the upper airways
- respiratory arrest
- cardiac arrest
- external bleeding
- thoracic injury

Once this has been done, certain basic actions can be taken on the spot:

- gathering up the injured
- evacuation of the injured on stretchers
- immobilization of broken bones
- compression to control bleeding
- clearing and protection of airways
- artificial respiration
- heart massage
- bandaging of wounds
- blood infusion
- antibiotic treatment
- sedation and pain relief
- prevention of tetanus

The decision as to which tasks can be performed on the scene of the injury will depend on:

- the rescue workers' level of training
- the sophistication of the equipment and materials at hand

**Generally speaking, first aid has an enormous impact on the survival rate of the wounded after a disaster or during an armed conflict.**[54]

## 2.2 Surgical Triage

Surgical "triage" can be defined as follows: "the process by which patients are sorted into categories according to the degree of severity of injury, such that PRIORITIES can be established in order to use the available facilities MOST EFFICIENTLY." [55]

"A disaster involves a large number of victims, and the disproportion between needs and immediately available means of treatment imposes a classification, a categorization, an act of triage." [56]

Triage is based on a combination of factors:

**a) Needs established on the basis of**

- the number of casualties
- the severity of the injuries
- the need for treatment

**b) The resources of the surgical unit to which the injured will be transferred from the sorting point**

- human resources
- material resources
  - operating rooms
  - surgical equipment

**c) Evacuation conditions**

- available means of transport
- duration of evacuation
- severity of the injury
- need for treatment

### *Practice of Triage*

When there is a flood of casualties, triage is the means of determining the order in which they will be evacuated to the surgical unit and the order in which they will be operated on. In this respect, two important points must be noted:

---

[54] "Early hospital admission for urgent surgery is not so important if there is adequate first aid beforehand". R. Coupland, "Epidemiological approch to surgical management of the casualties of war", *BMI*, vol. 308, 25 June 1994, p. 1683.

[55] Dufour *et al.*, *Surgery for Victims of War*, p. 27.

[56] R. Noto, P. Huguenard, and A. Larcan, *Médecine de catastrophe* (Ed. Masson, 1987), p. 239.

*Triage in the field must be carried out by experienced personnel, so that the real emergencies are evacuated first.*

Two pitfalls must be avoided here. First, no cases requiring emergency care should be delayed (triage sensitivity).[57] Second, non-urgent cases should not be evacuated, since they congest the surgical unit (triage specificity).[58]

*Triage must be a continuous process*

Initially, some of the wounded may be in stable condition, leading the triage team to postpone their evacuation to the surgical unit in favor of more urgent cases. However, the condition of some of these non-urgent cases may deteriorate, necessitating their immediate evacuation.

Practically speaking, this means that:

- in the triage area, those casualties who have already been classified should be re-examined periodically;
- in the hospital, those casualties initially set aside as not requiring immediate surgery should also be re-examined regularly.

There are a number of different methods for classifying the injured; the following system is given here as an example.[59]

| | |
|---|---|
| **Group T1:** | Lightly injured, able to manage for themselves. |
| **Group T2:** | Lightly injured, requiring assessment and treatment which can be provided on the spot or in the emergency room |
| **Group T3:** | Injured requiring assessment and surgical intervention. They can be subdivided into:<br>• Priority 1: cases requiring resuscitation and emergency treatment<br>• Priority 2: cases requiring early surgery<br>• Priority 3: cases requiring less urgent surgery |
| **Group T4:** | Wounded who will not survive their injuries |

57 Triage sensitivity: how well the triage detects the patients actually requiring care.
58 Triage specificity: how well the triage avoids the inclusion of non-emergency cases.
59 Dufour et al., Surgery for Victims of War, pp. 28-29.

## *Organizing Surgical Triage in the Field*[60]

### *Safety*

The spot chosen to sort the injured in the field should be reasonably safe.

### *Human Resources*

Triage is above all a decision-making process which demands experience on the part of those who assume this responsibility. The head of the team must not only be experienced, but must also exert a moral authority over the rest of the team so that his or her decisions will not be challenged. The decisions as to who does what should not be made in the field; all procedures and responsibilities should have been defined in advance in a contingency plan for receiving large numbers of casualties.

**Rules of Surgical Triage**

1. It must be carried out by competent and experienced personnel.
2. The most experienced person should be in complete control of the triage process.
3. Each member of the team should be responsible for a specific task.
4. Triage should conform to a system of categorization familiar to all the health-care personnel.
5. Triage is a continuous process: in the field, during evacuation, and at the hospital.
6. Measures should be taken to insure the safety of the wounded and the health-care personnel carrying out the triage.
7. The establishment of radio communications between the field and the facility of referral is essential to the success of the triage operation.

### *Material Resources*

Material resources are usually commensurate with the skill level of the triage team. They also depend on the remoteness of the scene of action and the conditions of evacuation (duration, types of transport, etc.). Equipment should be ready in advance so that triage teams lose no time during the emergency.

The injured should be "labeled" with standardized cards which are prepared in advance and familiar to all personnel, including the surgical unit.

### *Communication*

The establishment of a reliable channel of communication between the spot where the first triage is made and the surgical unit is indispensable in order to:

[60] Triage can also be used for medical and psychiatric cases.

- announce the arrival of casualties, their number, and the type of injuries;
- find out how many casualties the hospital can accommodate, and avoid sending too many at once, if the hospital is unable to care for them. Where several surgical units are available, the wounded can be channeled to one or another according to the material capacities of each.

## 2.3 Hospital Preparation

The second part of managing an influx of casualties is arranging for their reception by the surgical unit. In principle, the triage teams will have informed the latter of the imminent arrival of wounded, their number, and the type of injuries. At this point, the surgical unit will begin to implement its contingency plan for incoming casualties.

### *Contingency Plan for Incoming Casualties*

The contingency plan has several aspects.

#### *Preparing the Facility*

The hospital must be organized to receive an influx of casualties. The section designated for that purpose must be made operational immediately. The roads giving access to the hospital should be cleared to allow ambulances to pass.

#### *Preparing the Personnel*

The staff's duties in a situation of incoming casualties must be clearly defined in advance, so that no time is lost when the moment comes. The chief surgeon's job is to revise the operating schedule and to free beds occupied by patients who can be moved to other wards or facilities; the head nurse is usually responsible for supervising the preparation of equipment such as blood units, drugs, surgical supplies, etc. All the surgical staff should be in position, ready to assume the duties assigned to them. If preliminary information received from the triage team warrants it, reinforcements may be requested (off-duty personnel).

#### *Preparing the Equipment*

Every surgical unit should have emergency reserves permitting it to cope with large numbers of casualties, at least for a few days. This equipment must be prepared in advance, so that each type of item is immediately available. As at all levels of medical care, standardized equipment guarantees efficiency during emergencies.

#### *Preparing Medical Services*

A certain number of measures should be taken by the services directly involved in treating casualties. The operating bloc must be cleared and ready to go as soon as the first casualties arrive; the staff in charge of the blood bank must make sure that blood reserves are adequate. In wartime conditions, such as those in which the ICRC works, 25% of the wounded receive transfusions; each of them receives approximately three units of blood.

The intensive-care ward should transfer all patients whose condition permits to other wards. Beds should also be freed in other wards through the transfer of patients to departments that are not involved in emergencies, where their treatment can be continued. Similarly, other departments providing back-up services to the surgery department, notably the x-ray department and the laboratory, should be instructed to apply contingency procedures.

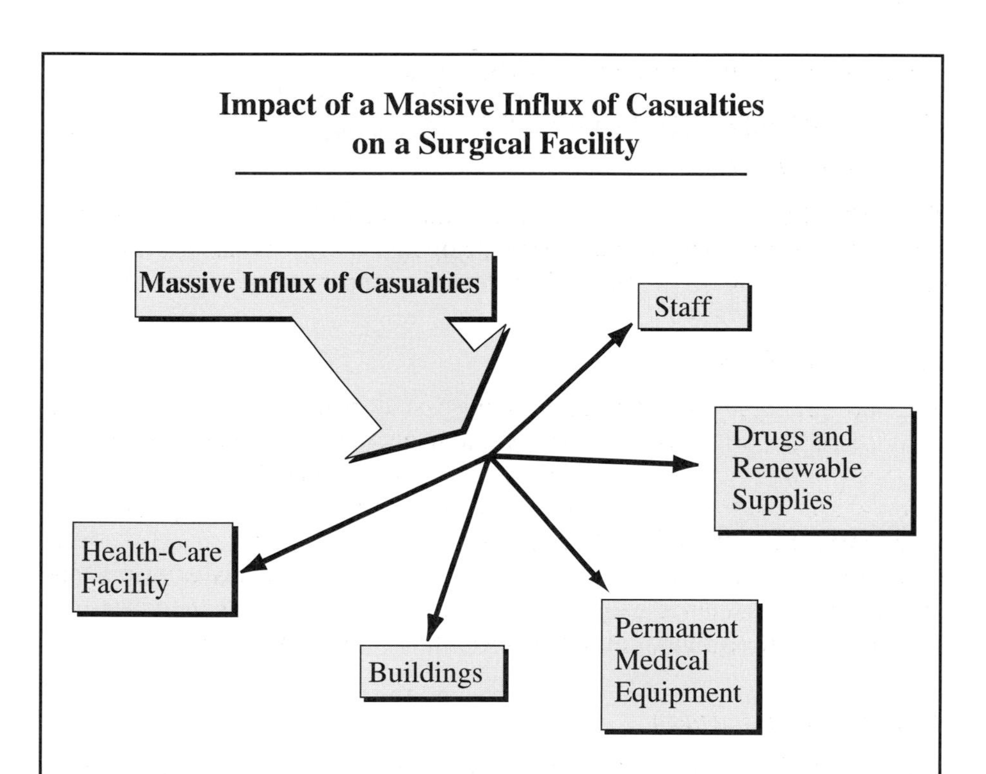


A contingency plan for this type of situation is required to:

- Give staff the capacity (number and skill) to treat the wounded
- Mobilize emergency stocks of supplies and drugs
- Free beds for urgent cases
- Prepare a triage area in the hospital.

### *Care of the Injured*

Casualty management within the hospital follows a specific procedure.

#### *Surgical Triage*

Upon arrival, the patients are all grouped together in the designated receiving area, which may be a platform at the entrance to the hospital, a tent, etc. If the triage team in the field have done their work well, each casualty will be accompanied by a medical chart (a simple, standard form) noting clinical signs, any treatment administered in the field, and the category of the injuries. The triage officer at the hospital must review these elements quickly and ascertain that the present condition of the patient conforms to the description on the chart. The condition of some of the patients may have deteriorated or improved during transport.

**The concept of constant review is important: it prevents the inadvertent neglect of patients whose condition has suddenly taken a turn for the worse.**

#### *Resuscitation*

Resuscitation is required for two major problems:

- asphyxiation due to:
  - airway obstruction
  - pneumothorax
  - hemothorax
- shock due to external or internal bleeding

#### *Surgical Procedures*

Another feature of wartime surgery is the type of lesions encountered, which necessitate a different therapeutic approach from that normally used. Wartime surgery requires a preliminary apprenticeship, for it has its own techniques.

The details of war-wound surgery are beyond the scope of this book; the main principles, however, are mentioned below:

- excision of wounds
- delayed primary closure
- early vascular repair
- judicious use of colostomy
- the avoidance of internal bone fixation

#### *Care in a Hospital Ward*

Hospital-ward care is the same as nursing care for ordinary surgery.

# 3. Institution of a Surgical Program in Wartime

## 3.1. Concept of the Chain of Care

Surgical care for the war-wounded is often restrictively equated with treatment by the surgical unit itself, or even by the operating theater alone. This highly reductionist view of the problem completely obscures the fact that the outcome of a surgical intervention depends on the functioning of a chain that begins with the first aid provided at the site of the injury, and ends with the rehabilitation measures designed to minimize a handicap. A chain is only as strong as its weakest link, the old saying goes — but as the cliché rightly indicates, operations to benefit the war-wounded must be conceived on a global scale.

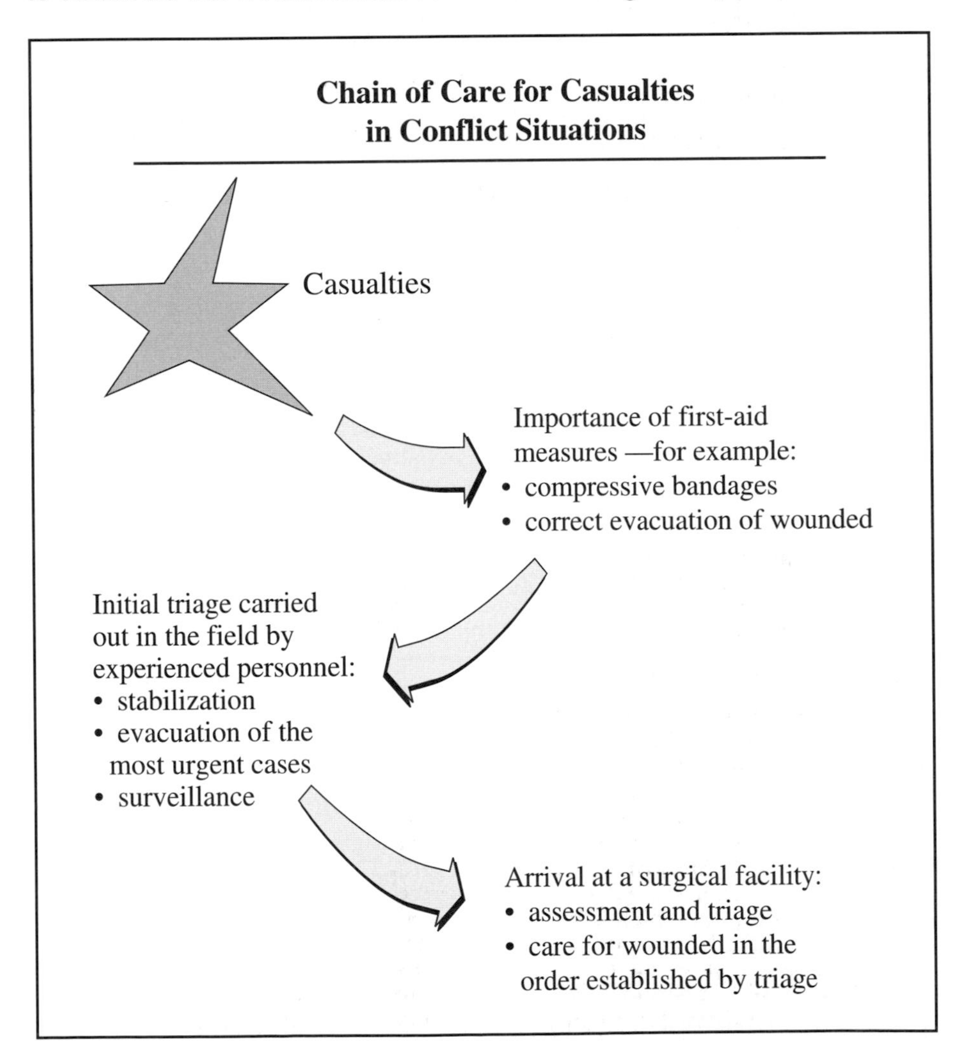

The absence or mediocrity of first aid will be reflected in:

- an increased number of deaths on the field of combat;
- an increased number of wounded who are suffering from shock (uncontrolled bleeding) when brought to the hospital;
- an increased number of infected wounds (if evacuation is slow).

The absence or mediocrity of an advance medical post and of means of medical transport will have the same effect.

The quality of surgical intervention definitely affects the survival rate of the most serious cases, as well as the degree to which a functional handicap can be reduced after the injury heals — that is, whether or not a hand, a limb, etc., can be used or not. In developing countries, where the mechanisms of mutual social aid do not facilitate reintegration into society, a handicap may doom its owner to begging for a living. Similarly, the quality of post-operative care is also essential to the survival of a certain number of casualties.

Consequently, when instituting a program to provide care for war-wounded, planners should take into account the possibilities and constraints involved at each link of the chain of care. In this way, the system set up will be coherent with the context in which it operates.

## 3.2 Autonomous Surgical Unit or Use of Existing Surgical Services?

In every situation involving war-wounded, the question arises whether to work with an autonomous surgical unit or to use existing surgical services. Making the right decision involves considering a whole set of parameters, such as the number of wounded, security, access to health-care services, and the quality of care. The procedure to follow is discussed in Chapter 7 ("The Health-Care System").

## 3.3 Level of Care

The level of care is conventionally defined in terms of a country's socioeconomic level. The facilities offered by the US army in Viet Nam, for example, have nothing in common with those of Angola, Ethiopia, etc.

The maximalist approach depends basically on the capacity to mobilize considerable resources in the form of personnel, logistic equipment (helicopters for evacuation, etc.), and so on. Only Western-type armies can afford this luxury.

The minimalist approach relies on the strict management of existing resources to achieve an optimal outcome with respect not only to survival, but also to functional recovery. Restrictions on logistic means and rapid access to the wounded, as well as the precariousness of the local surgical facilities, oblige relief agencies to think of the care chain in terms of its weakest link and to limit the triage criteria, among other adaptive responses.

### 3.4 Environment of a Surgical Unit

The establishment of a surgical facility must take the environment into account both physically (access to water and energy) and politically (security for both patients and staff).

# III. Rehabilitation of the Handicapped

## 1. Amputees

The use of anti-personnel mines, the frequently slow pace of evacuation, the ignorance of war surgery in the conventional surgical services — all help to explain the large number of amputees in evidence following armed conflicts.

Orthopedic appliances and aids should be constructed by means of a technique appropriate to the context. Factors to consider include:[61]

- the local availability of the primary materials necessary to fabricate prostheses;
- the possibility of procuring machines and basic tools locally;
- the availability of local technicians suitable for training;
- the nature of patients' wants in terms of the local economic and social context.

## 2. Paralytics

Although paralytics may be less common than amputees, their problem is much harder to comprehend. The construction of specialized centers satisfies immediate needs, but does not always solve the problem in the long run, especially in developing countries, where paralytics find social reintegration difficult.

## 3. Mental Trauma

Two groups of people are particularly vulnerable to mental trauma: the victims of a disaster and humanitarian workers.

[61] ICRC, *The International Committee of the Red Cross and the Disabled* (ICRC, 1986), p. 5.

### *Victims*

The causes of stress to victims are obvious — for example, the wait for aftershocks following the initial earthquake and the difficulties of daily life in the wake of a disaster (crowding, poor hygiene, the lack of elementary resources, etc.).[62] Refugee populations are particularly susceptible to psychosomatic complaints and psychological disturbances, owing to the disruption of their emotional, cultural, and economic environments, and to the feeling of being caught in an impasse. The material assistance provided to refugee populations is essential, but responsibility should not be taken away from the refugees; they must be allowed to make the decisions that will affect them. In conflict situations, stress factors are even greater: personal experience of traumatizing events, the persistence of danger, insecurity.[63] The effects of war have a particularly great impact on children.[64]

In war situations today, health services able to respond to psychological needs of this kind are frequently set up, so that despite adverse conditions, "mental health and psychiatric services have been maintained in many regions, and programs have been developed even under [...] conditions of war and economic difficulties."[65]

Those surgically triaged who are at greatest risk for mental health problems are those who have lost limbs, functions, or been deformed in some way.

### *Humanitarian Workers*

Humanitarian workers are often present during dramatic events such as bombings, faced with the sight of dead and injured people; they witness unbearable situations in which they are powerless, or are confided in by the victims of such horrifying violations of human rights as torture and rape. The resulting stress may manifest itself in three ways: "In increasing order of importance, basic stress, cumulative stress, including the specific stress

---

62 "Despite the widespread devastation, hope is generated from the expectation that the traumatic event is a temporary one." Frederick Burkle, "Neuropsychiatric Casualties" in F. Burkle, ed., *Disaster Medicine* (Medical Examination Publishing, 1984), p. 224.

63 "Of the 110 women interviewed, 87 had experienced traumatic events such as witnessing a murder, being tortured, threatened or humiliated by verbal abuse, injured as a result of political or miliary activity." M. McCallin, "Psychological Needs of Mozambican Refugees – A Community-Based Approach," *Tropical Doctor*, Supplement 1 (1991): 67.

64 "The psychological impact of war is harder to measure but cannot be overlooked. Witnessing atrocities committed against close relatives and scenes of plunder, being forcibly displaced and separated from one's family can cause either immediate or delayed changes in a child's psycho-social behaviour." *Children and War* (ICRC, 1994), p. 6.

65 Institute of Medicine/National Research Council, *The Impact of War on Child Health in the Countries of the Former Yugoslavia: A Report of the Workshop, March 27-30, 1994* (Washington, D.C.: National Academy Press, 1994), p. 30

associated with disasters, and traumatic stress."[66] Post-traumatic stress disorder (PTSD) merits special attention, owing to its seriousness: "This is a more serious condition, a complication of psychological stress, which could be compared to a wound that will not heal naturally."[67] PTSD is characterized by psychological disturbances and emotional reactions which appear after a certain period of latency following the traumatizing incident.

**Medical and surgical care are vital for the victims of emergency situations. Organizing such care requires attention to numerous parameters, ranging from political factors to locally available resources. Another imperative is that programs — and the tasks they comprise — be well-planned so that personnel will be effective at all levels of the care chain.**

[66] Barthold Bierens de Haan, "L'importance de la prévention du stress dans l'engagement humanitaire en zone de conflits: L'expérience du CICR," *Schweiz Z. Milit. Med.* 1995.72 (1): 6.

[67] *Humanitarian Action in Conflict Zones: Coping with Stress* (ICRC, Dec. 1994), p. 19.

Chapter 6

# EPIDEMIOLOGY

***This chapter will not attempt to cover all aspects of epidemiology, but will focus on those basic principles that are applicable in emergency situations. Accordingly, a general outline of epidemiology is provided here to identify the most commonly used epidemiological tools.***

# I. General Principles

Epidemiology encompasses the following:

1. information on health problems
2. identification of information sources
3. gathering of data
4. presentation of the data collected
5. statistical analysis of the data
6. synthesis of data
7. making decisions on the basis of the syntheses

### Concept of Epidemiology

The most commonly accepted definition of epidemiology is "the study of the distribution and determining factors of health problems[1] in the population as a whole and the application of this data to the control of these health problems." The study of the distribution of health problems is known as descriptive epidemiology, while the study of the causes of health problems is called analytical epidemiology.

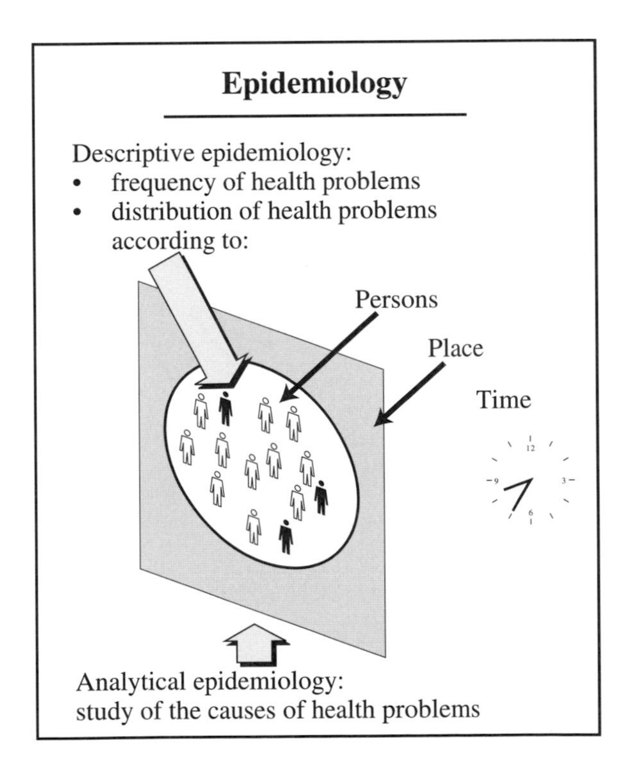


### Epidemiological Tools

- Definition of an indicator
- Criteria for selecting an indicator

[1] Epidemiology is not limited to the study of epidemics, but encompasses all health problems.

- Definition of incidence and prevalence
- Definition of the sensitivity, specificity, and positive predictive value of a test
- Relative risk and odds ratio
- Criteria for selecting a source of information
- Calculation of sample size
- Graphic tabulation with EPIINFO
- Definition of central tendency indices
- Definition of variability indices
- The chi-squared test
- The *t* test
- Definition of the *p* value

**Epidemiological Programs**

Epidemiological programs can be roughly divided into two categories:

- Epidemiological surveillance (routine systems)

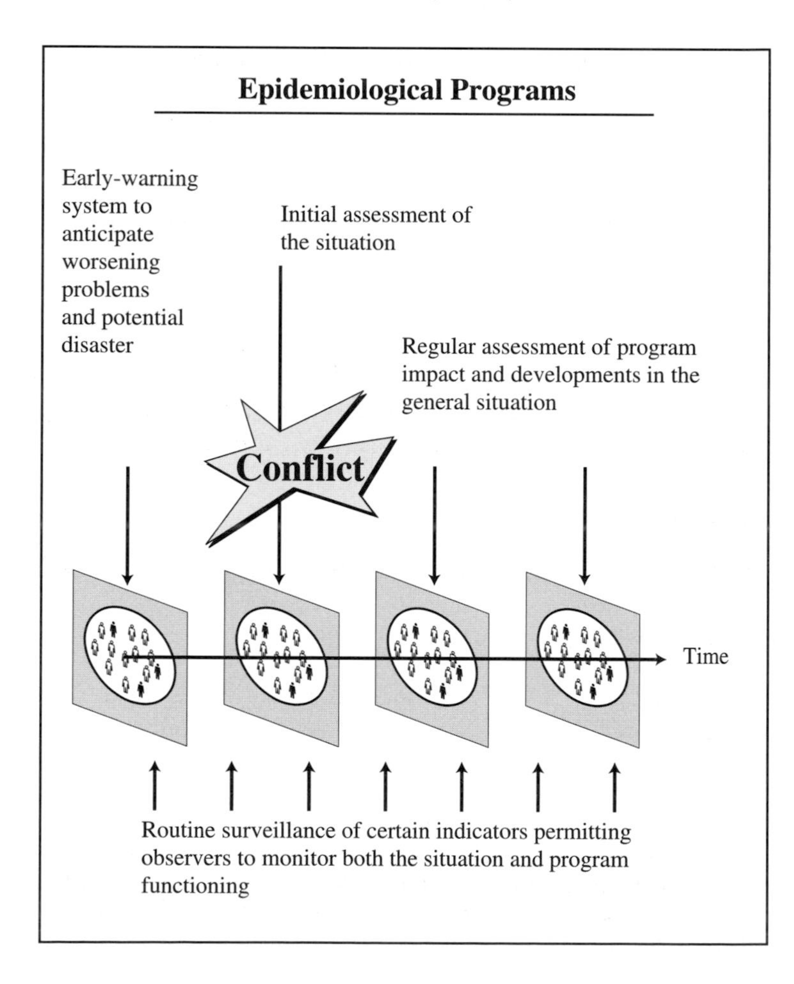

- regular surveillance of a health system
- early-warning systems

- Ad hoc investigations
  - initial assessment or survey
  - evaluation of an epidemic

# 1. Information on Health Problems

The list of information that can be assembled to follow the evolution of an emergency situation is particularly long. It is unrealistic to try to collect all the data possible, since that would require a great deal of time and a large staff, and the sheer volume of the data collected would make analysis difficult. The quest for information is best limited to certain health indicators, chosen for their relevance in describing a given situation or its evolution over time.

## 1.1 Indicators Directly Related to Health Status

Indicators directly related to health status are the following:

### *Mortality*

Disaster situations often involve very high mortality among the victims. Mortality rates are by far the most valuable indicator for measuring the impact of a relief operation.[2]

### *Morbidity*

Monitoring changes in morbidity allows epidemiologists to determine its main causes, to gauge the impact of preventive measures taken to benefit populations affected by a disaster, to sound the alarm when epidemics threaten, etc.

### *Nutritional Status*

Nutritional status is reflected by the rate of malnutrition and vitamin deficiencies.

## 1.2 Indicators Related to the Environment

Other indicators are related to the environment (in the broad sense). They can be subdivided as follows:

---

[2] "Death rates are the most specific indicators of the health status of a population; a community with high death rates cannot be deemed healthy." Michael Toole, "The Rapid Assessment of the Health Problems in Refugee and Displaced Populations," *Medicine and Global Survival* 1, No. 4 (Dec. 1994): 203.

### *The Condition of the Physical Environment*

- water resources
- housing
- climate

### *The Functioning of the Health-Care Services*

- number of consultations
- number of patients admitted to hospitals
- number of children immunized
- quality of the care provided

### *The Economic Environment*

An emergency situation should not be the cue to embark on a macroeconomic analysis of the country involved; at most, the country's economic profile may be sketched. A number of indicators can be used for this purpose which reflect the country's degree of dependence on the international economic environment.[3] On the local level, however, a microeconomic analysis of the mechanisms of access to food resources may be useful.

### *The Social Environment*

Dietary practices, the use of health services, and the physical environment all depend largely on the social context. These elements must be considered when the moment comes to choose the form that emergency relief will take. Social indicators, rarely quantified, are difficult to analyze, but remain relevant in an emergency situation.

### *The Political Environment*

In conflict situations, it is essential to consider indicators reflecting the political situation. Some political decisions have direct consequences for the victims' health status — for example, in the case of forced population displacements, or restrictions on access to food or medical services.

Having defined the type and number of indicators required, the epidemiologist must determine where the necessary data can be found.

---

[3] Including international aid, usually in bilateral form.

# 2. Sources of Information

Depending on the information sought, several sources are possible:

## 2.1 The Population

During the initial assessment, when the health services are not yet in a position to furnish precise data, the population itself is the only possible source of information. For the purposes of a surveillance system, however, it is still preferable to seek facts from the health services rather than the population, except in the case of research specifically concerning the latter.

## 2.2 The Administrative Services

The national ministries[4] and administrative services are good sources for socioeconomic and cultural data, censuses of the local population, etc.

## 2.3 The Community Health Services

Many health ministries run programs specifically oriented towards a particular problem, such as immunization, malaria control, diarrheal disease control, or tuberculosis control.

Information can be obtained not only on the characteristics of the country, but also on the policy followed in the areas mentioned above. This is particularly important, and means that a program to combat malaria within a refugee population, for example, can be coordinated with the local authorities.

## 2.4 The Health-Care Facilities

Health-care facilities (hospitals, clinics or dispensaries) are the best sources for data on morbidity (and, to some extent, on mortality). Medical files, consultation registers, and hospital admissions records are all sources of information.

## 2.5 The Humanitarian Agencies

When a surveillance system is set up at the beginning of a disaster, the voluntary agencies working in the area must be consulted for information on their activities. Depending on the relevance of their programs, this information may prove indispensable for a grasp of the development of the situation.

[4] The health ministry cannot be bypassed.

## 3. Collecting Data

Once epidemiologists have decided what information they want and where to find it, they must determine how to collect it: by going out to look for it, or by waiting for it to come to them.

If the population is the source, then the data must be sought in the field. If the source is the health-care services, for example, a system can be organized to transfer information regularly to the epidemiological center. In emergency situations, the following considerations will influence the choice of a data collection method:

- existence of a functional local system for data collection and analysis;
- time available for collecting data;
- physical access to sources of information;
- degree of reliability required;[5]
- necessity of establishing continuity in data collection.[6]

The volume of data to be collected for a given indicator raises the issue of sampling. To find out the level of malnutrition in a particular population, there is no need to examine all the children of a certain age group, since the results from a representative sample can be applied to all children of the age group selected.

The sampling method chosen will depend on such factors as geography (whether the population is widely dispersed or concentrated in one place). The size of the sample, too, depends on a group of factors: the degree of accuracy desired, the prevalence of the problem, and the confidence interval.[7]

## 4. Presentation of Results

The results obtained from a survey or by means of a surveillance system are difficult to interpret until they have been processed into a more digestible form. Converting them into percentages, rates, tables, and graphs facilitates the synthesis of data.

The way that results are to be presented will affect the way the data are collected. For example, if rates of anemia in a population are to be categorized by age groups, then age must be included in the data collected.

---

5 First-hand information is more reliable than second-hand.

6 The analysis of trends, based on the measurement of the same indicator at regular intervals, is often more instructive than the analysis of a single measurement.

7 These concepts are examined in detail later in the chapter.

# 5. Statistical Analysis of Results

The statistical analysis of data is based on the following concepts:

- data distribution
  - indices of central tendency
  - measures of variability
- sampling
- statistical comparison of the results for several populations:
  - relative risk
  - chi-squared test
  - comparison of two means (*t* test)
  - comparison of several means (variance analysis)
  - *p* value

The principles underlying these statistical procedures should be understood, but there is no need to demonstrate all the mathematical "machinery" by which they operate. At this point, epidemiology is above all a technical tool for obtaining a set of theoretically reliable and significant data concerning a particular population. However, compiling facts is useless unless those facts are to be interpreted and used as a basis for policy decisions.

# 6. Interpretation of the Results

Interpretation of the results begins with a systematic review to determine whether epidemiological tools have been properly used.

## 6.1 Critique of the Data Collecting Method

A good analysis requires reliable data.

- Were the indicators chosen relevant?
- Was the size of the sample adequate?
- Were the data recorded correctly?

## 6.2 Statistical Methods Used to Interpret the Data

- What confidence interval is used?
- What test is used?

# 7. Decision-Making

Epidemiologists can avoid relying on false data by following epidemiological procedures strictly; but just because the data are correct does not necessarily mean that the reasoning derived from them is correct. The facts must be critically interpreted within their context. For example, is a variation in the incidence of diarrheal diseases in a refugee camp due to a deterioration in hygiene in the camp, or is it a natural seasonal change? Is an increased malnutrition rate linked to inadequate feeding programs, or to the arrival of new refugees in the camp?

A study which is not followed up by policy decisions is a waste of resources and raises false hopes in the victims, since populations often consider a survey as the first step of an aid process. Accordingly, before launching any investigations, it is important to make sure that the people to be studied understand the study's goals and limits, and that whoever is commissioning the study has the means to act on the results.

The purpose of any inquiry is to provide the people concerned with the information they need to make decisions about the aid programs to be set up (initial assessment), about possible changes in a currently operating program, or about the measures to be taken in the case of an epidemic.

# II. Epidemiological Tools

Examining the tools of epidemiology in a few pages may seem an impossible task. A logical progression must be followed, each new stage using the concepts and terms studied in the previous stage.

## 1. Selecting Health Indicators

Health indicators are selected according to the following criteria.

- The indicator must be relevant to what the study is supposed to measure.
- The indicator can be precisely defined.
- The indicator can be analyzed in relation to other parameters.
- A test is available for the effective measurement of the indicator.

### 1.1 Relevance to the Factors to Be Measured

In situations where access to food is cut off, the rate of severe malnutrition should be measured as a way of assessing the urgency of the nutritional situation. This variable must be further refined, however; the aim must be to measure specifically the rate of severe, acute malnutrition of recent appearance, not the total rate, which includes both acute and chronic (associated with growth retardation) malnutrition.

### 1.2 Possibility of Defining the Indicator Precisely

Indicators must be defined precisely and unequivocally for data collectors in the field. Otherwise, there is a risk of combining, under a single label, data which have different meanings depending on their sources. For example, an episode of diarrhea may be precisely defined as "three liquid stools within a 24-hour period," while a malaria attack may be defined as "fever, chills, and headache," or else "fever with a positive malaria smear."

This clinical description, however, is not sufficient to characterize an indicator. Three more parameters must be added:

- *time*: On what date, or during what interval of time was the indicator recorded?
- *person*: What are the characteristics of the person for whom the indicator was recorded (age, sex, social group, etc.)? [8]
- *place*: Where was the indicator recorded (geographical area, name of dispensary)?

## 1.3 Possibility of Analyzing the Indicator in Relation to Other Parameters

For a specific health problem, a single indicator may turn out to be inadequate not only to describe the problem in question, but especially to permit a correct interpretation of the situation. If, for example, a famine is expected, efforts must be made to find out whether there is:

- a nutritional deficit;
- a food crisis;
- an agricultural crisis;
- an ecological crisis.

Anthropometric measurements allow epidemiologists to follow the development of a population's nutritional status and to detect any deterioration. If these are combined with the measurement of indicators reflecting access to food resources, a food crisis can be detected before it influences the population's nutritional status and the necessary measures can then be taken. Further back in the food chain, surveillance of agricultural activities will allow relief organizers to anticipate a crisis in access to food resources.

## 1.4 Availability of a Test Permitting Objective Measurement of a Given Indicator

Choosing a test is not as simple as it might appear. The following parameters must be taken into account:

[8] The word "person" is traditionally used in epidemiological manuals. Obviously, however, a health indicator may also correspond to objects, as in the study of the bacteria in a water source.

*Representativeness*

Representativeness is the concordance between the elements sought and those that the test actually finds. The indicators that may be chosen in an emergency are not necessarily the same that would be used in a normal situation. For example, the anthropometric measurements of weight for height and weight for age are used to detect conditions of severe malnutrition. Weight-for-height, however, is used to measure acute severe malnutrition, while weight-for-age can indicate both acute and chronic severe malnutrition. For this reason, the results obtained with the weight-for-age method are not representative of a problem of severe acute malnutrition which arises abruptly during a disaster.

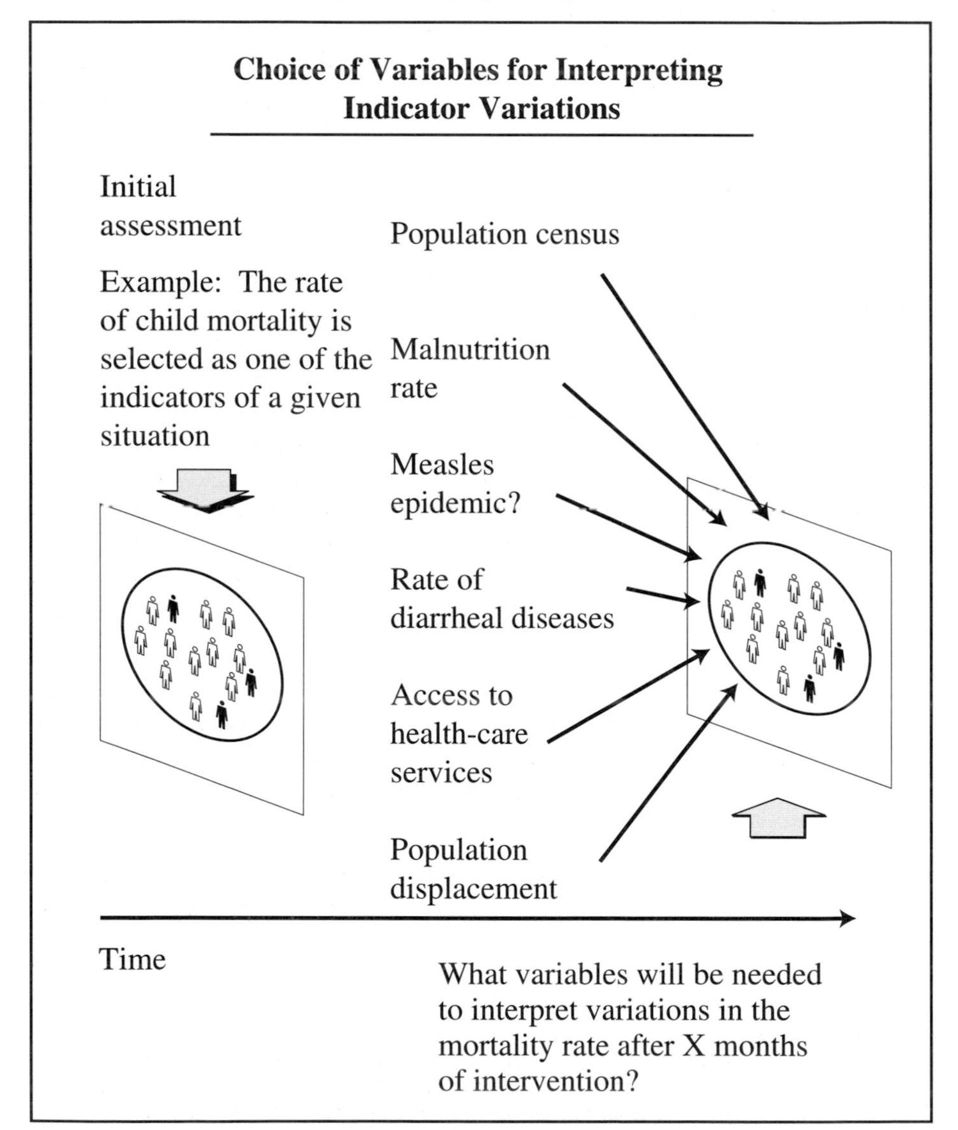

*Validity*

The validity of a test is characterized by two properties, sensitivity and specificity. *Sensitivity* is defined as "the proportion of true positives correctly identified by a test," while *specificity* is defined as "the proportion of true negatives correctly identified by a test."[9] The *positive predictive value* (PPV) of a test expresses the probability that an individual declared positive by the test actually has the disease.

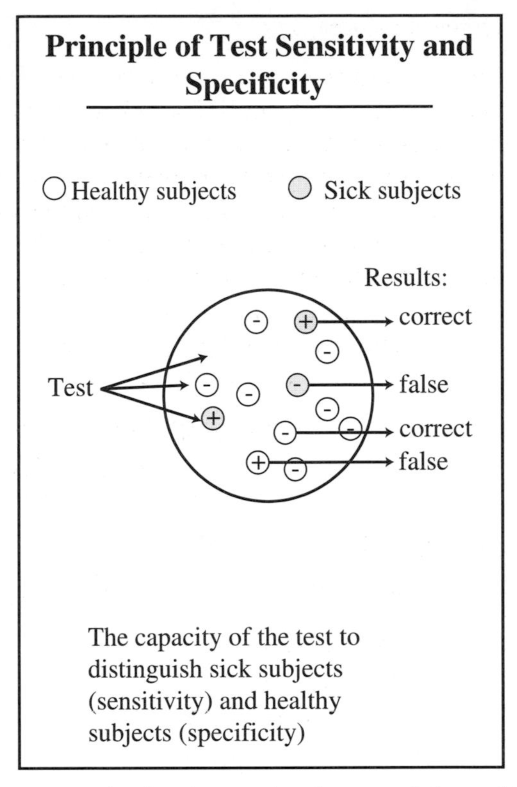


The capacity of the test to distinguish sick subjects (sensitivity) and healthy subjects (specificity)

*Implications for Emergency Situations*

In a region heavily infested with malaria, there is a danger that anyone showing up at the local clinic with a headache will be considered to be suffering an attack of malaria, if the indicator sought is the patient's complaint of "headaches." For greater exactitude, a more specific indicator must be used, such as fever (measured with a thermometer) and a positive blood test (analyzed in the laboratory).[10] The first indicator covers most cases of malaria and is therefore highly sensitive, but a number of cases thereby labeled as "malaria" are not actually malaria, meaning that this indicator has a weak positive predictive value.

If fever (temperature higher than 37.5°C) is taken as an indicator, the tendency will be towards a reduction of the proportion of negative cases labeled as positive by the first indicator (better specificity). At the same time, however, sensitivity will decline, in that a large proportion of genuine malaria cases will be labeled as not having the disease.

A test's positive predictive value varies according to the proportion of the selected indicator in the population. If the proportion of cases in the population is weak,

---

9 S.K. Lwanga and Cho-Yook Tye, *Teaching Health Statistics* (Geneva: WHO, 1986), p. 16.

10 The results of such a test can be accepted as fairly conclusive, although the fact that no parasites are detected in a microscopic examination does not formally rule out malarial infection.

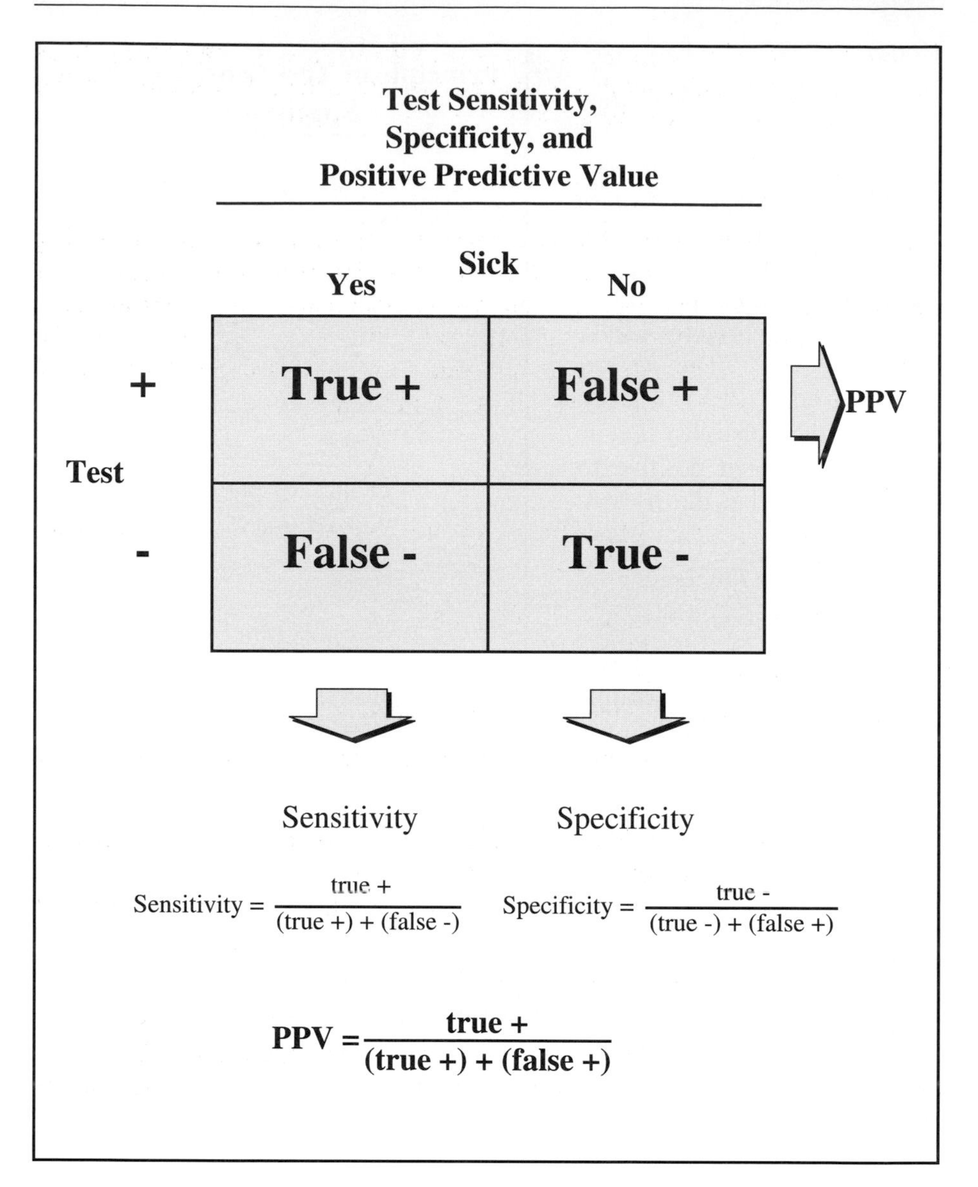


there is a high risk of attributing the indicator to subjects who are negative for the condition sought (weak PPV). Moreover, the prevalence of the condition sought changes after intervention takes place. Sensitivity and specificity may no longer correspond to original expectations. In this case, a different test may be needed.[11]

[11] C. Paquet and T. Ancelle, *Sensibilité et spécificité du CATT-test dans le dépistage de la trypanosomiase. Application à la situation du district de Moyo, Ouganda* (Epicentre/MSF, 1992).

In an emergency situation, the tendency is to try to treat as many subjects as possible by reducing the number of true positive cases tagged as negative by the test. This orientation gives sensitivity priority over specificity.

### *Standardization*

Except in cases of changed prevalence, as mentioned above, the same measuring method should be used for a given indicator so that data from different sources or collected at different times can be compared. The fact that humanitarian agencies work with different indicators and measurement tests does not favor the exchange of information. Similarly, humanitarian agencies should take note of the locally used methods and determine to what extent they should be used.

### *Reliability*

Reliability is defined as the capacity to furnish uniform results. The main elements influencing reliability are:

- variations in the measuring instrument itself;
- variations in the thing measured;
- variations in the observer;
- variations involving differences between observers.[12]

Several elements influence the reliability of the measures used in emergency situations:

- frequent changes in the expatriate health-care personnel, since that increases the risk of variations between different observers;
- rapid training of local personnel to perform simple tasks, increasing the risk of carelessness;
- lack of time to plan and execute measuring activities.

Simple tests are preferable, since although they may be scientifically less precise, they are also less apt to be vitiated by gross errors in application. To reduce distortions in the results, the procedures for applying the tests should be explained repeatedly.

### *Applicability*

A test's applicability means the ability to perform it.[13] In emergency situations, the lack of time and access to potential sources of information limit the choice of

---

[12] Lwanga and Tye, *Teaching Health Statistics*, p. 15.

[13] "Applicability is defined by:
- the test's acceptability to the population;
- cost;
- practical, logistic, and technological aspects." A. Rougemont and E. Brenner, "Evaluation epidémiologique," in Rougemont and Brunet-Jailly, eds., *La santé dans les pays tropicaux* (1989), p. 507.

indicators or else reduce their value, since they are thereby subject to distortions. Moreover, the available technical facilities are often limited. Therefore, relief teams must settle for simple indicators.

The selection of indicators is an important point, since it is a job that the health-care personnel out in the field are usually obliged to perform in order to monitor the progress of a relief operation. In the initial assessment of an emergency situation, a limited number of indicators are employed — enough to define the problems rapidly, but not always enough to monitor their evolution.

Accordingly, when a routine surveillance system is instituted, the choice of indicators must be fine-tuned to provide a better picture of the changing situation.

**Qualities Required in a Test or Data-Collecting Method for Emergency Situations**

Traditional qualities:

- Representativeness
- Validity
- Reliability

Qualities more specific to emergencies:

- Applicability
  - speed
  - simplicity
  - reproducibility
- Acceptability:
  - by the population
  - by the authorities

# 2. Criteria for Choosing Sources of Information

## 2.1 Quality of an Information Source

### *Quality of Information*

Information must be complete; data on cases of diarrhea or measles are hard to interpret if they are not linked to the age of the subjects.

### *Continuity*

While initial assessments tend to give a picture of the situation at a given moment, the purpose of surveillance is to juxtapose a succession of pictures in order to analyze the evolution, or trend, of a health problem. Information sources which send in data only half the time, for example, impede this kind of analysis.

*Uniformity*

All information sources must respect the same criteria for defining the indicators and the tests used.

## 2.2 Improving the Reliability of Information Sources

*Training*

Adequate training of the personnel commissioned to collect data and convey them to analysis centers is essential if quality information is to be obtained.

*Availability of Simple, Effective Means*

The danger of false, incomplete data increases with the complexity of the questionnaires that health-care personnel must fill out. Thus, it is preferable to make a correct analysis based on simple facts rather than to base the analysis on complex but false information. The use of computer programs (EPIINFO) to construct questionnaires is a quick and effective solution — provided you know how to run a computer program!

*Personnel Motivation*

Training helps motivate the staff, since it clarifies the purpose of collecting the data. Personnel should be informed of the results of analyses made on the basis of the data they collected, so that they will realize the significance of their daily work.

# 3. Presentation of Data

The way in which data are presented is important, and must answer two criteria:

- it must obey epidemiological norms;
- it must be clear enough so that decision-makers can interpret the data quickly.

## 3.1 Incidence and Prevalence

The *incidence* of a disease is the number of cases occurring during a given period of time, while the *prevalence* of a disease is the number of cases present at a particular moment or period.

The concept of incidence is important in the investigation of an epidemic, for the number of new cases per unit of time (days, weeks) gives some idea of the spread of the disease. The concept of prevalence is important for diseases of long duration, such as tuberculosis. It indicates the total number of patients during a given period (new cases plus cases that began before the period studied but which continue to develop during that period).[14] In the presentation of results, care should be taken to distinguish between incidence and prevalence.

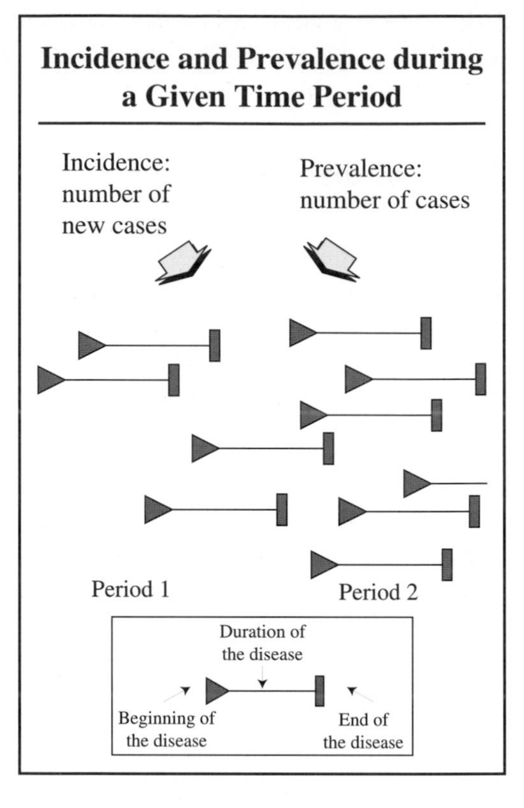


## 3.2 Rates

No conclusions can be drawn from the mere knowledge that there are 200 malnourished children in a particular population. This fact must be expressed in the form of a rate, defined by a numerator (the number of malnourished children) and a denominator (the total number of children in the age group examined). The significance of the malnutrition rate will vary depending on whether it is 400/5,000 (4%) or 200/1,000 (20%).

The rates most commonly used in emergency situations are:

- the mortality rate
- the malnutrition rate
- the rate of incidence of the most common diseases.[15]

Percentages are also used to describe the utilization of health services, as in the rate of occupation for hospital beds, or the rate of immunization coverage.

### *Difficulties in Emergency Situations*

In emergency situations, it is often difficult to determine the denominator, especially in widely dispersed, mobile populations. This problem is compounded by political manipulations reflected in the exaggeration or minimization of the estimated number of victims. Determining the numerator is hardly an easier task,

---

14 Prevalence depends on the incidence and duration of the disease (P = ID).

15 "It is not sufficient to know how much sickness is occurring and who are affected. The study will be much more meaningful if done in relation with the a) extent of impairment of bodily function, b) threat to life, c) extent of impairment of mobility, d) cost of burden or care of the sickness, and e) amount of pain produced." Remigio Mercado, *Biostatistics for the Health Administrator* (University of the Philippines, College of Public Health, 1990), p. 58.

given the unreliability of information sources; it is difficult to obtain exact estimations of the incidence of communicable diseases, the number of deaths, and other data.

### *Distribution of Data*

As mentioned previously, indicators must be defined in terms of three characteristic parameters: person, time, and space. The importance of this is reflected in the presentation of data, which shows the characteristics of the people studied (age, sex, ethnic group, social group), the time of data collection (season), and the geographical area (rural zone, urban zone, etc.). These elements provide the basis for calculating specific rates for certain population groups, such as:

- the mortality rate for children under one year of age;
- the mortality rate for children between the ages of one and five;
- the incidence of measles in children under nine months of age;
- the incidence of diarrheal diseases during the rainy season;
- the prevalence of tuberculosis in a nomadic population.

Different parameters can be combined as well — for example, the rate of child mortality in a rural environment, or the rate of malnutrition in female children under the age of five during the rainy season.

Thus, the evaluator can compare the results obtained according to specific categories defined by one or more characteristics, and determine whether there are any significant differences between them. This sort of analysis reveals which groups are most affected, so that priorities for action can be oriented accordingly.

For results to be comparable, the same denominator must be used for all the categories of people analyzed (for example, 1,000 as the denominator for mortality rates).

## 3.3 Graphic Presentation

A good graph is often more explicit than a five-page report. But it must include the components necessary to understand it — namely, the characteristics of persons, time, and place, and a definition of the indicator used.

Computer programs such as EPIINFO, Harvard Graphics, and Lotus facilitate the creation of graphic aids in such forms as:

- tables
- pie charts
- histograms
- scatter diagrams.

# 4. Statistical Analysis

Statistical analysis is often associated with epidemiology. Care must be taken, however, to avoid the pitfall of focusing on the mathematical foundations underlying the principles.

Statistical tools can be divided into three groups, depending on whether they relate to:

- data distribution
- sampling for data collection
- statistical analysis of data.

**Principal Causes of Mortality in Children under Five at the Khron Hospital in December, 1994**

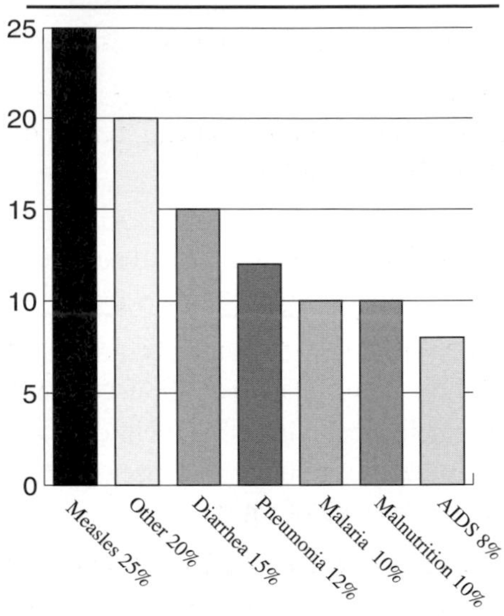

25
20
15
10
5
0
Measles 25%
Other 20%
Diarrhea 15%
Pneumonia 12%
Malaria 10%
Malnutrition 10%
AIDS 8%

## 4.1 Tools Relating to Data Distribution

The previous section showed the importance of characteristics in data distribution: persons, place, etc. Data distribution involves entire population groups which will subsequently be compared with each other.[16]

A way must be found of *distributing* individual data within each population group, to facilitate comparison between them. For a given population, the procedure is first to calculate the indices of central tendency (means), and then to establish the distribution of all the individuals in that population around the mean (index of dispersion). This, then, represents an individual distribution of data, as opposed to the distribution by population group studied previously.

On the basis of these indices, comparisons can be made using tests adapted to the data-collection method (significance tests).

### *Measures of Central Tendency*

Central tendency is calculated in the form of a mean. It defines the median axis around which are gathered the set of individual values in the population studied.

- The arithmetic *mean* (or average) of a set of observations is the sum of all the observations divided by the total number of observations.

[16] The method of paired comparisons, which consists in comparing matched series, will not be discussed here, since it is rarely used in emergency situations.

- The *median* of a set of observations is the value located "physically" in the middle of the set.
- The *mode* is the value that occurs most frequently in a set of observations.

*Applications in Emergency Situations*

Emergency situations are no different from normal situations as regards choosing an index of central tendency. The arithmetic mean is the most commonly used measure.[17]

## *Distribution Curve*

If all the individual values for a given population are represented on a graph, the result is the classic or "normal" distribution curve (Gaussian curve), with the arithmetic mean as its center. The individual values will be distributed around the mean, spreading out more or less in relation to the latter.

## *Measures of Variability*

In a given population, each individual value will be a different distance from the mean. On the basis of this fact, the degree to which these values vary from the mean can be determined by calculations of various kinds, ranging from the simplest to the most complex.[18] The basic measures of variability are:

- *the mean deviation*: the sum of the individual deviations (ignoring negative or positive signs) divided by the number of observations;
- *the variance*: the sum of the squares of individual deviations divided by the number of observations;[19]
- *the standard deviation:* the square root of the variance.[20]

Calculating the standard deviation is pointless unless it will lead to practical applications. The mean and the standard deviation represented on a Gaussian curve produce the following result:

- 68% of the individual values are situated within the limits constituted by the mean and $\pm 1$ standard deviation.
- 96% of the individual values are situated within the limits constituted by the mean and $\pm 2$ standard deviations.

---

[17] "The chief advantage of the arithmetic average is its amenability to mathematical treatment." Theodore Colton, *Statistics in Medicine* (Boston: Little, Brown and Company, 1974), p. 29.

[18] The *range*, which is the difference between the highest value and the lowest value, is seldom used.

[19] When population samples are used, the variance is the sum of the squares of the individual deviations, divided by the total number of values minus 1.

[20] The expression of the standard deviation in the form of the square root of the variance will produce the same units as the initial values.

If we take the example of the birth weights of a group of children where the arithmetic mean is 3 kilos and the standard deviation is 400 grams, 95% of the birth weights can be assumed to fall between 2.2 kilos and 3.8 kilos.

*Implications for Emergency Situations*

The standard deviation is the measure of variability most commonly used. The method of calculating the standard deviation should be properly understood, even though the EPIINFO computer program performs it automatically.

## *Measures of Comparison*

By comparing the values for two different populations, an evaluator can perceive possible differences between the two. Comparing raw data is useless; they can only be compared as rates or percentages (same denominator).

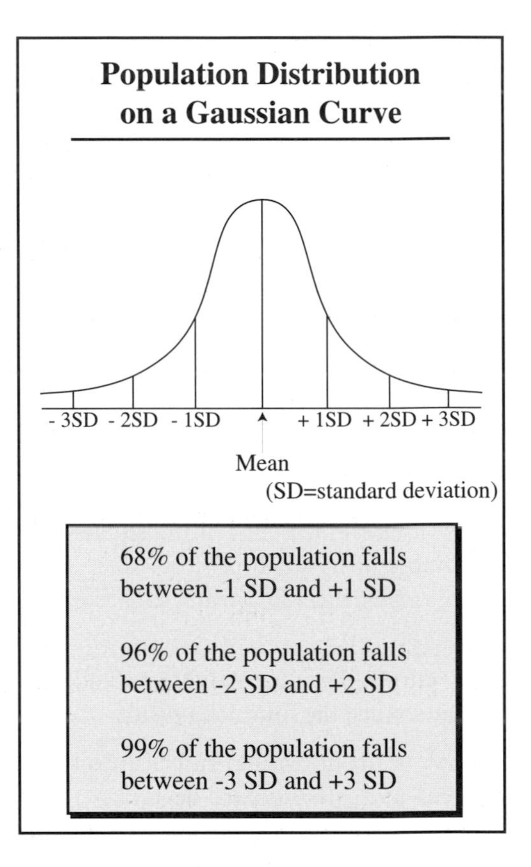


**Relative Risk**

Relative risk is a useful concept in analysis, since it is the ratio between the rates of a variable measured in two populations, in one of which the variable presents a risk. For example, in area A, the incidence of diarrheal diseases in children under the age of five is 12%, while it is 4% in area B. The relative risk is the relation between the two rates; in this case, population A has three times the probability of diarrheal diseases as population B. If the relative risk is close to 1, there is essentially no difference between the two populations. The measure of relative risk applies in particular to cohorts.

**Odds Ratio**

The odds ratio is based on the same principle. It is the ratio between the probability that a subject has been exposed to a risk factor and the probability that a control has been exposed to it. This test is used for controlled, unpaired studies, and is applied when a variable is measured for an entire population. Since an epidemiological investigation cannot usually be carried out on an entire population due to the constraints of time, cost, etc., it is common to use sampling techniques. In this case, the measures of comparison must take into account the errors inherent in the sampling process.

## 4.2 Sampling Tools

To be considered representative, a sample must adhere to the rule that "at the outset, all the subjects composing the target population must have the same probability of being included in the sample."[21]

### *Types of Sampling*

Various sampling methods are possible.

- *Simple random sampling*: For example, a number is given to each individual, and then the numbers are chosen at random by means of a random number table.
- *Stratified random sampling*: The population to be studied is first divided into groups according to certain characteristics: sex, area of residence, etc. Within each group, simple random sampling is carried out.
- *Systematic sampling*: Starting with an initial, randomly chosen unit, subsequent units are selected by adding a certain number to the first unit (10, 20, 50, depending on the size of the sample relative to the total population).
- *Cluster sampling*: The population is considered as a set of collective units, or *clusters*, chosen at random, after which all the subjects in these clusters are examined. This is the method that has been adopted for evaluating EPI coverage. In this application, it was calculated that 30 clusters were necessary, and that, in each cluster, it was sufficient to examine 7 children.[22] The geographical location of the clusters is determined on the basis of the sampling interval[23] and the cumulative list of the population present in each geographical location or area.

A sampling frame must be constructed for each of these methods. The sampling frame may consist in a list of all subjects (simple random sampling, systematic sampling), a list of all subjects by strata (stratified sampling), or a list of all the clusters (cluster sampling).

---

21 A. Rougemont and E. Brenner, "Evaluation epidémiologique," in Rougemont and Brunet-Jailly, eds., *La santé dans les pays tropicaux*, p. 483.

22 R.H. Henderson and T. Sundaresan, "Cluster Sampling to Assess Immunization Coverage: A Review of Experience with a Simplified Sampling Method," *Bulletin of the World Health Organization* 60, No. 2 (1982): 253-260.

23 The sampling interval is calculated by dividing the total population by the number of clusters provided for in the sample.

The choice between the different sampling methods will depend on various considerations:

- *geographical distribution of the population* — In a displaced-person camp where an entire, homogeneous population is concentrated in a restricted space, simple random sampling is adequate. If the population comprises subgroups with different characteristics (for example, ethnic or regional origin, date of arrival in the camp), stratified sampling is the method of choice. If small population groups are scattered over large areas, then cluster sampling is preferable.
- *cost of the evaluation* – In the case of widely dispersed populations, cluster sampling is less costly than other sampling methods, since it involves less moving around.
- *degree of accuracy* – Cluster sampling is statistically less precise than the other sampling methods.
- *constraints inherent in emergency situations* — The sampling method should take account of such constraints as lack of time, lack of qualified personnel, and lack of access to all the population groups affected by the emergency.

All this means that implementing correct sampling methods is often difficult in an emergency situation. The constraints involved give rise to distortions in the selection of subjects. If the purpose of the survey is to obtain some estimate, even a rough one, of mortality, morbidity, or malnutrition rates, the epidemiologist should take these distortions into account when analyzing the data.

### Sample Size

A sample should be as large as possible to reduce sampling errors to the minimum; it should be as small as possible to reduce the investment of operational resources to the minimum. In deciding on the right size for a sample, investigators must respect certain basic principles.

- *The concept of sampling error:* Where the entire population is surveyed and the mean is calculated, the result obtained is the true value of the mean (Xp). If, instead, sampling is employed and the mean (Xe) is calculated from the data collected from the sample, the value obtained will deviate more or less from the true mean. If the sampling process is repeated, each time with the same number of subjects, each time a mean ($Xe_1$, $Xe_2$, $Xe_3$, etc.) will be obtained that deviates $\pm$ from the true mean (Xp).

  If all the values $Xe_1$, $Xe_2$, $Xe_3$, and so forth are values representing individuals and arranged in a distribution pattern, the latter will have three main properties:[24]

[24] Colton, *Statistics in Medicine*, p. 101.

1. The mean (XE) obtained from the means of a series of identical samples is equal to the true mean (calculated on the basis of the entire population).
2. The standard deviation between the mean XE and the mean of each sample ($Xe_1$, $Xe_2$, etc.) is called the standard error.[25]
3. The distribution curve of the means $Xe_1$, $Xe_2$, etc., is a normal distribution curve.

It can be stated that 96% of the means found for a set of samples of identical size will fall between the value of the true mean and $\pm 2$ standard errors.

- *The confidence level:*
  Turning this reasoning around, it can be said that there is a 96% chance that the mean obtained from ONE sample will fall somewhere between $\pm 2$ standard errors and the true mean. In general, this reasoning works as follows:

**Distribution of Means of Repeated Samples Taken within the Same Population**

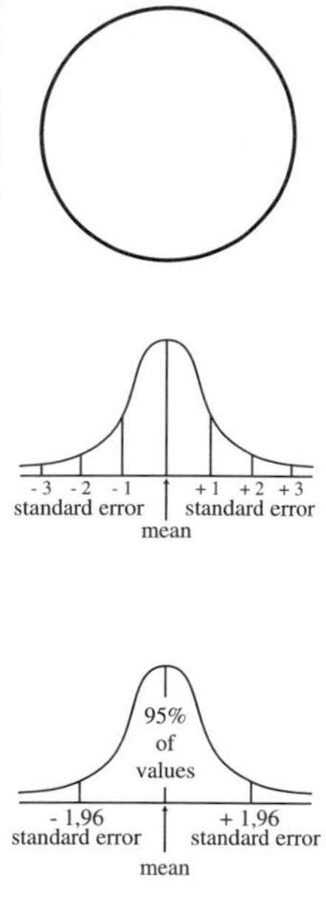


The average of the means found in repeated samples of the same population is equal to the true mean

The means found in successive samples follow a normal distribution curve and deviate from the true mean by the standard error

95% of the values found in successive samples in the same population fall between +1.96 and -1.96 standard errors

With a 95%[26] probability, the value found is sure to fall between $\pm 1.96$ standard errors relative to the true mean, or, from a pessimist's point of view, there will be a 5% risk that the value found in the sample will deviate by more than two standard errors from the true value (*x* errors). The formula $1.96 = z$ (where $z$ is the number of standard errors between the true mean and the sample mean) is important to remember, for it appears in numerous statistical calculations.

- *Confidence limits*:
  The confidence limits are equivalent to the degree of accuracy. This corresponds to the acceptable number of standard errors multiplied by the standard error itself: $d = z \times SE$. Since *SE* is unknown,

[25] The standard error is calculated as follows:

$$\text{Standard error} = \frac{\text{standard deviation (estimated by sample)}}{\text{square root of the size of the sample}}$$

[26] Values under 95% are not normally taken, but 99% can be taken as a confidence level. In this case, the number of standard errors must be altered (2.54 for 99%).

the global value of $d$ is estimated — that is, the sample must be large enough so that at 95% the value found by sampling is sure to fall $\pm d$ from the true mean.

- *Value of the variable:*
  The last concept involved in calculating sample size is the value of the variable sought. Since this value is unknown, it is estimated on the basis of previous data. If this cannot be done, for instance when the variable is a percentage, it is estimated at 50%.

### *Formulas for Calculating Sample Size*

A prerequisite[27] for calculating sample size is to determine:

- the confidence level — generally 95%, which gives a value of $z = 1.96$.[28]
- the degree of precision sought — expressed as $d$, which is the product of $z$ (x) SE. The smaller we want the standard error to be, the bigger the sample size must be.
- the value of the percentage sought.

The elements needed to calculate the size of a sample[29] are obtained as follows.

1. *Size of a sample to estimate a mean* in the framework of a random sample of an infinite population.

$$n = \frac{z^2 \,(x)\, \mathrm{SD}^2}{d^2}$$

For a sample of $n$ size, it is 95% certain that the value of the mean will fall between the established confidence limits.

2. *Size of a sample to estimate a proportion*[30] in the framework of a random sample for an infinite population.

---

27 These prerequisites are based on the following equation: the maximum value of the difference between the mean found in the sample and the true mean corresponds to the degree of precision established for the study. This value, d, is equal to z times the standard error (SE), or $d = z\,(x)\,\mathrm{SE}$. The standard error is equal to the ratio between the standard deviation (SD) and the square root of the sample size ($n$), or $\mathrm{SE} = \mathrm{SD}/\sqrt{n}$. Thus, $d = z\,(x)\,\mathrm{SD}/\sqrt{n}$

$$n = \frac{z^2 \,(x)\, \mathrm{SD}^2}{d^2}$$

28 This value can be rounded up to 2. Since $z$ will be part of the numerator of the formula for calculating the size of a sample, the size will be slightly increased — which helps rather than hurts.

29 According to Lwanga and Tye, "Estimating Population Values," in *Teaching Health Statistics,* pp. 68-70.

30 Proportions in the framework of a sample to study a proportion $p$ of subjects with the characteristic sought, in relation to the proportion $q$ (since they are proportions, $q = 1 - p$) of subjects who do not have that characteristic. In this case, the standard error is equal to the square root of the complex $pq/n$. The value of this proportion is unknown and must be estimated, although logical minds have trouble accepting the idea that the value to be calculated must be estimated in advance. If we have no idea of the value of $p$, we can take as our estimate $p = 50\%$, a figure which gives $pq$ its maximal value (0.25). Since this value is part of the numerator in the following formula, it gives the sample size its maximal value as well, taking into account accuracy and the confidence limits established.

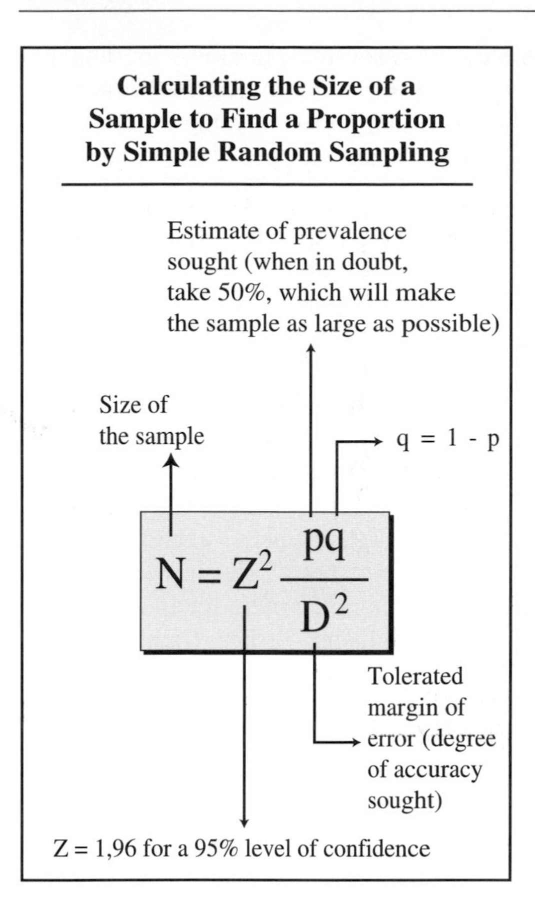


$$n = \frac{z^2 (x)\, pq}{d^2}$$

3. *Size of a sample from a finite population*[31]

$$nf = \frac{ni}{\dfrac{1+\text{ni}}{\text{N}}}$$

in which: $nf$ = the size of the sample of the finite population, and $ni$ = the size of the sample of an infinite population.[32]

4. *Size of a sample in cluster sampling* — Cluster sampling is used in particular for EPIs, to determine the percentage of children who have been immunized. In this case, then, sampling is oriented towards proportions. With a simple random sample and the following goals:

- proportion sought: 50%
- degree of accuracy: 10%
- confidence level: 95%

the result will be a sample size of 96.

---

[31] This is based on the following two formulas. For means:

$$\text{n} = \frac{z^2 (x)\, s^2}{\dfrac{d^2 (+)\, z^2 s^2}{\text{N}}}$$

For proportions:

$$\text{n} = \frac{z^2 (x)\, pq}{\dfrac{d^2 + z^2 pq}{\text{N}}}$$

[32] The size of a sample for an infinite population may be calculated with the formulas studied above, with due consideration to the parameters of accuracy and confidence. The value found will serve next for the calculation of the size of a sample representing a finite population.

Cluster sampling is known to be less accurate than simple random sampling, but this disadvantage can be offset by increasing the size of the sample. Experience has shown that doubling the sample size necessary for simple random sampling is sufficient to compensate for the statistical approximativeness inherent in cluster sampling.[33]

**Planning Procedure for Cluster Sampling**

1. Determine the size of the sample by using the same formula as for random sampling:

$$N = Z^2 \frac{pq}{D^2}$$

NOTE: The result must be multiplied by 2.

2. Determine the number of clusters — there should be at least 30.
3. Determine the size of each cluster by dividing the total size of the sample by the number of clusters.
4. Determine the geographical location of each cluster.

In the case given above, the size of the sample in cluster sampling would be 96 x 2 = 192. The minimum number of clusters must be 30. The size of the population from which the sample is drawn is in fact not very important, and it may not even be known. For a given sample size, it is better to choose a large number of clusters and a small number of individuals in each cluster rather than the contrary.[34] In our example, 7 children (6.4 rounded off to 7) will be examined in each cluster, giving a final total of 210 children.[35]

Let us take the example of measuring the prevalence of malnutrition in famine-stricken areas, with the following parameters:

- confidence level = 95%;
- estimated prevalence of < 80% weight-for-height = 20%;
- confidence limits = ±5%.

[33] This "2" factor (the design effect) is based on the ratio between the estimates of the two variances, the one produced by cluster sampling and the one that would be obtained using the simple random sampling method. In this case, the formula for calculating the size of a sample becomes:

$$n = \frac{Z^2\,(p)\,(1-q)}{d^2}\,(\mathrm{DEFF})$$

N. Birkin *et al.*, "Rapid Nutrition Surveys: How Many Clusters Are Enough?" *Disasters* 16, No. 2 (June 1992): 101.

[34] S. Bennet *et al.*, "A Simplified General Method for Cluster Sample Surveys of Health in Developing Countries," *WHO Statistics Quarterly* 44, No. 3 (1991): 100.

[35] WHO/EPI, *Training for Mid-Level Managers – Coverage Survey* (WHO, 1988).

A total of 400 children would have to be included in the study — either 30 clusters of 14 children or 50 clusters of 8 children. Increasing the number of subjects in each cluster will not significantly increase the accuracy of the results;[36] it is preferable to increase the number of clusters. In the example given here, the second option (50 clusters of 8 children) would provide greater accuracy.

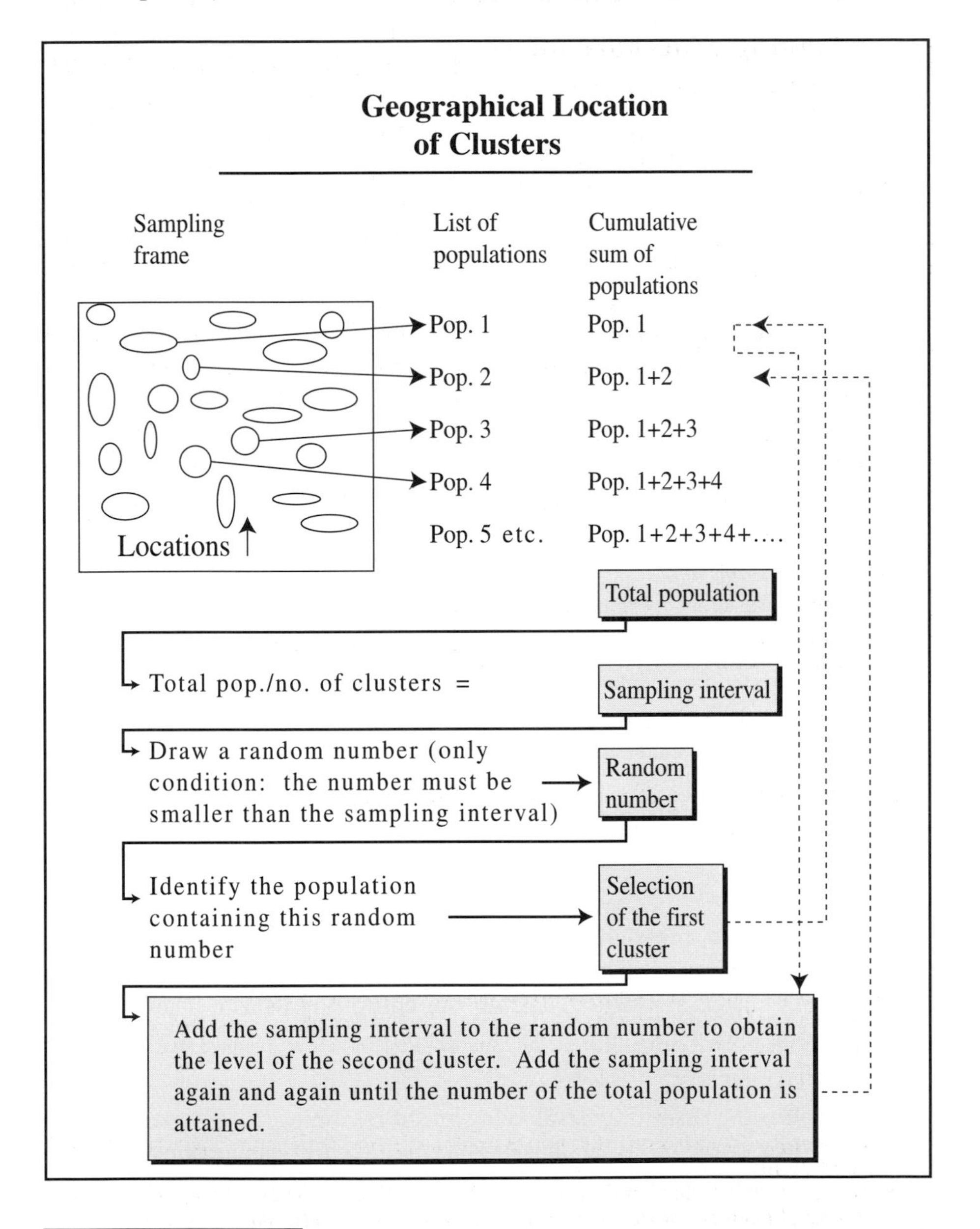


[36] N. Birkin *et al.*, *op. cit.*, p. 99.

### *Applications in Emergency Situations*

Emergency situations involving large populations provide ideal terrain for sampling of all kinds, whether the objective is to measure nutritional status, to study the incidence of basic medical problems, or to assess access to sources of potable water.

In such situations, an estimate is made of the value to be measured and the limits between which the result should fall. The confidence level of the result obtained will therefore correspond to the desired approximation to the true value.

It should be remembered that:

- usually, a proportion is sought;
- the choice of method depends on the distribution of the population:
  - displaced-person and refugee camps are best suited to simple random sampling or systematic sampling;
  - people dispersed in little groups over large areas are better suited to cluster sampling. In this case, the problem will be to obtain an estimate of the number of people by place of residence, a preliminary condition for calculating the cumulative populations and the sampling interval.

The EPIINFO computer program can be used to obtain the sample size automatically:

1. Select the function STATCALC.
2. Select the option "sample size."
3. Specify:
   - the size of the population (e.g. 5,000)
   - the estimated frequency of the condition sought (e.g. 15%)
   - the lower or higher limit (e.g. 10%)
4. Press F4 to obtain the result (e.g. 189).

## 4.3 Tools for the Statistical Analysis of Sample Data

### *Basic Principles*

As explained above, for a given population the means obtained from several samples of the same size will produce an average which will deviate more or less from the true mean, as calculated from the entire population. These sample means are distributed around the true mean so that 95% of them are within $\pm$ 1.96 times the standard error (SE).

This principle is the basis for the following line of reasoning. To compare a given variable in two populations, a sample must be taken in each population and compared with each other, to see whether they are similar or different. However, since these values were obtained from samples, they present a certain risk of error. In fact, a situation may arise where the true values for the two populations are similar, but the values found in the two samples deviate from each other to such a point that they are considered to be different. This sort of error is termed an "error of the first kind," or *type I* error.

For example, if we compare a control population in which variable X is 15%, while the true value of the variable in the population studied is 14%, we can say that the results are similar. However, since the study is based on samples, 95% of the values of the variable detected in a sample of $n$ size will fall between $\pm$ 1.96 standard errors. If, for example, the standard error is 2.95%, means found for samples of a given size $n$ will fall between 11% and 19%, corresponding to the limits of the 95% confidence interval ($z$ = 1.96). In this case, the two populations will be deemed similar, as long as the difference between the values of the control population and those of the studied population remains within the confidence interval. However, if the value for the surveyed population exceeds these limits, the two populations must be considered different with respect to the variable under examination. Yet this difference cannot be accepted as certain, since, in the example above, there is still a 5% probability that the populations are similar— even if the value of the population studied is outside the confidence interval, since this interval was defined with a confidence level of 95% ($z$ = 1.96).

The opposite situation involves two populations presenting different true means (for example, 8% and 17%). Due to sampling errors, the value obtained for the sample from the first population may be 12% (mean + $z$ SE), while the value for the sample from the second population is 13% (mean – SE). The two values are dangerously close, to the point where they are equated with each other. In this case, the affirmation that the two populations are identical is an "error of the second kind," or *type II* error.

The risk of error can be reduced by increasing the value of $z$. Thus, if $z$ = 2.58, the risk of the value falling outside the confidence interval would be 1%. In the preceding example, the limits of that interval would be 10% and 20% ($\pm$2.58 SE). This means that the value of the variable in the population studied must be more than 20% or less than 10% for the two populations to be declared different (with a 1% probability that the difference will be due to a sampling error). While the probability of type I errors is reduced by pushing back further and further the points at which the two populations are declared different, at the same time the probability of declaring different populations identical (type II error) increases.

Traditionally, the tendency is to control type I errors.[37] In this case, the initial hypothesis will be that the two populations are identical (null hypothesis). The

[37] "In fact, for a predetermined sample size, when we reduce the probability of making a type I error, we simultaneously increase the probability of making a type II error. In order to make both error probabilities arbitrarily low we would have to increase the sample size. For this reason we must choose which type of error we want to reduce; the convention has been to always control the probability of making a type I error." Michael Orkin and Richard Drogin, *Vital Statistics* (TMH, 1977), p. 122.

purpose of statistical tests is to calculate the difference between the values observed[38] for the two populations, and to estimate whether that difference is big enough to affirm that the populations are different (that is, to reject the null hypothesis). This must take account of the persistent risk of sampling errors; the error here would be rejecting the null hypothesis when it is in fact true. This risk is expressed as a probability, the *p* value. The difference between two populations is significant when the probability (*p*) of making a mistake is less than 5%, and highly significant when the probability is less than 1%.

## Statistical Tests

### Relative Risk

The measurement of relative risk is not, strictly speaking, a statistical test, since it involves merely simple calculations. However, since relative risk is directly linked to the value of the variable estimated from samples taken in two populations, it undergoes the same variations, based on the confidence level and the confidence limits. This is why the expression of the relative risk inherent in sample values takes the form of a confidence interval.

An exercise can be performed by means of the 2 x 2 table option of EPIINFO's STATCALC function.

### The Chi-Squared ($X^2$) Test

The chi-squared test is used for values expressing the number of individuals from two or more populations who possess or do not possess the characteristic sought. The purpose of the test is to show whether or not any difference found between the values from samples of the different population groups is significant.

The chi-squared test consists in computing the differences between the values observed and the one to be expected if there were no difference between the values.[39] To estimate these values, we must calculate the total number of subjects presenting the characteristic as a percentage of the entire population, and apply this percentage to the observed values of the number of cases. The values obtained are those that would appear if there were no differences in the number of cases in the different populations. The same procedure is carried out for the subjects who do not present the characteristic. The values obtained are those that

---

38 This difference is based on the calculation of the value of *z*, which is the number of standard errors between the true mean and the value found for the sample.

39 The premise here is that the null hypothesis is no difference between the populations.

would be obtained for the "non-cases" if there were no differences between the population groups.[40]

Thus, the test calculates the differences between the observed values and the values that ought to have been obtained if there were no difference. It expresses the result in the form of a numerical value. The magnitude of this value depends on the degree of difference between the values mentioned above. Empirically, the greater the chi-squared value, the greater the probability that the populations are different. If, for example, the chi-squared value is 3.841, the probability of error is 5%, and the two populations are affirmed to be different. The chi-squared value reaches 6.635 for an error rate of 1%, and so on. There are tables to determine, on the basis of the chi-squared value and the degree of freedom,[41] the probability of an erroneous rejection of the null hypothesis. Normally, the null hypothesis is not rejected if the error rate is more than 5%.

### *The t Test*

The *t* test is a method of comparing two means, measured from two samples taken from two populations. The starting point is the null hypothesis (no difference between the two populations). It is also possible to formulate this hypothesis by ruling that the means observed come from a single population. In this case, 95% of the means obtained from *n*-sized samples of that population fall into the interval between $\pm 1.96$ standard errors relative to the true mean. Accordingly, there is a 95% probability that the two means obtained will lie within this interval.

To try to prove or disprove this hypothesis, the *t* test establishes the relation between the difference between the two means observed and the standard error of the difference,[42] which is a combination of the two standard errors inherent in each average:

$$t = \frac{\text{Difference between the two means}}{\text{Standard error of the difference}}$$

---

[40] Value of chi squared: $X^2 = \frac{(O - A)2}{A}$

where O = values observed in sample and A = values expected if there were no differences between the population groups.

[41] *Degree of freedom*: When the number of values exceeds 4, we must take account of the degree of freedom, which is the number of values minus 1 in the column of tabulated values multiplied by the number of values minus 1 in the row of values.

[42] The standard error of the difference is calculated as follows:
Combined variance of the two variances of each sample

$$s = \frac{(n_1 - 1)\,(\text{variance } 1)^2 + (n_2 - 1)\,(\text{variance } 2)^2}{n_1 + n_2 - 2}$$

Standard error of the difference = $s\sqrt{1/n_1 + 1/n_2}$
The *t* test formula becomes:

$$t = \frac{\text{Difference between the two means}}{\text{Standard error of the difference}}$$

Logically, as the value of $t$ increases, so does the probability of exceeding the limits of the confidence interval (between which 95% of the means of a single population should fall), and so does the certainty that the means observed in fact belong to two different populations — although always with some probability of error.

The computation of this probability will depend on the value of $t$ and the degree of freedom. Tables are available for this. Thus, where $t = 2.179$ and the degree of freedom = 12, the probability of error is 5%, when the two populations are different. If the degree of freedom is 21 and $t = 3.819$, the probability of error is 1/1,000.

### *The p Value*

Epidemiological studies refer to the $p$ value, which is "the probability of obtaining, by pure chance, a difference greater than or equal to the one observed."[43] The norm is not to accept $p$ values higher than 0.05 (5% risk of rejecting a null hypothesis when it is true). Most authors prefer $p$ values under 0.01 (1% margin of error).

### *Correlation Coefficient*

Two variables may be positively associated (both evolving in the same direction) or negatively associated (developing in inverse ratio). This association is measured by the correlation coefficient,[44] which may vary between +1 (perfect positive correlation) and -1 (perfect negative correlation).

The statistical significance of a correlation coefficient can be determined as follows: "The correlation coefficient is multiplied by the square root of the number of pairs and, if the product is greater than 2, the correlation coefficient can be considered significant at the 5% threshold."[45]

### *Analysis of the Variance*

The test of the $F$ variance compares the results of several sets of data by examining the relation of the variability between the sets of measures and the variability within each of these sets. There are tables (Fisher & Yates) for calculating the value of $F$ for various degrees of freedom.

---

[43] R.F. Morton and J.R. Hebel, *Epidémiologie et Biostatistique* (Paris: Doin Editeurs, 1983), p. 109.

[44] The formula for calculating the coefficient of correlation is:

$$r = \frac{\Sigma\,(X - Xm)\,(Y - Ym)}{\sqrt{\Sigma\,(X - Xm)^2\,\Sigma\,(Y - Ym)^2}}$$

[45] A. Rougemont, "Méthodes statistiques élémentaires pour l'analyse des données épidémiologiques," in Rougemont and Brunet-Jailly, eds., *La santé dans les pays tropicaux*, p. 561.

# 5. Interpretation of Results

The interpretation of results is not, strictly speaking, an "epidemiological tool." Nevertheless, a critical analysis of results is essential, especially in emergency situations, when the risk of erroneous or tendentious information — or even disinformation — is great. Nowadays, health-care personnel handle statistical tools with greater expertise, samples are correct, and the *p* value is correctly analyzed. There is a tendency, however, to overestimate the value of initial information and consequently to make correct statistical calculations on the basis of false data — which leads to interpretations and recommendations that are hazardous, to say the least.[46] In such cases, the entire process must be reviewed in the original order, to see whether the procedure followed was correct.

## 5.1 Pertinence of Data

Is the information sought pertinent in an emergency situation? The mortality rate is; but the rate of prevalence of intestinal parasitic infestations, in contrast, is not, at least not in the initial phase of the emergency. An intervention to control intestinal parasitic infestations will not have a dramatic impact on reducing mortality, and other information is more important at this stage (diarrheal diseases, malaria, etc.). Nonetheless, after the initial phase the prevalence of intestinal parasitic infestations can become a significant element in studies on the impact of sanitation programs.

## 5.2 Adequacy of Data Collected to Describe the Situation Objectively

In an emergency situation, the main difficulties are to obtain information from all the population groups concerned (access to information) and to obtain reliable responses in a conflict situation (reliability of information).[47]

## 5.3 Statistical Analysis of Results

Was sampling done correctly, using an appropriate method and a sufficiently large sample? Is the statistical interpretation of the data obtained correct, coherent and based on an appropriate analysis method?

## 5.4 Interpreting Results in Context

Mere statistical interpretation is not an adequate basis for forming an opinion. When analyzing results, researchers should take into account:

---

[46] Garbage in –> garbage out!

[47] Hence the importance of comparing information from several different sources.

- *the local climate.* An increase in the number of malaria cases at the beginning of the rainy season, and an increased rate of malnutrition in the months before the new harvest are not unusual phenomena.
- *the sociocultural context.* The difference between two population groups in the prevalence of diarrheal diseases may be linked to a difference in water-supply sources, but it may also be linked to behavioral differences in the use of the water.

### 5.5 Interpreting Results Based on Total Information

A reduced rate of malnutrition may be linked to correctly implemented food aid; but it may also be due to an increase in mortality rates among the people most affected by malnutrition. An increased malnutrition rate may be linked to insufficient food aid, but also to an increase in the number of victims. In both cases, the combined analysis of all available information is essential for judging the value and impact of food aid.

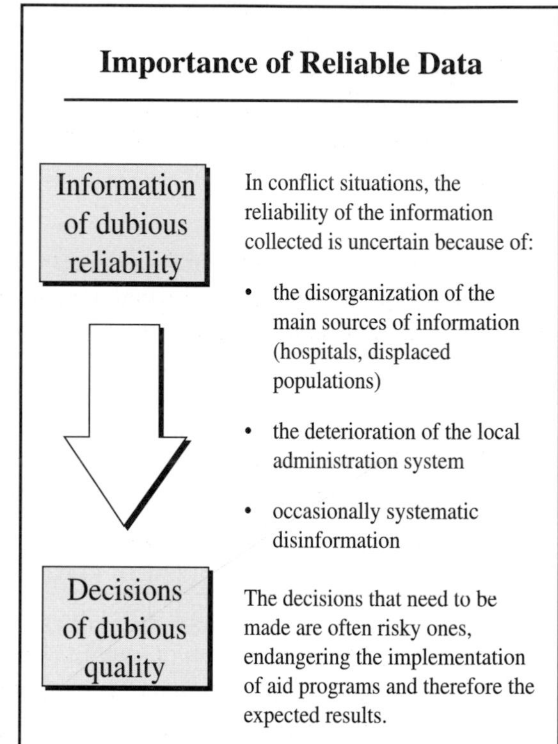


## 6. Decision-Making

Epidemiological studies implemented during emergencies must be, above all, operational — that is, they must facilitate fast decisions about what to do.

The decision may be:

- to do nothing;
- to carry out more specific investigations;
- to repeat the same study within a given period of time;
- to intervene immediately.

Proposals for action should be clearly stated in all epidemiological studies.

**The Epidemiological Approach to Armed-Conflict Situations Improves the Quality of Decision-Making**

1. A quantitative and qualitative approach to health problems, permitting the establishment of clear priorities

2. An analytical approach to health problems which identifies their causes and thereby facilitates the promotion of a preventive approach

3. A permanent approach to health problems, which involves monitoring their development and measuring the effects of humanitarian interventions

4. A systematic epidemiological approach to armed-conflict situations which, by permitting comparative analyses, provides general information

# III. Epidemiological Programs

Epidemiological programs are viewed here in the general context of emergency situations. The first goal of epidemiological programs is to foresee — before the crisis — the advent of problems that will demand intervention. Action should be taken before the crisis has attained such proportions that the victims are seriously affected. Early-warning systems serve as epidemiological instruments to detect problems such as a potential famine.

Once the crisis arrives, epidemiologists must respond to the following question: Are local resources adequate to meet the victims' needs? If they are, outside intervention is unnecessary. Some situations pose no immediate need, but deterioration can be expected within a certain time period. In this case, epidemiologists must decide whether immediate intervention is required to minimize the effects of a future disaster — for example, preventive action against a threat of famine. If local resources are inadequate, immediate intervention is required.

After the crisis, epidemiologists must answer another question: Did the humanitarian aid provided during the crisis indeed serve its purpose? The institution of an epidemiological surveillance program will make it possible to determine the impact on the victims' health status, the effectiveness of the services provided, and the way the inputs provided were used.

Epidemiology's role extends to other phases of intervention as well, notably those of rehabilitation and reconstruction. In this book, the study of epidemiological programs will be limited to those phases involved in crisis situations, specifically the following:

1. initial assessment of an emergency situation
2. assessment of an epidemic
3. organization of a surveillance system
4. organization of an early-warning system.

# 1. Initial Assessment

## 1.1 Principles of an Initial Assessment

The basic concept of an initial assessment (already described in Chapter 1) is the necessity of determining whether there is a patent imbalance between victims' vital needs and the local facilities normally responsible for meeting them. A distinction must be made between the imbalance directly caused by the circumstances of the crisis and any chronic structural imbalance between needs and services.[48] No analysis of the first kind of imbalance, however, will make much sense unless it takes the second kind into account. In short, besides the factors triggering the crisis, the underlying causes of the imbalance must be examined. This approach may have a fundamental influence on the choice of intervention type and *modus operandi.*

Some organizations have a very specific mandate for a particular type of action, such as feeding and nutrition, aid to the handicapped, etc., or for a particular

[48] *Assisting in Emergencies* (UNICEF), p. 29.

category of victim, such as women and children (UNICEF), war victims (ICRC), or refugees (UNHCR).

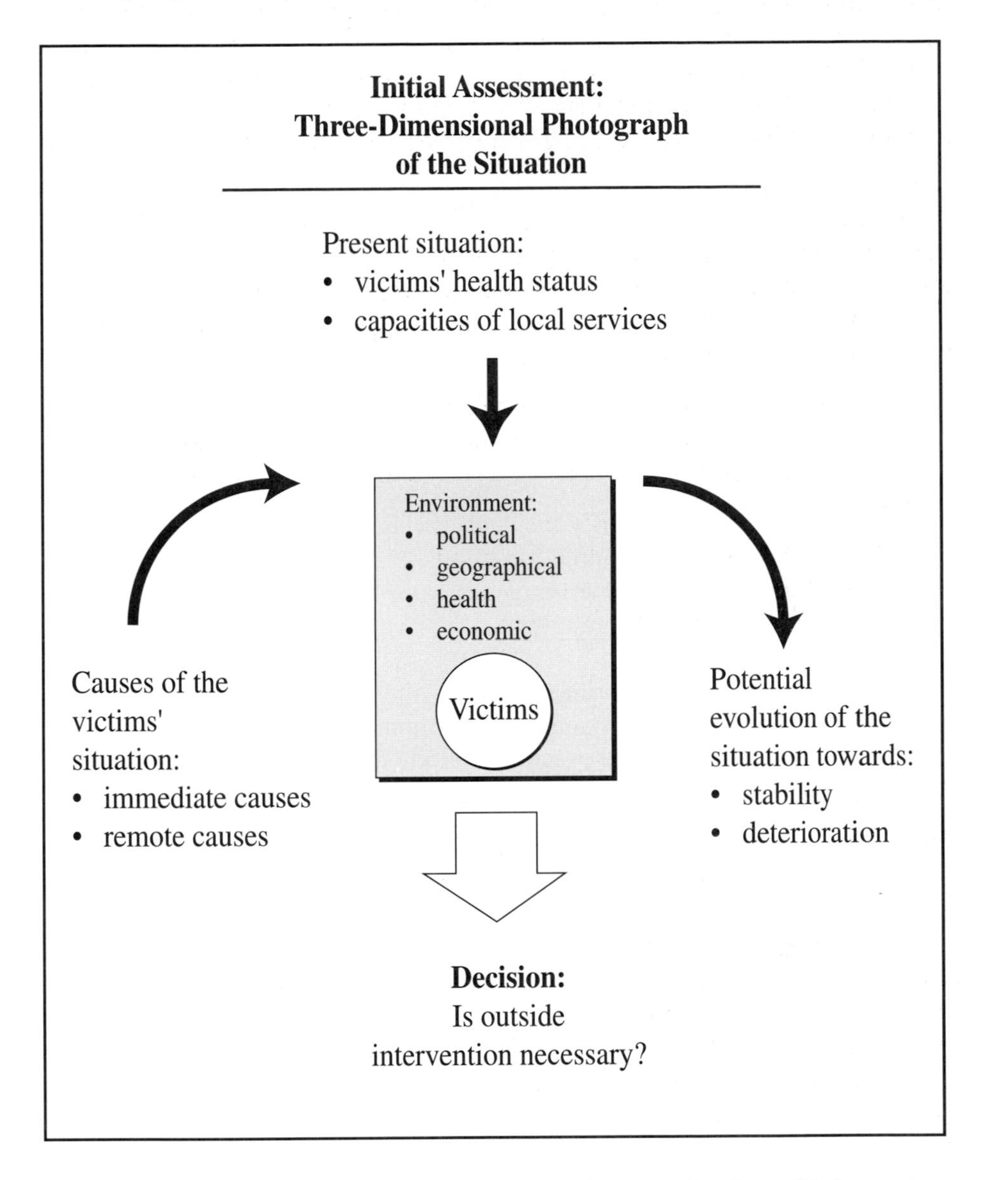


An initial assessment should not be considered as a collection of information gleaned at random in the field. On the other hand, although the assessment should reflect a systematic quest for data following a pre-established plan, that plan should not become an excuse for neglecting opportunities that may arise in the course of the assessment. Spontaneously acquired information of this kind may help to define problems and identify possibilities for immediate action.

The initial assessment in an emergency situation should aim at clarifying as quickly as possible those major health problems that pose a vital risk to the population affected.

## *Indicators*

### *Types of Indicator*

Depending on the situation, indicators should include:

- factors reflecting the victims' needs
  - population census
  - number of sick
  - number of malnourished
- local resources
  - number of hospitals
  - agricultural production
- circumstantial factors
  - political situation (security incidents, belligerents' attitudes towards the civilian population in conflict situations)
  - ecological situation (for example, in cases of drought, measurement of rainfall in the preceding months)
- structural factors
  - evidence of a chronic incapacity in the local services to meet the population's needs (for example, weak immunization coverage)
  - evidence of sociocultural practices that are harmful to health

The choice of indicators depends on the level of analysis desired. If the goal is to define a serious crisis affecting the population, studies should be restricted to the main indicators capable of demonstrating the existence of a major crisis: mortality rate, malnutrition rate, prevalence of communicable diseases, access to medical care, access to food resources. If the goal is to determine the underlying causes of a crisis, indicators must be selected which will outline the major infrastructural systems: agriculture, health, social services, etc.

### *Check Lists*

Generally, relief agencies want check lists for the information needed in an emergency situation to be as complete as possible. The ideal list does not exist, however. Lists can be established on the basis of:

- the original problem
  - assessment of health needs following floods and hurricanes[49]

---

[49] "Technical Paper No. 11," PAHO.

  - initial assessment of health problems in famine situations[50]

- the type of victim
  - assessment of health problems during sudden population movements[51]
  - assessment of the problems of war-wounded

- a specific technical problem
  - assessment of a water-supply point[52]
  - assessment of the bacterial quality of water[53]

- assessment of a hospital
  - structure
  - buildings
  - provision of water
  - provision of energy, etc.

- assessment of resources
  - personnel
  - equipment and drugs in stock

- quantitative assessment of activities
  - number of hospital admissions or services for a given unit of time
  - average hospital stay

- qualitative assessment of the work carried out
  - type of procedures employed[54]
  - type of prescriptions (standardization)

Rather than seek the ideal, all-purpose list, it is preferable to define the field to be covered and to take that as a basis for outlining an initial assessment, drawing on specific data that already exists.[55]

### *Information Sources*

Information sources are diverse:

#### *Population*

In principle, the population itself is the most reliable source of information. It is not always accessible, however, and several factors must be taken into consideration:

---

50 ERO/EPR/90.1.8, WHO.
51 ERO/EPR/90.1.7, WHO.
52 ICRC, *Evaluation d'un point d'eau* (1988).
53 WHO, *Guidelines for Drinking Water Quality* (1985).
54 Bone fixation in fractures due to war injuries!
55 There is no point in trying to reinvent the wheel in all spheres.

- the absence of a census
- the mobility of populations
- the identification of people actually affected by the crisis
- changes in the number of people involved
- changes in population structure relative to a normal population

Assessing a population's health status will require the use of the main epidemiological tools studied previously: sampling, tests, questionnaires, etc.

*Existing Surveillance Systems*

Where infrastructural services (social services, health care, agriculture) are equipped for systematic data collection, they must be consulted. Nevertheless, the unreliability and irregularity of the data should be taken into account.

## *Analysis of Results*

Analyzing the information collected is the crucial point of every initial assessment, since it leads to the decision-making process. An incorrect appraisal of the situation may have disastrous consequences.

Three cardinal rules must be respected:

*Data analysis must be multisectoral*

- rate of diarrheal diseases and water supply
- rate of malnutrition and communicable discases
- number of hospital admissions and rate of avoidable diseases

*Data must be analyzed in context*

- rate of malnutrition and season of the year
- access to food resources and political context
- quality of care and level of development

*Data should serve as a basis for projections over time*

Projection over time is the most difficult level of analysis. A given situation will often develop haphazardly, even over a short time span. For this reason it is difficult to say whether the victims will be able to manage without external aid.

## *Decision-Making*

Paradoxically, decisions are easy when everything is going either badly or well. There is no need to wonder whether food aid is necessary for populations decimated by drought, as in Ethiopia in 1984, or whether help is required by war wounded if there are no hospitals to treat them. At the other end of the spectrum, an earthquake in California does not mobilize the international community, given the region's high level of preparation and relief organization for cases of disaster.

The difficulty arises in those gray areas where the victims are not in a catastrophic state, but deterioration is probable or possible. This is the kind of situation that involves risky decisions.[56]

In such cases, there are two options:

- institute a surveillance system in order to detect future problems;
- undertake preemptive measures to prevent the crisis from worsening.[57]

The principle of preventive interventions is difficult to promote; the international community rarely mobilizes to intervene in situations that have not yet produced their quota of horrors, and the leaders of humanitarian organizations hesitate to commit themselves to relief operations that may later prove to have been unnecessary.

To facilitate the decision-making process, organizations tend to adopt specific quantitative criteria for intervention, such as a death rate higher than 2/10,000 per day or a malnutrition rate that is considerably higher than normal. These parameters define situations that are already much deteriorated and that urgently require intervention. Clearly, however, organizations should not wait until health status has reached this point; far better to intervene with preventive measures when mortality and malnutrition levels are still within acceptable limits. Timely intervention costs much less than resorting to emergency air transport, purchases made under pressure without the opportunity to issue tenders, etc. Humanitarian organizations should base their decisions on common sense rather than precise intervention criteria, and accept the necessity of making risky decisions.

Finally, every assessment arouses in the population involved expectations of some kind of assistance. For this reason, assessments should be avoided if it has been decided in advance that no action will be undertaken in any case.

## 1.2 Organizing an Initial Assessment

Organizing an initial assessment is complicated. Not only do the technical aspects mentioned above have to be taken into account, but also:

---

[56] That is, the risk of making the wrong decision — for example, providing aid that later proves not to have been really necessary.

[57] Why wait for a high malnutrition rate before intervening?

- *political constraints* (access to the victims) — long months of negotiations may be necessary before authorization to make an initial assessment can be obtained.
- *logistic support* – difficulties in transport, fuel supply, etc.
- *human resources* — training local personnel to take measurements, carry out population surveys, collect data, etc.

# 2. Planning a Surveillance System

The purpose of a surveillance system is to collect on a regular basis a set of data selected for their usefulness in:

- describing developments in a population's health status, in the functioning of the health-care services, in access to food resources, and in the water supply;
- detecting epidemics;
- facilitating decisions concerning the conduct of operations.

This section will discuss the principles of organizing a surveillance system in the framework of a relief action.

## 2.1 Basic Principles

An effective surveillance system is based on the following conditions:

- *Standardization of indicators, tests, sources, and methods of analysis*
  - With no standardization, there is a danger of comparing variables that are defined differently according to their source. Similarly, if tests are not standardized, it is difficult to compare results obtained by different organizations working in the same region.
- *Continuity in data collection*
  - Trend analysis will be all the more cogent if data are gathered at regular intervals and over a fairly long period.
- *Simplicity of operation*
  - The health-care personnel given the task of feeding a surveillance system with

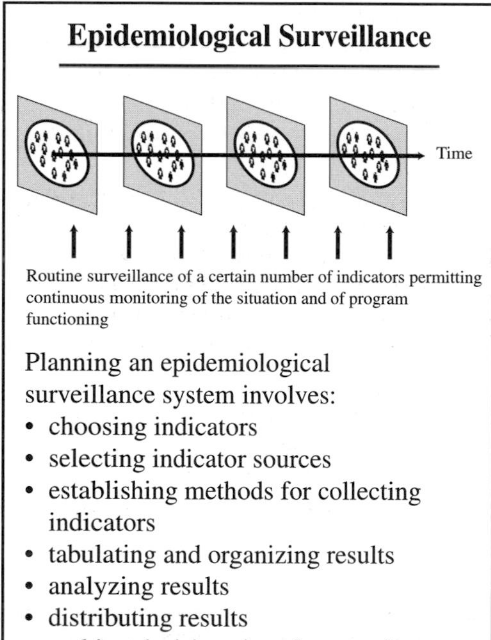


Routine surveillance of a certain number of indicators permitting continuous monitoring of the situation and of program functioning

Planning an epidemiological surveillance system involves:
- choosing indicators
- selecting indicator sources
- establishing methods for collecting indicators
- tabulating and organizing results
- analyzing results
- distributing results
- making decisions based on results

basic data will perceive this as an extra burden on top of their daily care-providing activities. The simpler the system, the more likely it is to function correctly.

### *Indicators*

The selection of indicators is much easier if precise operational objectives have been set at the beginning of the relief action, such as:

- immunize 90% of children under five years of age within three months;
- guarantee a food intake of 2,400 kcal per day for the entire population within one month;
- provide a minimum of 20 liters of potable water per person per day;
- treat all cases of malaria[58] with a standard anti-malarial regime;
- reduce the malnutrition rate from 15% to 5% in children under age five within one month.

Operational objectives such as these provide a basis for determining the indicators that will serve as a gauge of achievement:

- immunization coverage after three months;
- food ration distributed;
- number of people with access to food distribution;
- quantity of water distributed;
- rate of malnutrition after one month.

**Choice of Indicators for Epidemiological Surveillance**

Three kinds of factors must be considered in the choice of indicators:

**1. Technical factors:**
- Indicator relevance: What is being measured? Program functioning, health status, etc.
- Reliability of information sources
- Possibility of systematic data collection

**2. Coordination:**
- Link with the indicators specified at the time of the initial assessment
- Link with the operational objectives
- Standardization among the indicators collected by the different people or groups involved in the humanitarian intervention

**3. Political factors:**
- Are the information sources free to furnish the necessary data?
- Is regular access guaranteed?

### *Selection of Indicators*

It is important to avoid the danger of choosing too many indicators,[59] the collection and analysis of which will prove

[58] The possible definitions of what constitutes a case of malaria were studied in the previous chapter and in section II-1.2 of this chapter.

[59] In its manual on evaluating national programs for the control of diarrheal diseases, WHO proposes a choice of 13 indicators. CDD, *Programme Management, A Training Course* (1988), p. 31.

impossible. Too few indicators, however, may be just as bad, permitting only a very basic level of analysis.[60]

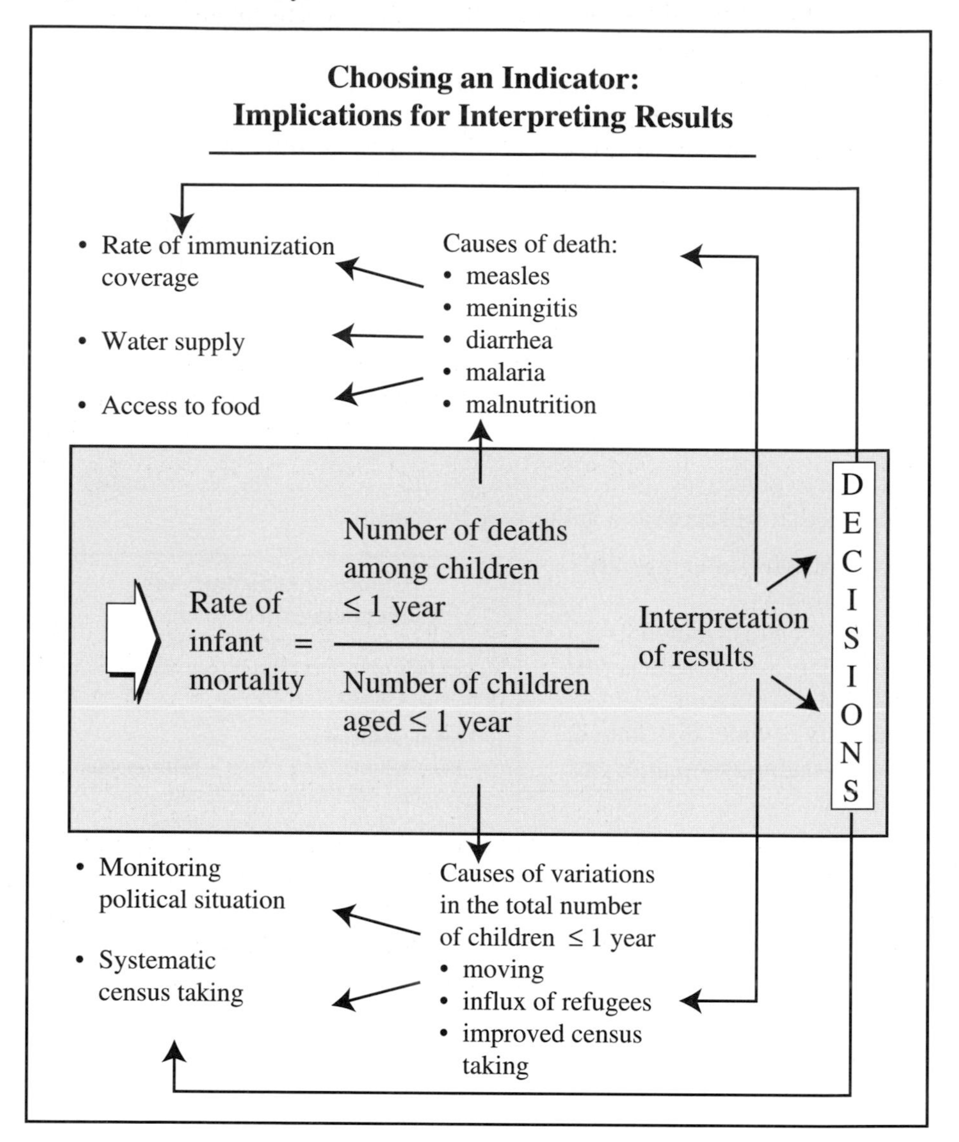


Certain indicators are indispensable:

- *indicators concerning population status*
  - number of people covered by the intervention

[60] Monitoring the rate of malnutrition will permit conclusions as to whether malnutrition is stable, rising, or falling, but not more precise ones such as whether the increase in malnutrition corresponds to an increase in new refugees, or whether a decrease in malnutrition corresponds to the food input furnished (rather than to increased mortality in the age group considered).

- rate and causes of mortality
- rate of morbidity for diseases of particular importance for public health (malaria, diarrheal diseases, respiratory infections, meningitis, etc.)
- rate of malnutrition

■ *indicators concerning the functioning of services*
- immunization coverage
- number of admissions to health facilities
- number of food rations distributed
- number of latrines built
- number of shelters built

### Sources of Information

Health-care facilities should be able to furnish routine information on a regular basis. If there are too many of them, a few should be selected to play the role of "sentinels," or reporters. The rate of malnutrition should be monitored within the population, an important source of information, and not from the cases of malnutrition referred to the health-care facilities.

### Data-Collecting Systems

There are two ways of collecting data. A routine surveillance system can be set up, through which the collected data are channeled every day, week, or month to the appropriate person or center for analysis. This is the "passive" system, which consists in waiting for the information to arrive.

The second method involves starting an "ad hoc" survey. This kind of evaluation may be repetitive — for example, measuring a population's nutritional status at regular intervals. It may also be initiated following an alert by the routine surveillance system. One example would be investigating the quality of the water provided by various sources following a significant increase in the rate of diarrheal diseases diagnosed by the health facilities. This is the "active" system, which consists in going out and collecting the information.

### Data Analysis

Information on several levels may be analyzed.

- *Impact on the population's health*: This is the most important level, at least for health-care personnel. To assess a population's health status, various points of reference must be used — for example, the previous level of health. The main criterion is still the mortality rate.
- *Quality and quantity of services provided*: This level involves evaluating the operation and organization of the inputs provided. For example, the evaluation of a medical consultation should take into account the following:
  - number of consultations (quantitative aspect)

- quality of the organization of resources. A medical consultation involves the combined action of a care provider, a health-care facility, equipment, and drugs. Are treatments correct?
- quality of relations with the patient

Data analysis should also cover:

- *the relation between the services provided and their impact on health.*
- *the relation between the services provided to victims and those accessible to the resident population.* All too often, this relation is evaluated in terms of the victims' level of health, an approach which does not take into account sociocultural differences between the two population groups. These differences may explain notable gaps between the health levels of the two populations, despite similar care. In such a case, it is better to compare the level of health-care services offered to each population and to adapt them to the particular community, to avoid creating friction between the two.
- *the mobilization of resources.* That favored domain of administrators, the surveillance of mobilized resources (material, human, and financial), should provide the answer to the question: Were the mobilized resources sent where they should have been? Paradoxically, it is surveillance of resource mobilization which mobilizes the most resources. This can be attributed to the fact that the humanitarian agencies are obligated to report to their donors. And what is most important to donors is knowing whether the aid they financed did indeed reach its destination. The impact on the victims' health status appears to be of secondary interest.

### *Decisions*

By collecting data, a surveillance system helps the administrators of intervention operations to make decisions concerning:

- *the functioning of programs*
  - decision to increase the medical coverage of a population;
  - decision to phase out a therapeutic feeding program when indicators (malnutrition rate, access to food) give the "go-ahead";
  - decision to initiate operational research on a particular issue;
  - decision to begin a study of food consumption within the family to discover the reason for persistent malnutrition in certain groups of children.
- *the management of resources*
  - modification of lists of available drugs to fit the pathology better;
  - replacement of expatriate personnel by locally trained staff.
- *the purpose of the intervention itself*
  The surveillance system should allow administrators to judge, on the basis of technical information (local services' level of self-sufficiency) and political information (opportunities to return to normal life), whether aid should be

continued or stopped within a certain time limit. This idea is important, since it obliges program planners to establish criteria defining the limits of the intervention at the outset. These criteria might consist in:

- the re-establishment of the conditions that prevailed prior to the crisis;
- a liaison with long-term programs designed to increase the level of development.

### *Research*

If the surveillance system detects a problem with no immediate solution, it is not at all utopian to contemplate a study on the subject, if such a study will help provide a practical response to the problem. Thus, a study on the resistance of *Plasmodium falciparum* to drugs, intended to improve the performance of treatment regimens, should be immediately considered if a resistance to the traditional treatment is suspected.[61]

## 2.2 Organizing a Surveillance System

Organizing a surveillance system is more than just carrying out a few ad hoc assessments among the population and compiling statistics from health facilities. To be effective, a surveillance system must:

- be planned in conjunction with the relief activities;[62]
- integrate all the components of the intervention.[63]

The organization of a surveillance system requires:

- a definition of what is to be monitored;
- a definition of the norms governing data collection;
- provision of the forms on which information will be recorded (data-recording sheets in dispensaries, hospitals, etc.);
- the establishment of mechanisms by which information will be transferred (postal service, visits to data-collection centers, telephones, fax machines, etc.);
- the establishment of a facility to process and analyze information (epidemiological center);[64]
- the establishment of a mechanism to transmit analyses to decision-making centers and to the providers of the raw data;[65]

---

[61] A. Schapira, "Malaria Unit," SOS course, WHO (Geneva, June 1992).

[62] This also makes it more likely that indicators will be linked with the operational objectives.

[63] Thus facilitating linkage between different data and increasing the likelihood of correct decisions.

[64] An initial analysis can be carried out directly by the people collecting the information. An epidemiological center is justified only for large-scale interventions, in which the volume of data and the dispersion of collection centers demand a centralization of all information in order to detect general tendencies.

[65] It is essential that the people who furnish the raw data get "feedback" in the form of analyses. It will be difficult to maintain their motivation for paperwork if they never see what it is used for.

- the integration of new decisions in the surveillance system.

The following conclusions, formulated in the wake of flooding in Khartoum in 1988, nicely sum up what can be expected of a surveillance system:

"Simple symptom-oriented case definitions for diarrhoeal disease, measles, respiratory disease, malaria, and jaundice were included on the report form used to collect daily counts of outpatients in a sample of both temporary and permanent clinics located in areas of the city most affected by the flood. In addition, special surveys collected information unobtainable from health facilities. Sentinel clinic surveillance data indicated that diarrheal disease accounted for the greatest number of clinic visits, while malaria was the second most common reason for seeking medical attention." [66]

# 3. Investigating an Epidemic

## 3.1 "Epidemic" Risk in Emergency Situations

The word "epidemic" is a constant of disaster situations. The first reports of such situations almost invariably speak of incipient epidemics. This myth must be eradicated once and for all: "Epidemics do not occur spontaneously after a disaster and dead bodies will not necessarily cause catastrophic outbreaks of disease."[67]

Some situations, of course, have indeed given rise to genuine epidemics, such as the 1964 malaria epidemic in Haiti following Hurricane Flora. The main danger of an epidemic developing, however, is attributable not to the disaster itself, but rather to the consequences of the disaster. These consequences can be divided into two categories:

- *population concentrations* — the often precarious hygiene conditions obtaining in camps or other densely populated locations may pose the threat of epidemics.[68] However, several conditions must be present simultaneously (infectious agents, vulnerable population, vector) if an epidemic is to take hold. Thus, a population that moves out of a cholera-free region into another cholera-free region runs no particular risk of contracting this disease, whereas an epidemic of malaria is almost inevitable in a non-immune population arriving in an area where malaria is hyperendemic — unless appropriate measures are taken.

---

66 B.A Woodruff, M. Toole, *et al.*, "Disease Surveillance and Control After a Flood: Khartoum, Sudan, 1988," *Disasters* 14, No. 2 (1990): 151.

67 C. de Ville de Goyet, "International Health Assistance in Relief Operations: Preparing the Local Health Personnel to Meet the Challenge," *International Review of the Red Cross* (Sept.-Oct. 1991): 515.

68 One more reason to avoid setting up camps.

- *deterioration of prevention services* — the destruction of the means of communication, the reorientation of activities in response to the emergency, and insecurity are a few factors which explain the deterioration of the health-care services, particularly those concerned with preventive care. The result is an increased incidence of communicable diseases, which may reach the epidemic threshold.

### *The Epidemic Threshold*

An epidemic may be defined as an indisputable increase in the number of cases of a disease compared to its usual rate. This definition should reflect the norms for individual disease prevalence in a given geographical area. In Burkina Faso, meningitis is considered to have reached epidemic proportions when the rate of meningococcal meningitis is greater than 15 cases per 100,000 people per week for two consecutive weeks. Similarly, a 20% increase in the number of cholera cases in Bangladesh is business as usual, but a single case of smallpox is the beginning of an epidemic!

### *The Alarm Signal*

The alarm may be sounded by:

- *the population itself*, which notices spontaneously an unusual number of deaths following fever (malaria), rash (measles), diarrhea (cholera), or other symptoms.
- *the surveillance system*, which shows a significant increase in the number of cases of a particular pathology;
- *rumors* of unknown origin to the effect that people are dying.

The reliability of such an alarm depends on its origin. By definition, information furnished by a surveillance system is more credible than rumors. Whatever the source of the alarm, however, an investigation will have to be undertaken to confirm or disprove the initial reports.

## 3.2 Organizing the Investigation of an Epidemic

Investigating an epidemic involves several stages.

### *Confirming the Epidemic*

An investigation undertaken to confirm an epidemic must adopt a two-pronged approach, both defining cases and confirming the increase in the number of cases.

**Defining Cases**

1. Establish with certainty the presence of cases of communicable diseases — for example, meningitis, cholera, and measles. Rumors should not be a basis for instituting a whole set of emergency measures, and in the case of such diseases as meningitis and cholera, bacteriological confirmation must be obtained.
2. Establish the link between the duly documented cases and the beginning of an epidemic. There may be a number of sporadic cases but no confirmation of an epidemic.
3. Once the cases have been documented and their epidemic character has been confirmed, subsequent cases will be diagnosed and treated solely on the basis of clinical criteria.

### *Defining Cases*

Diagnosing cases is relatively simple when the patients have been admitted to a health-care facility. It is easy to visit the facility and talk to the nursing staff. If the alarm has been raised at an early stage, some of the patients will probably still be in the hospital, where they can be examined. If not, their files must be consulted. Depending on the reliability and specificity of the tests conducted (clinical examination, bacteriological tests), the patients admitted may or may not prove to have been infected with meningococcal meningitis, measles, typhoid fever, cholera, or whatever disease was suspected.

When initial reports are based on rumors, in contrast, it is much more difficult to ascertain the truth of the matter. The source of the rumors must be sought so that the original cases can be found. The patients may be:

- cured — in which case the patient history may help establish a diagnosis;
- still sick — a clinical examination and, if necessary, biological tests[69] will make diagnosis possible;
- dead or absent — the sole possibility in this case is to question the patient's family or friends.

If doubts persist, new cases must be sought. If there is no longer any doubt, a case profile will have been defined which will serve as a basis for identifying subsequent cases.[70]

[69] There are lists of available equipment for taking specimens under satisfactory conditions. See P. Brés, *Public Health Action in Emergencies Caused by Epidemics* (WHO, 1989). As soon as a hypothesis regarding possible diagnoses has been formed, possibilities for testing must be investigated: What laboratory is equipped to look for *vibrios*? What laboratory is able to identify meningococcus?

[70] For example, WHO proposes the following guidelines for identifying cholera: "A case of cholera should be suspected when:
- in an area where the disease is not known to be present, a patient aged 5 years or more develops severe dehydration or dies from acute watery diarrhoea
- in an area where there is a cholera epidemic, a patient aged 5 or more develops acute watery diarrhoea with or without vomiting.

A case of cholera is confirmed when
- *Vibrio Cholerae 01* is isolated from any patient with diarrhoea." WHO, *Guidelines for Cholera Control* (1993), p. 15.

### *Confirming an Abnormal Increase in the Number of Cases*

The other step in confirming an epidemic consists in verifying that there is indeed an abnormal increase in the incidence of cases. It has already been noted that for some diseases — meningitis, for example — epidemic thresholds can be established. For other diseases, the local context must be used as a reference. The cases will be inventoried on the basis of the data collected by the health-care facilities, or from cases found among the population. The information recorded for each case should reflect:

- the profile established for the case — for example, clinical signs such as fever, vomiting, diarrhea, etc.
- the requirements of future analysis concerning:
  - the group of people most affected (for which data on age, sex, occupation, etc., will be needed);
  - the geographical areas most affected (origin of cases);
  - the onset of the disease and the date of contact with other cases.

  These three aspects constitute the traditional bases for a descriptive analysis of the epidemic: person, place, time.[71]

The epidemiologist's role is not only to confirm an epidemic once it has spread, but to predict such a spread on the basis of a few declared cases. The identification of risk factors is therefore essential:

- size of the population groups susceptible to infection;
- way of life (overcrowding or widely scattered populations);
- malnutrition;
- unhealthy environment.

If an epidemic has not been openly declared, but a strong epidemic potential is present, it may be necessary to take control measures very quickly.[72] These measures will determine whether the disease has epidemic potential and whether an epidemic or the risk of one exists.

### *Surveying the Measures Taken and Local Resource Potential*

Have the health-care services already taken steps to control the epidemic? Do they have the resources required to implement the measures planned?

---

[71] If this information is not collected at the outset, it will be difficult to find later.

[72] In displaced-person camps, mass measures of control must be taken much more quickly than in normal settings, due to the high epidemic potential.

## *Data Analysis*

### *Epidemiological Data*

- *Persons:*
  What group or groups are affected? The rate of infection must be measured for different population groups. Similarly, the rate of mortality specific to the disease in question must be determined for each of the groups affected.
- *Space:*
  Where did the epidemic begin? Which regions are most affected? Both the rate of infection and the mortality rate must be determined by geographical area.
- *Time:*
  When were the first cases identified? An epidemic curve should be constructed to show the number of cases in relation to time.

### *Risk Factors*

The risk factors are:

- salubrity of the environment
- nutritional status
- housing conditions
- level of health education
- deterioration of health-care services
- insecurity
- size of the group at risk

Are these factors strong enough to contribute to the outbreak of the epidemic?

## *Determining a Strategy for Action*

The strategy for action consists in reviewing all the stages of the communicable-disease cycle[73] and making a list of possible actions. Examples include:

- Prophylactic action against the pathogenic agent
  - treatment of healthy carriers
- Vector control
  - destruction of vectors
  - action to eliminate breeding grounds
- Active protection
  - immunization
- Passive protection
  - chemoprophylaxis

[73] See Chapter 4 ("Communicable Diseases").

- Early screening for cases
  - putting health facilities on alert
  - promoting public awareness (through the media)
  - actively seeking out cases within the population
- Treatment of diagnosed cases
  - reinforcement of health-care personnel's technical expertise
  - provision of necessary equipment
- Removal and cremation or burial of bodies

Next, the activities best suited to the situation[74] must be selected, following two lines of action: one to flatten the epidemic curve — essentially through preventive measures — and the other to reduce mortality, by curative measures.

Trying to decide which of these two lines should take priority is unrealistic; they are mutually dependent. Prophylactic measures such as improved personal hygiene cannot be proposed if no solution is offered to the people already diagnosed with the disease. Similarly, merely treating the sick is not enough; efforts must be made at the same time to control the spread of the disease.

### *Determining Whether Outside Aid Is Necessary*

The local health-care services do not always have the necessary resources to cope with an epidemic. This includes material resources, the technical expertise for making the initial diagnosis, and logistic support. International aid may prove necessary.

### *Gaining Support for the Recommended Measures*

#### *Support from the Political Authorities*

Epidemics are a sensitive subject for health and political authorities. The political authorities must understand the health-care personnel's proposals before they will agree to assist in the institution of control measures. The political authorities tend to minimize or deny the existence of an epidemic because of the negative image that such news projects to the outside world, or because of its repercussions on tourism. Where refugee populations are concerned, an epidemic may serve as an argument for reinforcing coercive measures against them.

#### *Support from the Population*

The population, too, must be clearly informed about:

[74] It should be remembered that an appropriate action is one which combines an acceptable rate of effectiveness with an acceptable degree of feasibility.

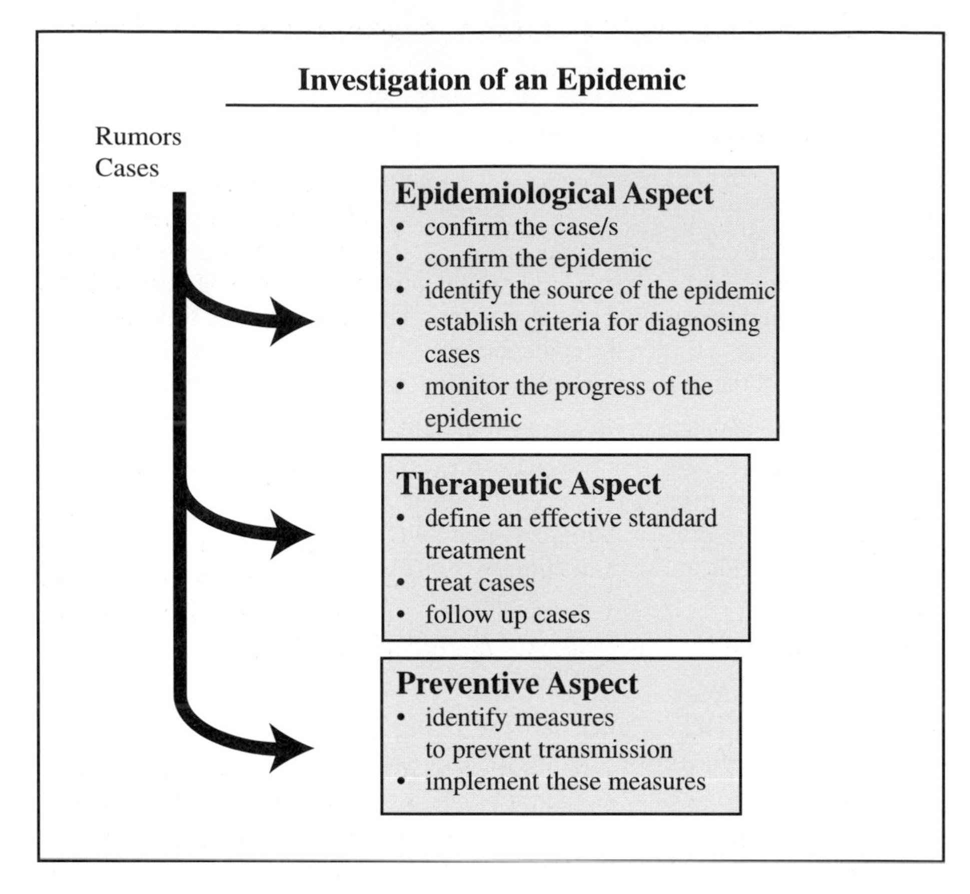


- the clinical manifestations of the disease which permit early detection;
- the risks involved;
- precautions that can be taken;
- means of treatment.

### *Evaluating and Adapting the Measures Already Implemented*

The set of measures already being implemented, adapted to the problem and the urgency of the epidemic, constitutes a kind of surveillance system in itself, particularly in terms of organization.

## 4. Early-Warning Systems

Early-warning systems (EWSs) are a variant of surveillance systems, designed to anticipate a disaster and limit its effects. There is a tendency to confuse EWSs and the use of space technology (satellite photos). In fact, the concept of EWS is not new. In ancient cities crossed by rivers, the inhabitants used to measure the water level regularly in order to see when the danger level had been reached. At that point they would begin to take steps to protect themselves against the rising waters.

## 4.1 Basic Principles

Theoretically, all disasters could be predicted by EWSs, which would report preliminary signs of conflict — social instability, disturbances between ethnic groups, political conflicts, etc. — and early signs of natural disasters, such as the results of seismological, volcanic, and hydrological surveillance. However, trials of EWSs have been confined mostly to drought prediction, for the following reasons.

### *Ease of Prediction*

Droughts are easy to predict compared with disasters that develop extremely quickly, such as earthquakes and cyclones. There are two reasons for this. First, droughts develop slowly, allowing time (theoretically) to take preventive measures in case of alert. Second, the indicators that permit observers to predict a drought, or at least its initial consequences for a population (migration) and the economy (market prices), are relatively simple and reliable.

### *Seriousness*

Drought is very serious for a population. Of course, a drought does not appear to kill as many people as the immediate effects of an earthquake, since it is a slowly developing phenomenon which does not have the suddenness of an earthquake. The death rates per 10,000 people affected by an earthquake or a drought are, respectively, 150 and 8.[75] Nonetheless, of all the disasters, drought is in first place due to the size of the populations affected[76] and the mortality associated with it (the number of deaths is often underestimated).

## 4.2 EWSs in Drought-Prone Areas

### *The Choice of Indicators*

The choice of indicators depends on the probable causes of drought. Although these indicators are interwoven in a complex manner, a certain hierarchy among them can be established, based not on their power to precipitate the problem, but on their capacity to reflect the seriousness of the situation. This approach is

[75] International Federation of Red Cross and Red Crescent Societies, *World Disasters Report* (1993), pp. 103-104.

[76] In 1992, an estimated 100 million people were affected by famine in Africa.

particularly warranted for humanitarian organizations working in emergency situations. Their problem is deciding to intervene early enough to prevent the disaster from reaching its ultimate stage (dramatic malnutrition and mortality). For example, very generally speaking, surveillance may be:

- ecological (pluviometry),
- agronomical (state of the crops),
- economic (state of market prices, migration of workers),
- social (population movements — migration),
- nutritional (changes in the malnutrition rate),
- monitoring the mortality rate.

A major decrease in measured rainfall compared with the usual norms will not call forth immediate food aid. It warrants, however, closer surveillance of subsequent, related phenomena.

### *Levels of Intervention*

An EWS is pointless unless the alarm it sounds gives rise to an intervention. Alerts prompted by threatened floods, volcanic eruptions, or earthquakes give rise to population evacuation. Emergency measures are all the more effective if prepared in advance.

In cases of drought, decisions to intervene are more difficult. Intervention must take place before the beginning of great migratory movements, which are usually accompanied by high mortality. Migration in fact begins when the crisis is already serious, and the migration is in itself an additional source of stress for the physiologically most vulnerable groups.

Theoretically, then, it is at the moment when the EWSs begin to produce signs of agricultural and economic crises that aid interventions should be planned. The implementation of this principle, however, is hindered by several obstacles:

- *Indicator unreliability*
  Locally recorded agronomical indicators are fairly reliable, but give a geographically limited view of the scope of the problem. In contrast, a satellite picture of the region gives an overall view, but does not lend itself to accurate analysis.
- *Lack of resources*
  Anticipating disasters is not high on governments' priority lists; they prefer to focus resources on programs that have an immediate impact, rather than on EWSs, the utility of which is less obvious.
- *Political difficulties*
  Political leaders are loath to admit that a crisis is near, and tend to downplay its extent. Only in a serious nutritional crisis will they admit the truth.

- *The unwieldy nature of interventions*
  Relief interventions are generally logistically ponderous, and decision-makers prefer to wait for solid evidence[77] before putting them into motion.

Under such circumstances, EWSs have a limited value, unless their predictive value is improved in future and decision-makers' mentalities change.

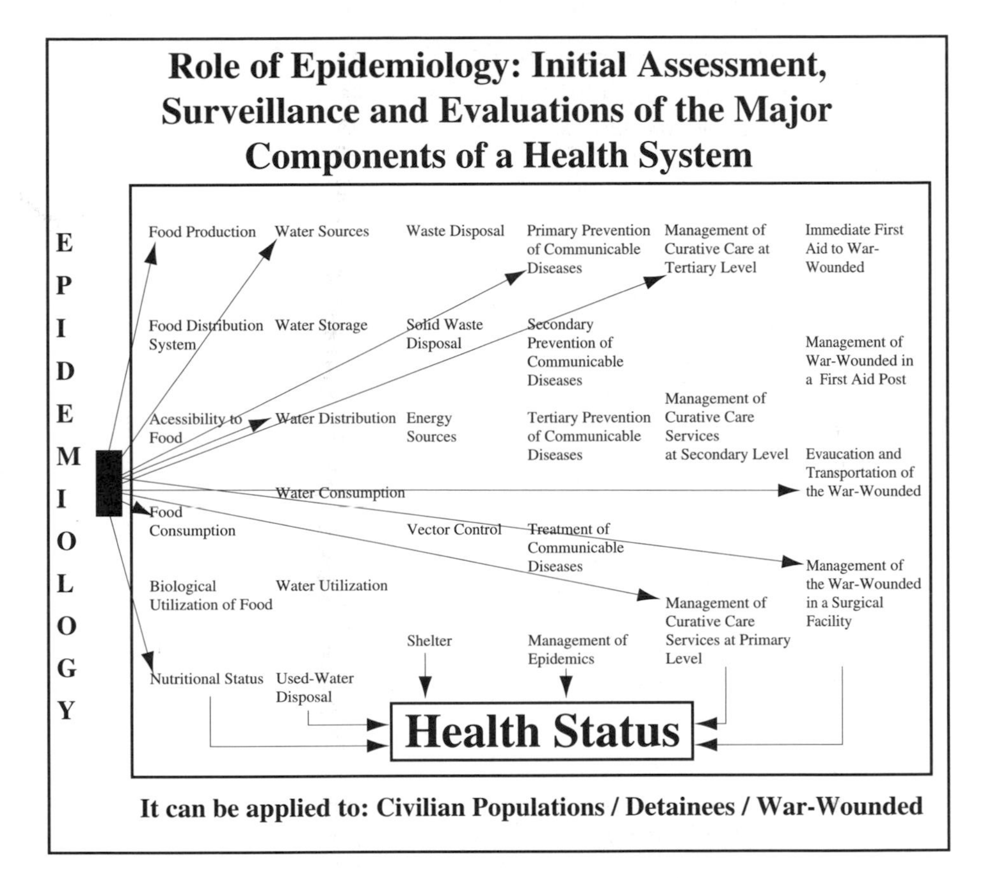


**Epidemiology is an important component of relief actions. Epidemiological tools are necessary in all fields: nutrition, environmental hygiene, communicable diseases, curative medicine. Moreover, their integration in the framework of epidemiological programs permits a global approach to crisis situations (initial assessment) as well as providing the opportunity to monitor crisis evolution (epidemiological surveillance).**

---

77 Today's mentality considers "evidence" to be a high mortality rate.

# Chapter 7

# THE HEALTH-CARE SYSTEM

***The goal of this chapter is to map out the creation of a health-care system according to the general principles applicable in normal situations, while making allowance for the specific constraints and criteria obtaining in emergency situations.***

***In particular, this chapter will examine the bases of health-care systems in general, as well as the similarities and differences between systems established for normal purposes and those set up for emergencies, and the relations between the two types in a given situation.***

# I. General Remarks

A health-care system may be defined as the organization of health-care services in a designated geographical entity — country, province, district, or the like. A relief organization operating in an emergency situation rarely has to cover the entire national territory of a country;[1] emergency operations are usually limited to certain regions. The health-care systems used for relief operations are similar to those which normally function at the district level.

Health-care systems for refugee camps are organized on the principle of geographic decentralization. The governmental authorities of the country in question delegate the responsibility for health care either to their own representatives or to a humanitarian agency or consortium of agencies. Humanitarian agencies are generally allowed enough freedom of maneuver to undertake this responsibility themselves. It should be remembered, too, that health-care systems are closely tied to the political and economic systems, particularly with respect to financing.

The proper functioning of any health-care service depends on its capacity to deal with whatever specific problems arise.

## 1. Health Problems

### 1.1 Increased Needs

Medical needs in emergency situations are similar to those present in normal times. The difference lies mainly in their extent and the speed with which they arise. In a newly created camp for displaced people, medical needs are multiplied two or three times over.

[1] There have been a few cases where the national health-care system completely collapsed — for example, in Cambodia in 1979 and in Somalia in 1991.

### 1.2 The Distinction between "Wants" and "Needs"

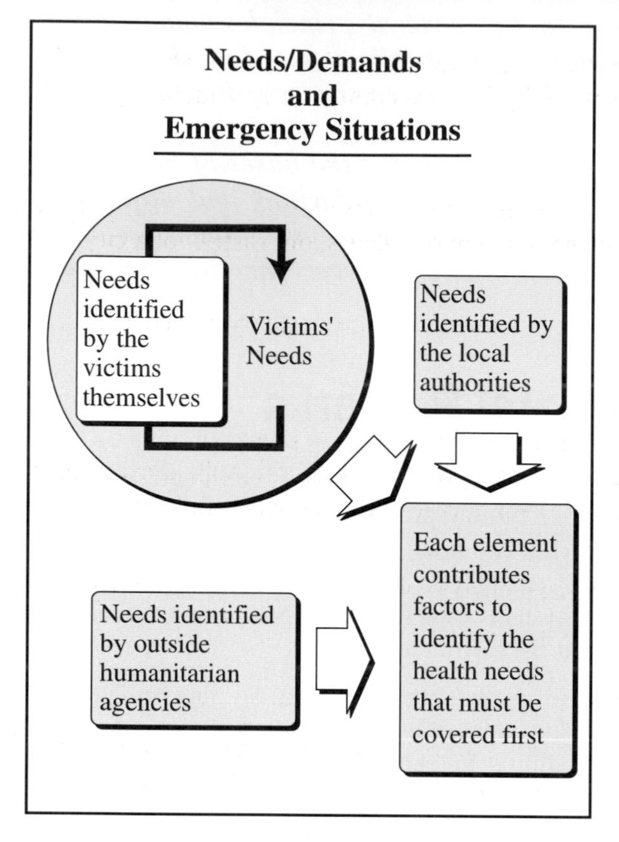


A distinction must be made between:

- *wants*, the expression of what the victims themselves want from the health-care services; and
- *needs*, the care and services that the health-care personnel consider necessary for the victims.

In normal situations, the health-care facilities generally take both these factors into account, offering the population services that correspond to both their wants and their "real" needs as defined by health-care professionals. There should be a concurrence between real needs, experienced needs (wants), and the technically and financially possible responses.

In times of disaster, the effort to reconcile "needs" and "wants" is usually cut short. Humanitarian organizations tend to impose a health-care system that will cover the victims' immediate needs. This approach should not be considered as a form of humanitarian imperialism; it is dictated by the urgency of meeting the victims' vital needs, by the know-how acquired in previous crisis experience, and, especially, by the human and financial resources that the agencies are able to muster.

Although the imperative of quick action should not obscure the importance of considering the victims' wants, in this respect there is a major difference between emergency situations and normal situations.

## 2. Levels of Health Care

There are several levels of health care.

## 2.1 Structural Levels

- *The family level:*
  A certain amount of health care, both preventive and curative, can be provided within the family itself, by family members or by community health workers.[2]
- *The community level:*
  The community level corresponds to a population unit defined by geographical features: a village, a group of villages, one district of a city.[3]
- *The dispensary level:*
  The dispensary level combines all types of ambulatory care provided in health-care facilities.
- *The rural or district hospital:*
  Rural and district hospitals are classified with the first level of hospital care; this is also the level usually assigned to units specially built during relief operations to provide general hospital care to the civilian population.
- *The referral hospital:*
  Referral hospitals are the second-line facilities — provincial hospitals, specialized hospitals, etc.

## 2.2 Health-Care Providers

Each of the levels described above features a particular type of "health-care personnel," whose training must correspond to what is expected of them:

- mothers
- community health workers (CHWs)
- nursing staff
- doctors
- specialists

Health-care providers work on several levels. The CHWs, for example, are supposed to go from household to household, receive patients at their health stations, and go regularly to the dispensary on which they depend for further information. Similarly, doctors and nurses, besides the care they provide, play an organizational role in dispensaries and hospitals, and, in some cases, directly in the community.

---

[2] Such care includes health education, personal hygiene, introduction to prophylactic measures (immunization), guided weaning, family-planning advice, treatment of diarrhea, management of a family medicine chest, introduction to health services, etc.

[3] This level involves health-related activities that can be undertaken at the family level but extend beyond the framework of individual health due to factors such as environmental hygiene, water supply, food production, the organization of immunization campaigns, etc.

The financial and technological resources allocated to a health-care system shape its activities. If, in a disaster-stricken country, hospitals and the training of high-level medical personnel are given priority, to the detriment of the grassroots levels (dispensaries, community, family), the result will be essentially a European type of health-care system.

Balancing the distribution of financial and human resources between primary health-care (PHC) programs and medical-care programs in health-care facilities should be the ultimate goal, so that everyone has access to the care he or she requires, regardless of social class. In conflict situations, access to medical care must not be allowed to depend on political, ethnic, or military affiliations.

# II. Primary Health-Care Strategy

Depending on the way it operates, a health-care system can have a "big head" or "big feet." In the first instance, most of the system's resources are channeled into the operation of high-level health-care facilities such as hospitals, while in the second case, the orientation is to decentralize the health-care system towards the periphery, the goal being a better adaptation of health services to the population's needs. The strategy of the first approach is based on the so-called "trickle-down" effect, in which resources directed towards the top of the health-care pyramid are supposed to spread down towards the base. The second approach demands a strategy based on primary health care.

One approach does not exclude the other; a happy medium must be found between the two, the main idea being to prevent and/or resolve medical problems to the extent possible. The second strategy is essential, but does not eliminate the necessity of dealing with serious medical needs in the framework of hospital facilities. The same balance can be sought in emergency situations.

PHC involves three aspects.

## 1. The Political Aspect

The basis of the political aspect of PHC was enunciated in the declaration of Alma-Ata:

"[...] international commitment to primary health care should be oriented to support national primary health care programmes by creating a positive climate of opinion; by facilitating the exchange of expertise, technology and information through technical cooperation among developing countries and between industrialized and developing countries; and by encouraging proper orientation of financial resources. However, all international agencies, non-governmental agencies and countries providing support have to be aware that the purpose of their efforts is in the long run to enable countries themselves to apply primary health care as part of their overall development and in the spirit of self-reliance."[4]

Primary health care is a strategic option aimed at achieving the objectives established by the Conference of Alma-Ata:[5]

"Primary health care forms an integral part of the country health system, of which it is the central function and main agent for delivering health care. It is also an integral part of the overall social and economic development of the community."[6]

WHO has distilled from this approach the basic principles for the development of a health-care system:

"– The system should encompass the entire population on the basis of equality and reciprocity.

- The system should include components from the health sector and from other sectors whose interrelated actions contribute to health.
- Primary health care should consist of at least the essential elements enunciated in the Declaration of Alma-Ata.
- The other elements of the health system should support the first contact level of primary health care to permit it to provide these essential elements on a continuing basis.
- At intermediate levels, more complex problems should be dealt with, more skilled and specialized care as well as logistic support should be provided, and more highly trained staff should provide continuing training to primary health care workers — as well as guidance to communities and community health workers on practical problems arising in connection with all aspects of primary health care.
- The central level should coordinate all parts of the system and provide planning and management expertise in aspects that are common to all institutions in the country."[7]

---

4 WHO, *Alma Ata,* A Joint Report of WHO and UNICEF (1978), p. 79.

5 Declaration made at the conclusion of the international conference held in Alma-Ata (USSR) on 12 September 1978, which marked a turning point in health service organization with regard to achieving a more equitable distribution of care. This conference gave rise to the WHO slogan "health for all by the year 2000."

6 WHO, *Formulating Strategies for Health for All by the Year 2000: Guiding Principles and Essential Issues*, Health for All Series, No. 2 (Geneva: WHO, 1979), p. 12.

7 WHO, "Implementation of the Global Strategy for Health for All by the Year 2000, Second Evaluation," *Eighth Report on the World Health Situation*, Vol. 1: *Global Review* (Geneva: WHO, 1989), p. 37.

The decision to orient a health-care system towards PHC obviously represents a political stand on the part of the government. In emergency situations, however, this political dimension is absent, except when the governments of donor countries or humanitarian agencies try to impose a hospital for high-level care during a disaster situation, in order to "look good."

## 2. The Management Aspect

Two principles are important with respect to management, the participation of the population and self-management. One of the basic principles of PHC is maximal delegation of responsibility to the population itself. In theory, this principle also applies in emergency situations: from the beginning of an intervention, the displaced or refugee population should be called upon to help take charge of its own health problems. It must be recognized, however, that on many occasions solutions are simply imposed upon the victims. There is thus a notorious difference between emergency situations and the practice of PHC under normal circumstances.[8]

The ultimate goal is self-management of PHC programs by the population itself; the population furnishes the financial and human resources, and therefore decides the program's orientation. In such a case, PHC becomes a genuine process of development.

The situation in this respect is markedly different in an emergency, when the health-care system functions almost exclusively thanks to outside help.

## 3. The Technical Aspect

WHO recommends that PHC include at least the following activities:

- education about health problems
- promotion of good nutrition
- adequate provision of safe water and basic sanitation measures
- preventive care for mothers and infants
- immunization
- prevention and control of local endemics
- treatment of common diseases and lesions
- provision of essential drugs

By analogy, a list of programs[9] can be drawn up for situations involving displaced or refugee populations.

[8] Even though here, too, solutions are often imposed by the hierarchy, and the people are not consulted.

[9] Such programs may be implemented by local health-care systems, humanitarian agencies, or a combination of the two.

- food provision
- supplementary feeding program[10]
- supply of potable water
- waste removal program
- housing program
- vector control program
- immunization program
- communicable disease control program
- health education program
- ambulatory care program
- hospital care program[11]

Thus, the same types of programs are adopted in both kinds of situation.

## 4. Appraisal of the Three Aspects of PHC

In an article comparing primary health care under normal circumstances with that dispensed in an emergency situation, authors from various academic circles (the London School of Hygiene and Tropical Medicine, the University of California at Los Angeles, the National Council for International Health in Washington, Lousiana State University at New Orleans), as well as Oxfam and the High Commissioner for Refugees strongly emphasize that:

"emergency medical aid must be considered as a means of intervention similar to long-term medical and sanitary action, implying the community-based, participatory approach of PHC.

This concern to avoid cutting emergency medical-health interventions (EMHIs) off from long-term action is intended, on one hand, to counter the main criticisms of emergency medical aid, and, on the other, to take account of the fact that the needs of refugee populations are not essentially different from the everyday health needs of developing countries." [12]

Specific health interventions are offered as an alternative to PHC services, which are judged to be utopian and expensive. These specific interventions are designed to focus exclusively on health priorities, which are technically defined according to the following criteria:

- the prevalence of the health problem;

[10] If necessary, nutrition rehabilitation programs.

[11] If necessary, care for war-wounded.

[12] D. Grodos, "De l'aide d'urgence aux soins de santé primaires," *Médecine tropicale* 48, No. 1 (1988): 53.

- its morbidity and mortality;
- its susceptibility to a treatment that can be easily applied to large groups.

Thus, specific health interventions are intended to free individuals and communities from their principal health scourges and to save the most vulnerable lives. This definition has the merit of distinguishing emergency actions from true PHC. The most common types of intervention concern the following:

- access to food resources;
- access to potable water;
- waste disposal;
- access to shelter and eventually to proper housing;
- protection against the cold (shelter, blankets, clothes);
- immunization;
- measures against communicable diseases;
- provision of essential drugs.[13]

PHC and EMHIs have similar purposes: to offer populations a health status that conforms to norms reflecting local conditions. EMHIs are not directly related to satisfactory social and economic development. In fact, EMHIs are usually artificially based: financial, logistic, technical, and managerial supports[14] are usually external, particularly when the implementation of the programs has no connection whatsoever with the local authorities. The danger with EMHIs is that they are apt to leave nothing behind when they and the outside aid come to an end. In this sense, PHC and EMHIs are different.

The two approaches use a similar strategy, however. Access to health services must be as broad and as easy as possible, and the emphasis is on preventive measures. One difference, however, is that in emergency situations, results are expected within a couple of weeks, while results from PHC are part of the strategy of "health for all by the year 2000."

A second difference lies in the population's preliminary involvement in selecting the intervention programs. Taking the "wants/needs" formulated by the population into account is imperative in the framework of PHC, whereas in emergency situations, health measures are usually imposed by humanitarian agencies.

On occasion, however, a synthesis of the two different approaches may be possible. Emergency actions may then be considered as a group of specific

---

[13] Within the framework of the ambulatory care program.

[14] The financial aspect is particularly important, since in emergency situations, the entire financial burden is borne by the local services or by humanitarian agencies (either directly or through aid to the local services). In normal situations, one of the main requirements for a successful PHC program is that the community takes at least partial financial responsibility for it.

interventions which, despite everything, are coordinated to a certain degree. The victims should participate in their planning and implementation as much as possible. In this way, disaster-stricken populations will be able to survive in acceptable conditions in the short term, and, in the long term, they will retain certain benefits that can be applied to development activities. When such activities evolve from the emergency situation itself, the link between EMHIs and PHC is clear, since emergency activities thereby gain a "developmental" dimension.

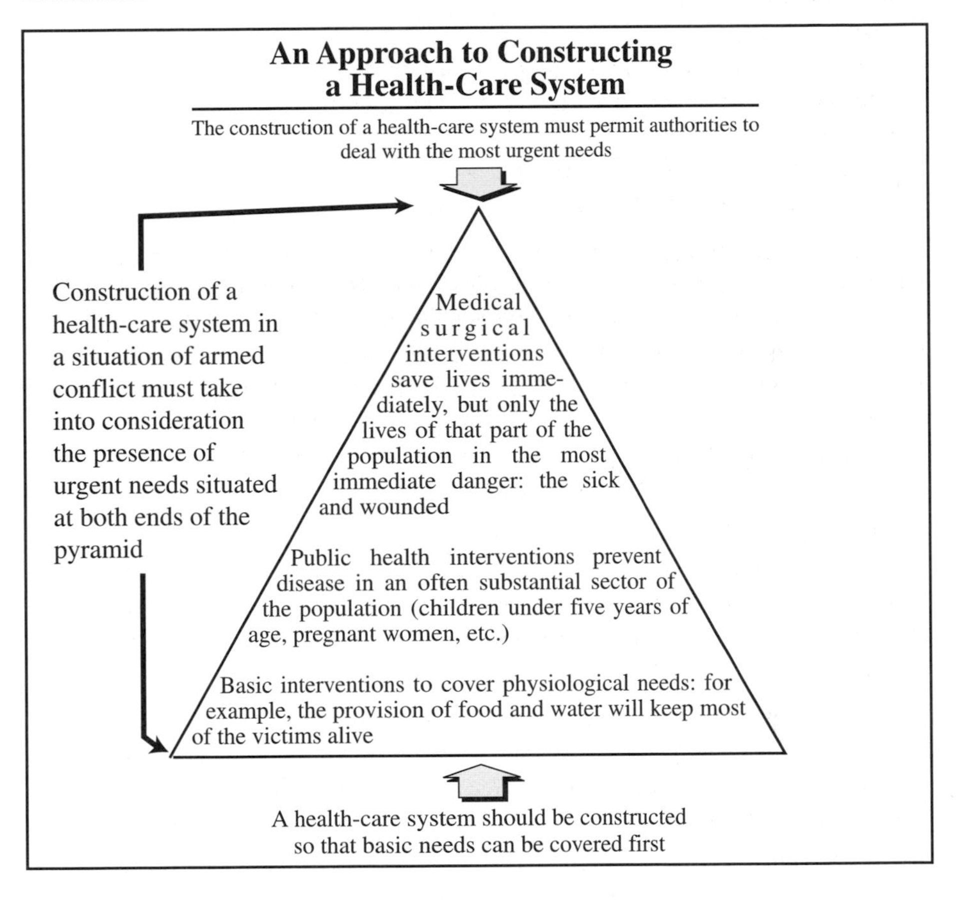


# III. Functioning of a Health-Care System

The overall functioning of a health-care system is judged by:

- the coordination between the services offered and the needs of the population;
- the equitable distribution of services;
- the accessibility of care.

These three criteria are also valid for emergency situations — with, however, variable connotations.

# 1. Coordination between Services and Population

The match between the services offered and the population's needs is based on four principles:

- decentralization of the health-care services
- coordination between the systems involved
- pyramidal organization of the health-care services
- coordination between the partners involved.

## 1.1 Decentralization of Services

As noted earlier, the skills of the care providers, whether family members or medical personnel, must be suited to the tasks they are supposed to perform. This principle works in both directions: on one hand, the civilian health-care systems may not be prepared for difficult medical cases (insufficient skills); on the other, health-care personnel may be performing tasks that could be executed at the lowest levels by people who are medically less qualified but who are closer to the population.

The decentralization of health-care services should in any case further the essential goal, which is to give populations direct access to the primary level of health care. Decentralization can be defined in two ways:[15]

- *functional decentralization* — Certain tasks are delegated to the periphery for example, the treatment of diarrheal diseases, respiratory infections, and fevers is delegated to CHWs. The procedures for diagnosis and treatment are laid down by the medical hierarchy.

- *geographical decentralization* — The responsibility for organizing health-care systems is delegated to the officials in charge of an entire geographical area. They can decide how dispensaries will function, how to organize public health measures, etc.

In refugee camps, the responsibility for running the health services often devolves on humanitarian agencies, with greater or lesser participation and control by the country's ministry of health. Inside the camp, the issue of decentralizing health services is not as pressing as in normal situations. The population is concentrated in a restricted space and is not usually occupied by daily work; consequently,

[15] A. Mills, J.P. Vaughan, D.L. Smith, and I. Tabibzadeh, *Health System Decentralization* (WHO, 1990) p. 15.

access to health-care services is easy. A certain concentration of services in the central medical facilities can therefore be tolerated. Nonetheless, the implementation of preventive measures (immunization, health education, hygiene measures) still requires a decentralized approach.

## 1.2 Coordination between Health-Related Systems

As shown, health depends only partially on the health-care services. Other factors, such as agriculture, environment, and social structures, are also strong influences. In an emergency situation, the concept of health-related systems is replaced by the more specific one of programs for feeding and nutrition, water, environmental hygiene, and the like.

### *Prevention Programs*

In each of the areas discussed below (nutrition, environmental hygiene, prevention), aid organizations may establish programs with a specific objective, defined by the target population they are trying to cover (children under five, pregnant women, etc.) and by the high selectivity of the intervention. These are isolated programs such as emergency mass immunization campaigns, nutritional rehabilitation programs, water supply projects, and so on.

Such programs respond to a vital need, such as the immediate immunization of all vulnerable subjects against measles, the provision of drinking water to a population as quickly as possible, or the treatment of malnourished people to keep them alive. However, if such programs are not part of an integrated system, they may miss their mark. A nutrition rehabilitation program does not solve the problem of malnutrition, if households do not have access to food resources. Similarly, the establishment of a water-supply system goes hand in hand with waste removal, since otherwise the waste is liable to contaminate the water sources.

Clearly, these programs are complementary. The cold induces an additional expenditure of individual energy, while food intake is usually inadequate. The distribution of clothing and blankets and the provision of satisfactory housing therefore "cover" nutritional needs to some degree.

Health-education programs, set up during the acute phase of emergency situations, are essential at all levels of prevention, if the population is to derive maximal benefit from them.[16]

[16] These programs are better described as a set of more or less coercive measures than as training designed to modify the behavior of the population. In fact, the authoritarian measures taken at the beginning of a crisis in order to reduce health risks as much as possible are usually replaced at a later stage by true education programs.

### *Curative Programs*

The interaction of curative programs is a concept familiar to health-care personnel. Medical services are constituted by facilities for ambulatory care and facilities for hospital care, with a communication network (ambulances) between them.

Once the most urgent medical problems have been defined, a decision must be made as to what level of the health-care system will treat these problems. This implies that the exact skills of the health-care personnel at each level are known, including those of any community health workers.[17]

Delegating standardized tasks on the basis of skills is an essential integrational activity at the beginning of an intervention. This, of course, can be done only if diagnostic and therapeutic procedures and criteria for inter-level transfer have been rationalized, standardized, and well-formulated in advance.

### *Integration of the Preventive and Curative Levels*

Primarily curative activities are unlikely to influence the health status of a disaster-stricken population. They will save a certain number of victims, of course, and the media will have the opportunity to present dramatic features about "the fantastic work done by medical teams working under horrifying conditions"; but, overall, the health situation will not change much.

On the other hand, an exclusively preventive approach will run up against incomprehension on the part of the victims — who will not understand why no one is taking care of their sick — and on the part of the media, who will immediately interpret this policy as a criminal failure to render assistance to people in danger.

> Integration between preventive and curative measures is technically necessary and politically desirable.

The value of curative care is unquestionable. Nonetheless, curative measures are merely a palliative for the medical problems most frequently encountered in disaster situations. They improve individual cases to some extent, but do not provide reasonable solutions in the medium term. A purely curative approach leads to a vicious circle which is difficult to break.

---

[17] If there are no community health workers, the definition of the tasks that they would assume will serve as a basis for a training program.

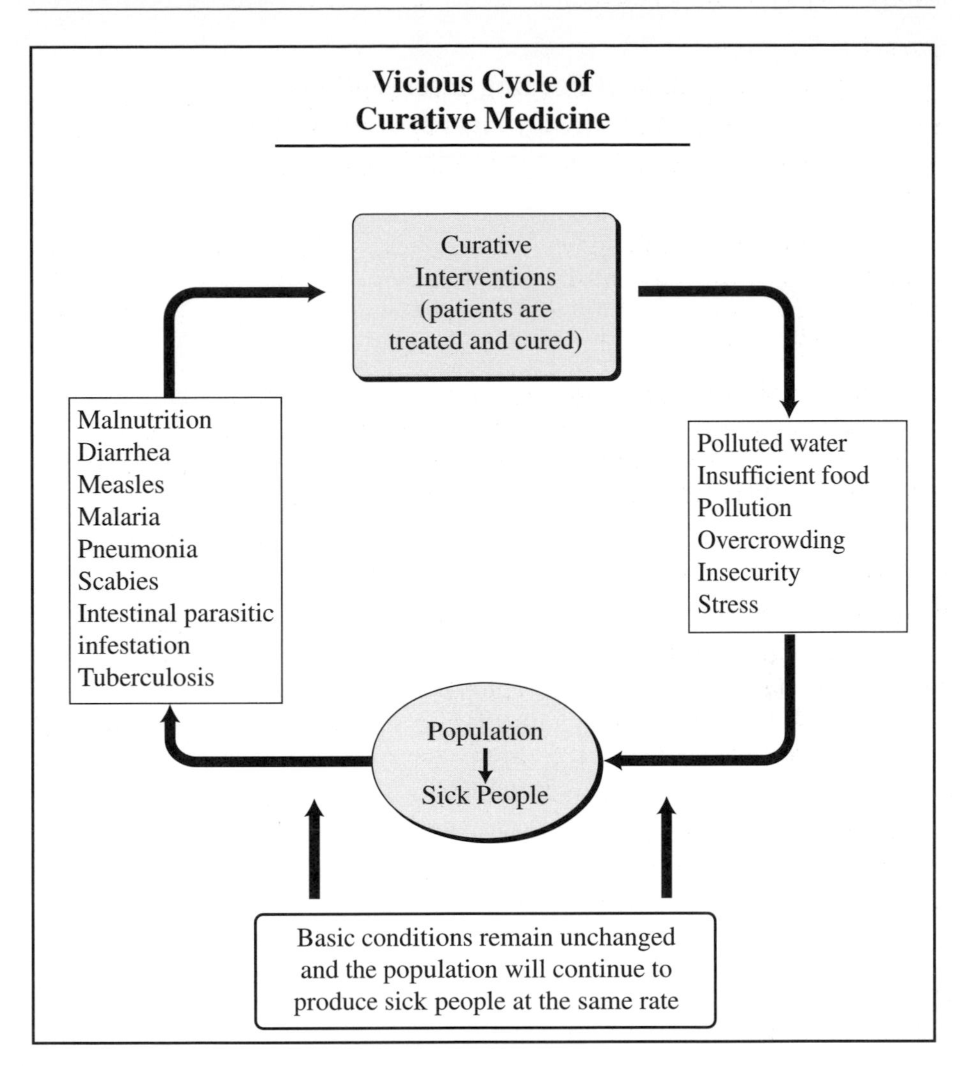


If priority is given to the problem of lack of food, by facilitating access to food resources or directly providing victims with the food that they need, not only will the prevalence of malnutrition decrease, but also that of the medical problems that are generally closely linked to it.

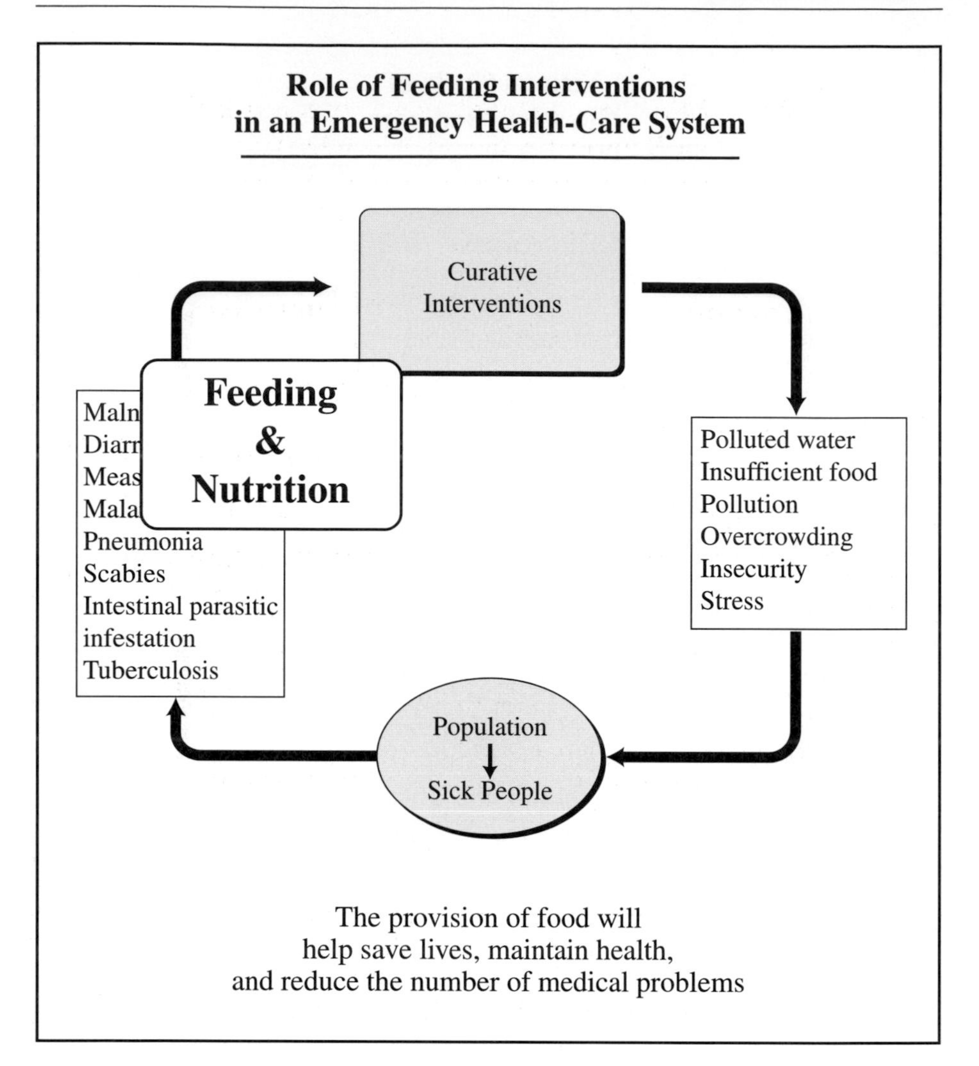


Similarly, supplying the victims with sufficient quantities of clean water will contribute to a notable improvement in the health status of the entire population, mainly by reducing the prevalence of diarrheal diseases.

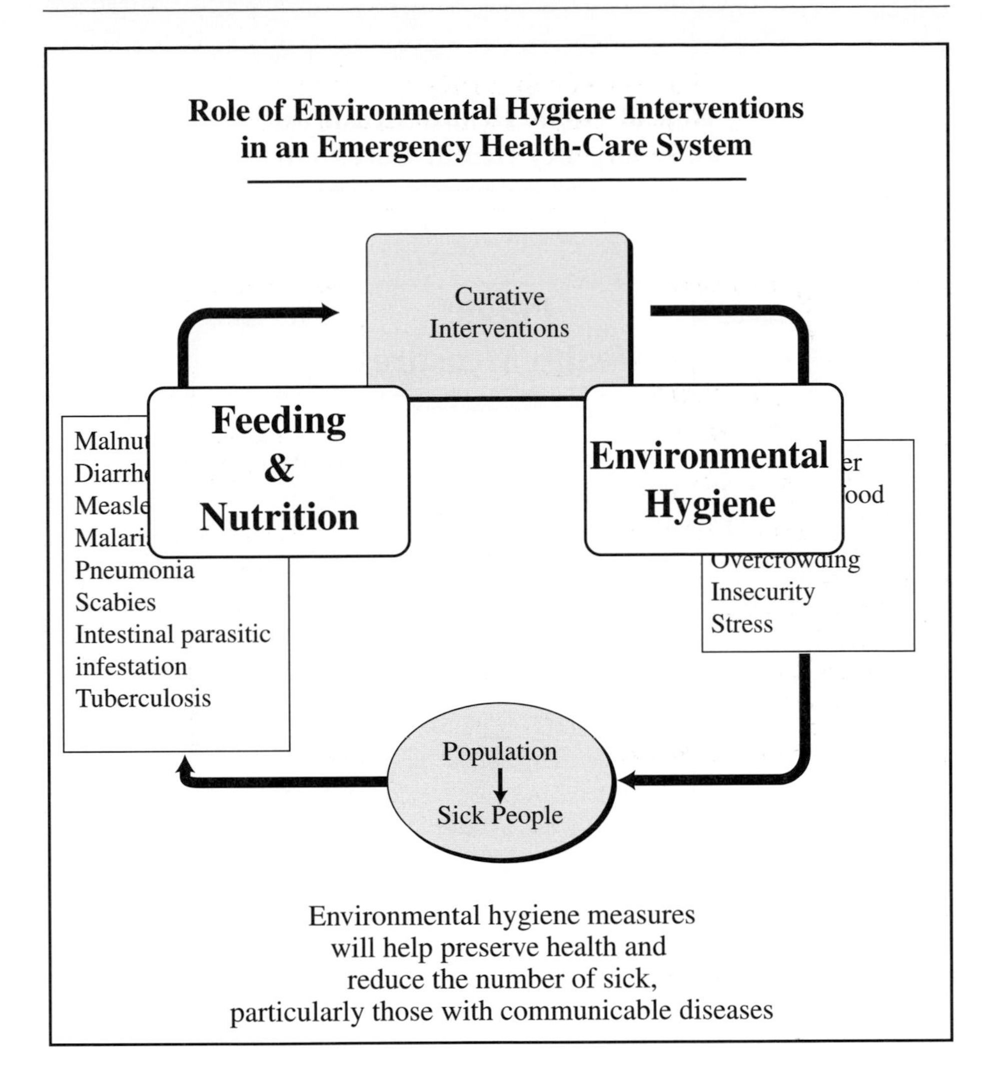


Other measures are also important in reducing mortality — for example, immunization against measles and the promotion of oral rehydration.

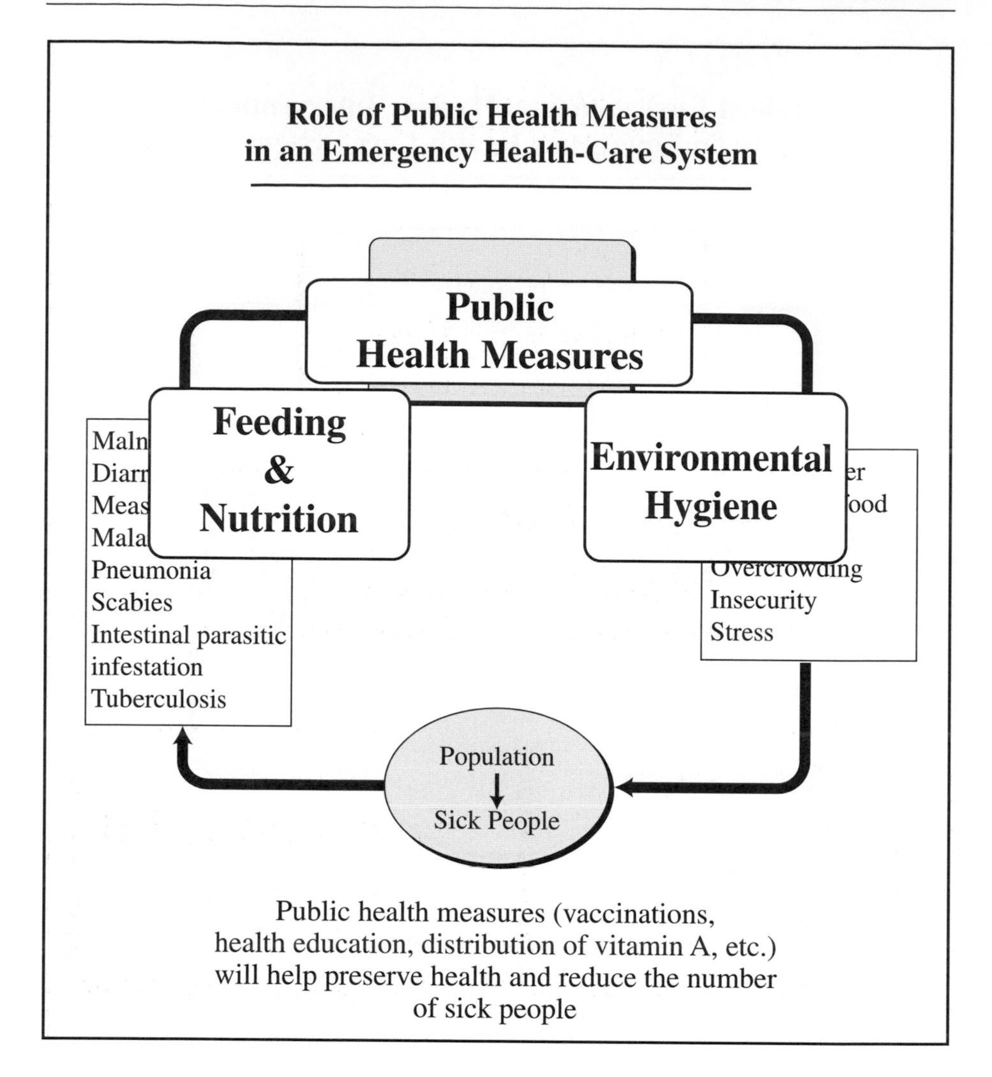


Public health measures (vaccinations, health education, distribution of vitamin A, etc.) will help preserve health and reduce the number of sick people

The purpose of all these programs is to promote and preserve health. They should be the basis of any health-care system on which curative-oriented services will depend; from the very beginning of an action, a multisectoral approach to health problems should be envisioned.

## 1.3 The Health-Care Pyramid

The health-care systems proposed for emergency situations are structured like a pyramid, the base being the keystones of health: access to food resources, access to clean water, and proper environmental hygiene. On this base rest public health measures such as immunization, health education, control of epidemics, routine care, etc. On top of that comes medical care *per se*.

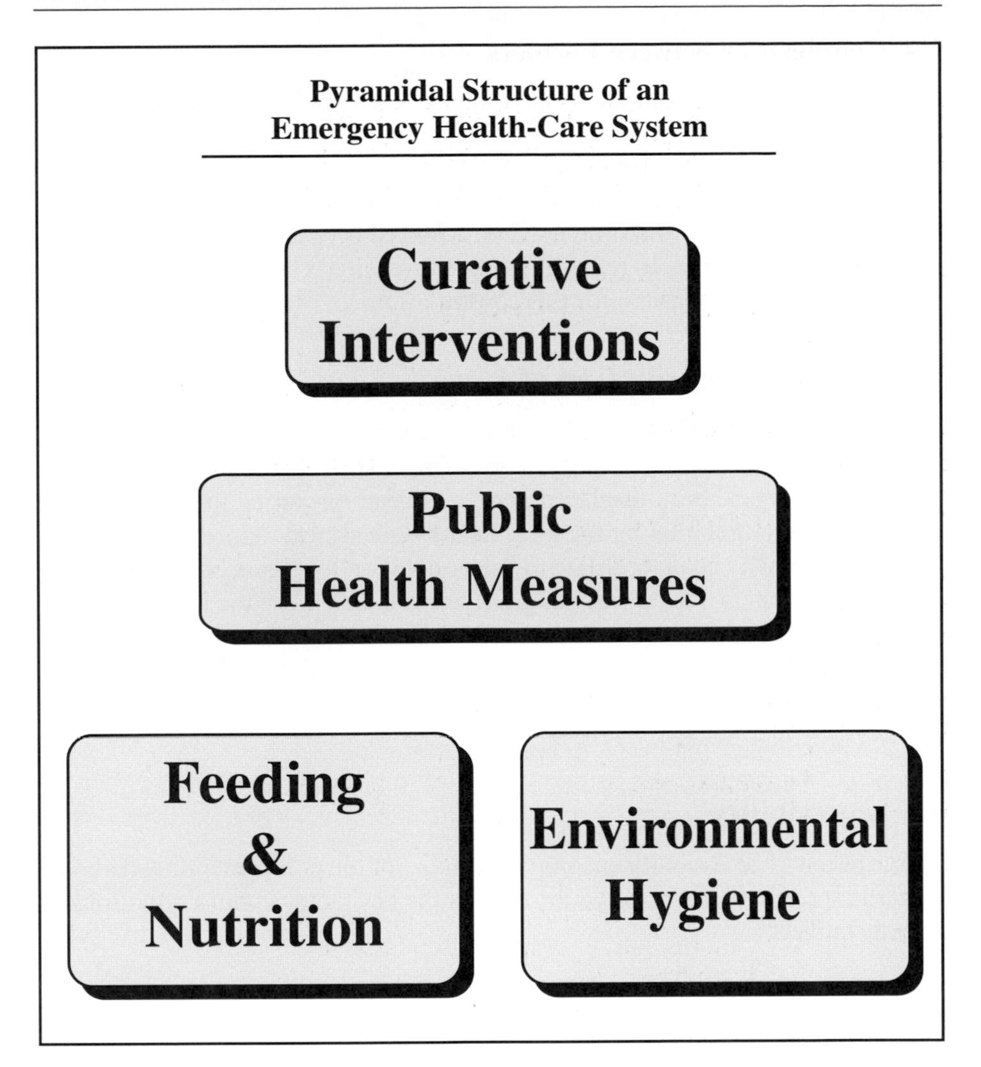


**Is it realistic to try to follow this principle to the letter?**

In practice, a certain flexibility is required in strategies for action; the order in which programs are set up does not have to follow the established principles strictly. Prevention-oriented programs are generally more unwieldy than curative ones, and there is no need to wait until all the preventive measures have been instituted before beginning to plan and implement curative programs. The essential thing is to maintain an overall view of the health-care system that is to be instituted, and to integrate the programs into it as they are implemented. Without this global vision, health-care systems established in emergency situations usually remain chaotic.

### 1.4 Coordination between Partners

Organizing a health-care system is complex, even though certain aspects of emergency conditions facilitate its establishment. One factor is that financial resources are available through international aid; another assist is the limited geographical area that is usually involved. Nonetheless, for the system to function well, solid coordination must be achieved between the different parties involved in its operation. In refugee camps, the country's health ministry and the HCR are usually responsible for this coordination.

## 2. Equitable Distribution of Care

The geographical distribution of health services should cover the majority of the population. The issue of equity also arises when the care provided by humanitarian agencies to displaced people is clearly superior to that provided to the resident population by the local health-care system. Moreover, the local health services may be inaccessible to the population for financial reasons (high cost or lack of social security coverage). This, too, may raise the issue of equity, insofar as the emergency health services are free. Discriminatory provision of health care is a major problem in situations of armed conflict. Depending on their affiliation to one side or the other, victims may be denied access to health-care services.

## 3. Accessibility

The criterion of accessibility encompasses many of the points mentioned above. It merits special attention, however, for it is the key factor in most situations of armed conflict.[18]

### 3.1 Accessibility and Geographical Location

The farther away health services are from the population, the less they are used.[19] In developing countries, installing health-care facilities such as dispensaries or hospitals in immediate proximity to the homes of all the potential patients is a utopian dream. In these countries, the remoteness of health centers is a problem difficult to surmount. In disaster situations, when communications are even more trouble-ridden than usual, the gap between health facilities and victims becomes even wider.

A few comments should be made about the institution of mobile teams which visit villages and displaced-person camps every two to four weeks for a more direct

---

[18] Accessibility is also a problem in natural disasters, where it may be reduced (owing to the severance of communication routes) or complicated (owing to the chaotic influx of all the humanitarian agencies).

[19] M. King, *Medical Care in Developing Countries* (Nairobi: Oxford University Press, 1966).

access to victims. This approach is indicated for prophylactic activities such as immunizations and hygiene programs, which do not require daily follow-up. Mobile teams that deliver medical care, in contrast, do nothing to control serious cases of disease, because access to the population is too sporadic. A child's chances of being saved will depend on whether he comes down with pneumonia a few hours before or a few hours after the team passes through. Access to the victims is not only a matter of contact at regular intervals, but also of continuity in the relations between the health-care services and those who need them. The mobile teams move on, the patients remain.

### 3.2 Accessibility and Economic Restrictions

Many health services, particularly curative services, are accessible only to paying patients. A situation of conflict aggravates preexisting economic differences and tends to reduce equitable access to health services. This factor may be one of the reasons that the victims of conflict tend to congregate in places where health services are accessible.

### 3.3 Accessibility and Security

Unsafe conditions may prevent access to a population's usual services, for example, to health facilities. They may also restrict an entire population's access to its immediate environment. For example, the placement of antipersonnel mines in the fields around a village tends to reduce the land normally available for cultivation, and, as a result, the population's agricultural and food resources. The destruction of communication routes (bridges, for example) may also cut off access to local services.

To these direct consequences of conflict must be added the political practices obtaining in most countries. The distribution of health facilities, for example, is notoriously subject to political pressures: a particular hospital will be built in the geographical district controlled by a politically influential man.

In conflict situations, political accessibility is especially important for several reasons. At best, the authorities will try to direct aid to politically favorable regions; usually they will hinder or even forbid the establishment of health-care facilities in areas they do not control.

### 3.4 Accessibility and Social or Ethnic Origin, or Affiliation with a Political Group

Accessibility is also significant in emergency situations where several population groups of very different social and ethnic origins are thrown together. The use of services, particularly those involving personal hygiene (baths, latrines, etc.), depends largely on their cultural acceptability to these populations. Similarly, if the makeup of food rations does not take the beneficiaries' dietary habits into

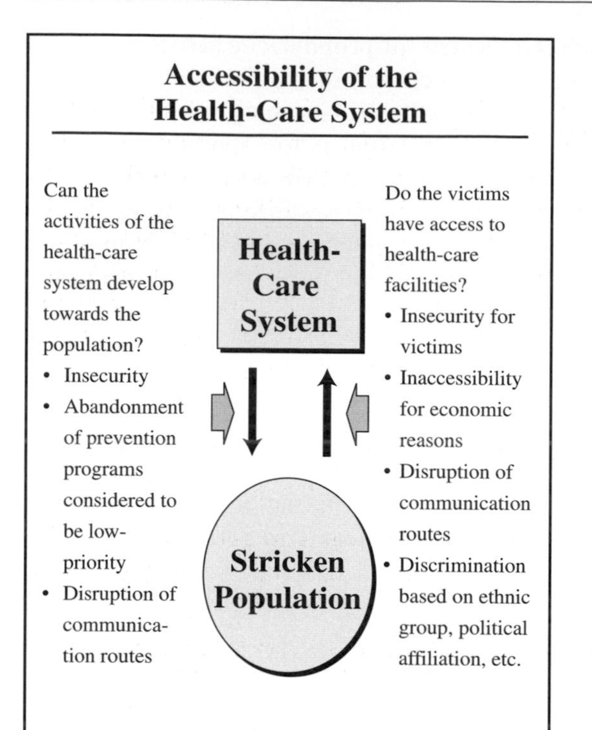


account, distributed food will not be eaten but rather sold, exchanged,[20] or, worse, thrown away.

In situations of armed conflict, the principle of accessibility is the key to organizing an equitable health-care system.

The conditions for the proper functioning of a health-care system having been laid down, two questions remain to be answered: To what degree are the local health-care systems able to respond to the requirements of the situation? When must international relief intervene?

# IV. International Humanitarian Assistance and Local Health Systems

To clarify the relations between international humanitarian aid and local health-care systems, two questions must be answered:

- Is international humanitarian aid necessary?
- If so, in what form?

The answers depend on an analysis of the local health-care system's capacity to cope with the situation.[21] Too much space would be required to analyze all the facets of a health-care system here; this section will be limited to medical facilities and how they can be analyzed with the help of a flow chart.

[20] Within certain limits, this is perfectly acceptable.

[21] In some situations, moreover, the local health-care systems, for political and/or economic reasons, refuse to take responsibility for refugee populations, leaving them to humanitarian agencies.

# 1. The Basic Problem

In developing countries, most of the health-care services are insufficient to respond to the needs of the population. This is the reason, for example, for the congestion of health-care facilities and the long waiting lines at water distribution points. This problem leads to dysfunction in these facilities and a lack of motivation in health-care personnel, who are swamped by a demand they cannot satisfy, and in the populations themselves, who hesitate to turn to the health-care services. In an emergency situation, demand is especially great, and without rational organization, services[22] are quickly overwhelmed. Certainly, a doubling of the population in the space of a few weeks in a city of average size often strains the capacity of hospital facilities intolerably.

Nor is the quantitative aspect the only issue; emergency situations are often characterized by the presence of needs, particularly medical ones, which differ from conventional medical needs. One example is war wounds, which require a particular approach involving triage, special operating procedures, and so on. The quality of the care provided by the local services is difficult to evaluate. The rule, insofar as one exists, is to make sure that the procedures followed are not contrary to the interests of the victims. As to their effectiveness, this must be defined in terms of the local context, which serves as the basis of reference. Distributions of powdered milk to a displaced population, for example, clearly contravene universally recognized rules. Similarly, the use of conventional surgical procedures to treat war wounds causes secondary complications, such as infections, which the techniques of war surgery can prevent.

**Imbalance between the Victims' Needs and the Services Available**

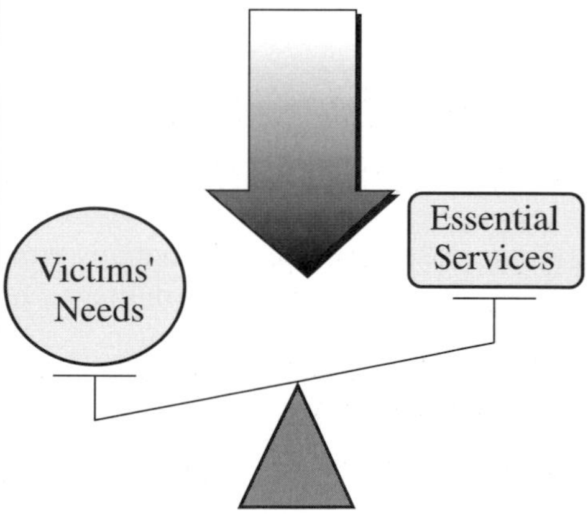

Victims' Needs

Essential Services

A strategy of action can be defined for humanitarian agencies. Actually, the smooth functioning of the local services and their accessibility to the victims of a

[22] Basically the health-care facilities.

disaster may seem to indicate that humanitarian aid is not required. But in fact things are never that simple. The pressure exerted by local services taking advantage of the crisis to launch apparently unfounded appeals for aid, together with the pressure of donors who want to help, even if help is not needed, singularly complicate the process of deciding when and how to provide external assistance.

In the face of these difficulties, the flow chart that follows is a useful way of defining the possible forms that humanitarian aid may take, based on the criteria of the capacity and accessibility of the local services.[23]

## 2. Starting Point for the Flow Chart

**Take as a starting point the criterion of accessibility, and answer the question: Are the local services accessible to the victims? YES/NO**

YES: Move to the next criterion -> capacities of the local services

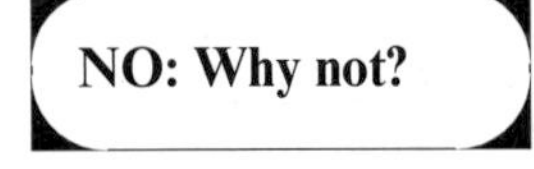


a) *Physical or geographical inaccessibility*: The health-care services are too far away from the displaced population; there are no means of transport. This kind of problem is not specific to emergency situations; rural populations are usually very far away from health-care facilities.
b) *Financial inaccessibility*: Civilians wounded in the course of a conflict, for example, may not have the money to pay the hospital, even though the latter has the capacity to treat them.
c) *Social inaccessibility*: This may be exacerbated by the increased demand during a crisis; the most deprived social classes may be denied access to health-care facilities.
d) *Political inaccessibility*: This is very specific to conflict situations. Discrimination may be based on various factors, such as membership in a political party, an armed band, or an ethnic group. In addition, security problems keep victims from reaching health-care facilities, or preventive programs (immunization, mosquito-control programs, etc.) from reaching certain regions.

---

[23] "Success in reorganizing and expanding the health system must be assessed in terms of access to, and coverage by, at least the essential services — and assessing not only their utilization, but also their quality. There is no universally satisfactory indicator for assessing 'coverage'; the general concept must be broken down into measurement of accessibility, availability, and utilization." WHO, "Evaluation of the Strategy for Health for All by the Year 2000," *Seventh Report on the World Health Situation, Global Review*, Vol. 1 (Geneva: WHO, 1987), p. 37.

e) *A combination of different kinds of inaccessibility*: The displacement of populations to a region far removed from any medical infrastructure because of their political, ethnic, or other affiliations exemplifies a combination of geographic, financial, and political factors.

A certain number of decisions must already be made at this stage, depending on whether the inaccessibility can be reduced or not:

- Can the displaced population be returned home?
- Is it possible to negotiate non-discriminatory health care for all the victims of a conflict, whatever their political affiliation?
- Is it possible to negotiate free access to health services for the disaster victims?

When problems cannot be resolved by local means, external aid[24] must be contemplated in the form of:

- financial aid, to give victims access to the local health-care services;
- ICRC protection, to preserve the local health-care services' access to the populations they serve;[25]
- making a hospital neutral ground, in order to guarantee safe access to it;[26]
- establishing parallel facilities to take the place of the local services. This is a last resort, when everything else has been tried to no avail.[27]

**The accessibility of local services is established or guaranteed. Are they able to meet the victims' needs in addition to their usual work?**

The health-care services' capacity to cope with an emergency situation can be analyzed on the basis of two subsidiary criteria — which may, in fact, be combined:

- the potential to furnish the quantity of services required by the emergency situation;
- the potential to adjust the quality of the services to accommodate certain specific requirements of emergency situations.

**1. Quantitative aspect: Are the local services able to furnish the quantity of services necessary?**

[24] "External aid" means aid from outside the system directly affected; it may be regional, national, or international.

[25] For example, the ICRC provided protection for health ministry teams in El Salvador so that they could continue their immunization campaign in combat zones.

[26] The ICRC neutralized the Jaffna hospital in Sri Lanka in this way, so that all the victims of the conflict would have access to it.

[27] On the Thai border in 1979, for example, Khmer refugees had very limited access to Thai hospital services. There it was necessary from the start to erect autonomous hospital facilities for this population.

YES: In this case, verify the quality of the service.

**NO: Why not?**

The inability may be due to:

- **Lack of material means**

This problem is almost a constant of all emergency situations, particularly in developing countries. It comes on top of a usually chronic lack of means that exists even in the absence of any acute crisis, and includes in particular:

- a lack of drugs;
- a lack of bandages;
- a lack of spare parts to repair water pumps;
- a lack of food stocks;
- a lack of vaccines.

- **Lack of personnel**

Over the last 20 years, personnel have become less of a problem. In many African countries, of course, shortages are still acute, but in Latin America, the Asian countries,[28] and the European countries, health-care personnel are sufficiently numerous to deal with emergency situations.

- **Lack of facilities**

Medical facilities are usually designed to meet the normal needs of a population. If for some reason that population doubles, such facilities are immediately overwhelmed. When displaced populations settle in regions completely without infrastructure, the lack of facilities is conspicuous.

- **Lack of logistic support**

In many cases facilities exist and staff are available, but supplies and equipment are not where they ought to be. The problems of drug and medical equipment supply are well-known; for example, deliveries from the central depot to the district hospitals, although scheduled for four times a year, are actually made only twice a year due to lack of transport.

- **Lack of financial means**

A lack of financial means may be the common denominator of all the other shortages mentioned above. The use of local resources (personnel, material resources), though they may be available on the spot, requires the mobilization of specific financial resources — which may be lacking.

The role of humanitarian relief is to mitigate these deficiencies.

[28] Except in Cambodia, which lost almost all its health-care personnel between 1975 and 1979.

- **Financial means**

As mentioned, this factor is often the common denominator of all the others. However, direct financial aid in cases of disaster is not as common as might be imagined. Indeed, to apply financial means immediately to urgent needs, the necessary resources (material, logistic, and personnel) must be available in the country — something which is by no means always the case. Donors prefer to import the necessary resources directly, both for reasons of efficiency and in their own interests, rather than to give local authorities the financial wherewithal to buy abroad and import what they lack.

Nonetheless, the humanitarian agencies do employ this means of intervention, on a limited scale. They may, for example, undertake to pay the salaries of the local personnel recruited for the emergency situation. Another possibility is meeting the needs of the victims by providing them with direct financial support.[29] This option is often used on a case-by-case basis to help individuals or families through a difficult period.

There have been few instances, however, of direct financial interventions[30] within a population. This approach is worth examining, if the material resources the victims lack are available on the spot. In most emergency situations, it is in fact the loss of purchasing power that is the victims' main problem, staple goods being available elsewhere in the country.[31]

- **Material means**

Material aid may have unfortunate economic or ethical consequences.

- *Economic consequences* — Mass food distributions in a still-productive agricultural environment cause a drop in food prices. This drop benefits neither the victims[32] nor the local farmers, since the latter can no longer sell their produce at a reasonable price. Buying large quantities of food products locally can have the opposite effect, by creating shortages on the local market.
- *Ethical consequences* — The procedures to be followed in sending supplies have been sufficiently publicized;[33] the dispatch of inappropriate goods (past expiry date or unsuited to needs), or of material not requested by the organizers of the emergency action is now a matter of humanitarian ethics more than ignorance. Similarly, when humanitarian agencies provide highly sophisticated medical equipment, they help create new habits among the local health-care personnel — habits the latter will not be able to maintain in the long run due to lack of money, absence of technical upkeep, etc.

---

29 More advanced studies should be done on the use of this method of intervention.

30 Distribution of money to entire populations, on the model of food distributions.

31 This statement does not apply, of course, to major droughts that recur several years in a row, making food products scarce. In such cases, money is of little use.

32 The market value of the products given them decreases.

33 See the ICRC publication *Red Cross Cargo* (Geneva: ICRC, 1994).

- **Human resources**

The factor of human resources is becoming increasingly important. On one hand, many countries now have enough health-care personnel to employ them in emergency situations. On the other hand, in the donor countries a real market has developed for "humanitarian personnel," who would like nothing better than to get out in the field. Choosing between these two types of human resources is now a real dilemma. They must be compared on the basis of various criteria:

- technological skills
- acceptability to the victims
- influence with local authorities
- cost
- knowledge of the sociocultural environment
- possibility of linkage with development activities
- impact on local services[34]

A crisis does not necessarily mean that specialized expatriate personnel must be sent in!

- **Aid to infrastructure**

It is essentially the health-care infrastructures that are under pressure during an emergency: hospitals may be forced to cope with a flood of wounded; the water supply system and dispensaries may have to accommodate a displaced population. Along with the shortage of supplies and personnel, the facilities themselves may be physically inadequate to meet the demand. Humanitarian agencies then have a choice between several options:

- not to modify infrastructures, but to maintain them by temporary means for example, tents to house the wounded in a hospital;
- to expand the capacity of the infrastructures by constructing new buildings where most needed;
- to erect a new facility — that is, to build a new hospital.[35]

The choice between these options depends on various factors:

- *the urgency of the needs* — A flood of wounded who cannot be properly referred to a surgical unit is grounds for considering the installation of a field hospital.[36]
- *the extent of the needs* — A nutrition rehabilitation program will be set up differently depending on whether it is supposed to treat a dozen severely malnourished children or several hundreds. In the first case, patients can be

[34] That is, the impact of diverting local human resources away from routine health-care facilities to emergency facilities.

[35] In this case, the material supplies and equipment, human resources, and logistical supports required to run it will also have to be provided.

[36] Either an imported surgical unit or one built from structures (not necessarily medical ones) already existing in the area.

treated in an existing facility;[37] in the second case, it may be wise to create an infrastructure (for example, a nutrition rehabilitation center) especially for the program.

- *the long-term implications* — Increasing the capacity of an existing facility (or, more often, reconditioning it in the context of an emergency situation) fulfills a real need, not merely to respond to the new "demand," but also afterwards, when the emergency has passed. Nonetheless, existing health-care facilities should not be made into medical complexes that are too expensive to maintain once the financial windfall from the emergency has ended. This is laying the local resources open to problems of "mis-development."

**2. Qualitative aspect: Do the local health-care facilities furnish services that are suited to the victims' needs?**

If the answer is YES, then the local services are accessible, capable of providing services in sufficient quantity and of a quality suited to victims' needs. The role of external aid will be to maintain contact with the local health facilities involved in the relief effort, and, if their capacities become strained, to take the necessary steps of the procedure used in cases where local services are inadequate.

**NO: Why not?**

- **Inadequate technical means**

Quite often emergency situations demand specific equipment that is unavailable in many countries.[38] Whether such gaps should be filled with a tailored, limited external aid depends on the need (how urgent it is, whether there is an alternative), the cost, and the long-term repercussions. One solution is to supply the needed equipment for the duration of the emergency and then take it back. Such plans often fall foul of reluctant local authorities who, by means of red tape, prevent the reexport of the equipment to its country of origin.

- **Lack of technical skills**

Personnel may be present, but not necessarily trained to cope with the technical problems generated by emergencies. The most common example is war surgery, which requires the use of specific procedures unfamiliar to civilian surgeons. International aid can offer local surgeons appropriate training during the period of the emergency.[39]

---

37 For example, the pediatric ward of a hospital.

38 During the Gulf war, the ICRC sent machines to Baghdad that produced plastic bags of drinking water directly from water taken from unprotected sources.

39 Obviously, this sort of training is best provided *before* an armed conflict begins.

- **Lack of organizational skills**

This problem involves essentially a lack of the skills needed to manage problems created by a sudden surge in demand, where resources are sufficient in quantity — for example, the organization of a hospital to cope with an influx of casualties,[40] or the management of logistical resources. The presence of WHO experts in national ministries answers this need.

## Impact of Support Measures on the Overall Functioning of a Health-Care Facility

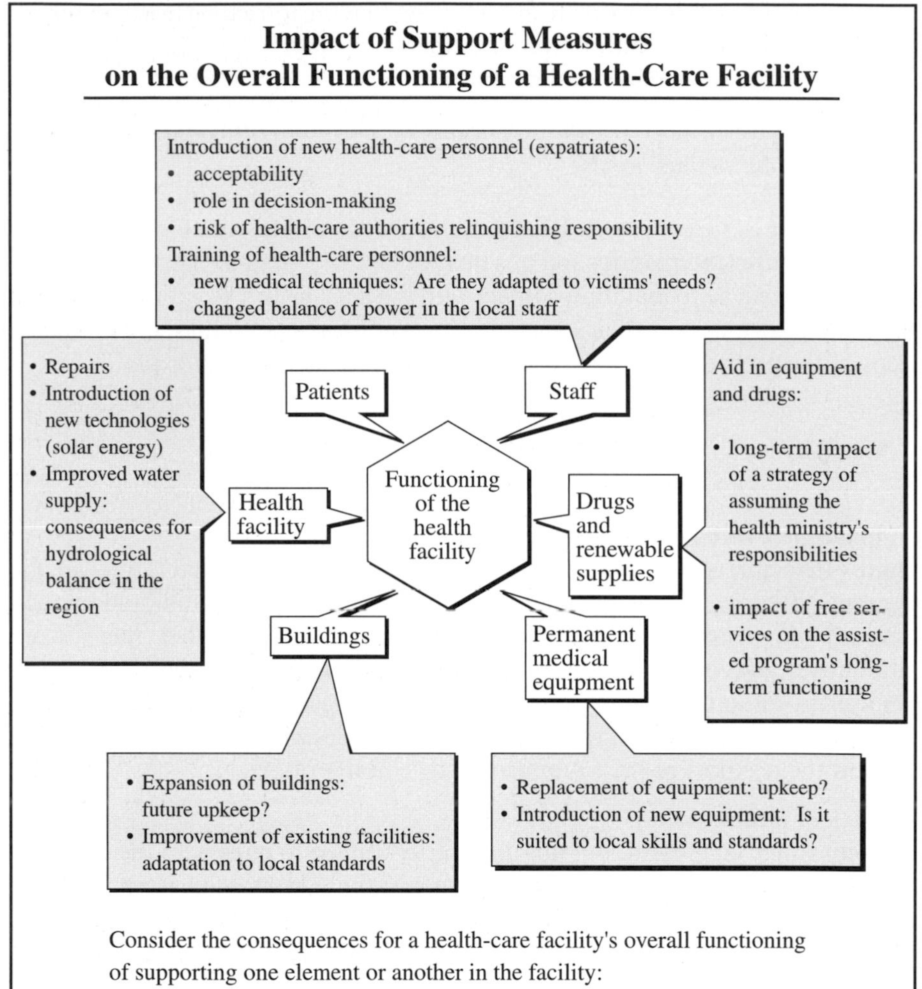


Consider the consequences for a health-care facility's overall functioning of supporting one element or another in the facility:

- impact of providing new equipment;
- impact of the presence of expatriate personnel;
- impact of expanding the buildings.

[40] Hence the usefulness of hospital contingency plans for emergencies, designed and tested before the crisis.

# 3. Synthesis

It is always difficult, presumptuous, and arrogant to judge the quality of the work supplied by local sources. Every judgment is based on norms. Initially, the terms of reference must be defined: international norms, customary local norms. The latter should take priority — as long as they meet a certain criterion of effectiveness, since it would be ethically questionable to base an intervention on erroneous local norms. For example, an immunization program against cholera should not be introduced even if the laws in force recommend it.

In certain situations, the constraints involved are so complex that it is difficult to follow any norms. From a pragmatic point of view, the choice is sometimes between abstention or an external intervention which, although possibly outside the acknowledged norms, nevertheless brings a certain relief to the victims. In this case, the terms of reference should not be norms, but rather what the alternatives would be.

A good study of the ways that humanitarian relief agencies deal with local health-care facilities[41] identified four approaches used in Ethiopia by non-governmental organizations, noting the problems characteristic of each:

- *direct management of the facility by the humanitarian agencies*: Effectiveness is greater when the expatriate personnel are present; foreign personnel tend to resort to treatments that are not standard for the country.
- *material support of local facilities*: Local habits may be modified by reliance on outside aid, depending on the type of resources supplied.
- *the multisectoral approach*: The institution of large-scale programs requires a major investment in personnel to cover all the sectors linked to health — agriculture, education, etc.
- *the "trickle-down" approach*: Resources are given directly to the health ministry, which redistributes them; the great risk is losing control of the distribution and use of the resources.

**Relief agencies should work as much as possible through the local system, not only repairing or replacing weak elements (both material and human), but also proposing, if necessary, improvements in the management and organization of the facility's resources.**

[41] J. Walley *et al.*, "Integrating Health Services: The Experience of NGOs in Ethiopia," *Health Policy and Planning* 6, No. 4: 327-335.

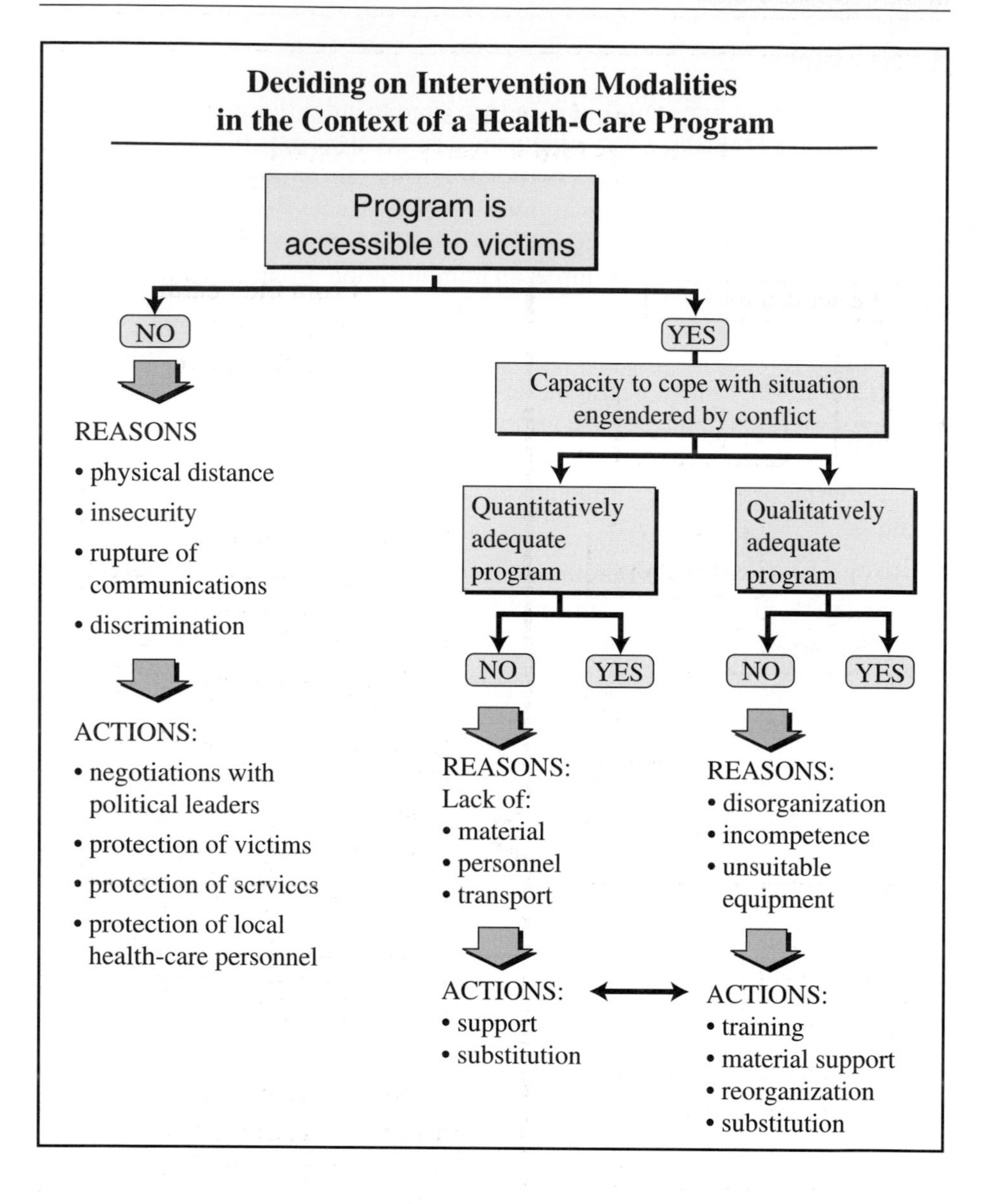
Deciding on Intervention Modalities
in the Context of a Health-Care Program
Program is accessible to victims
NO
REASONS
• physical distance
• insecurity
• rupture of communications
• discrimination
ACTIONS:
• negotiations with political leaders
• protection of victims
• protection of services
• protection of local health-care personnel
YES
Capacity to cope with situation engendered by conflict
Quantitatively adequate program
Qualitatively adequate program
NO
YES
NO
YES
REASONS:
Lack of:
• material
• personnel
• transport
ACTIONS:
• support
• substitution
REASONS:
• disorganization
• incompetence
• unsuitable equipment
ACTIONS:
• training
• material support
• reorganization
• substitution

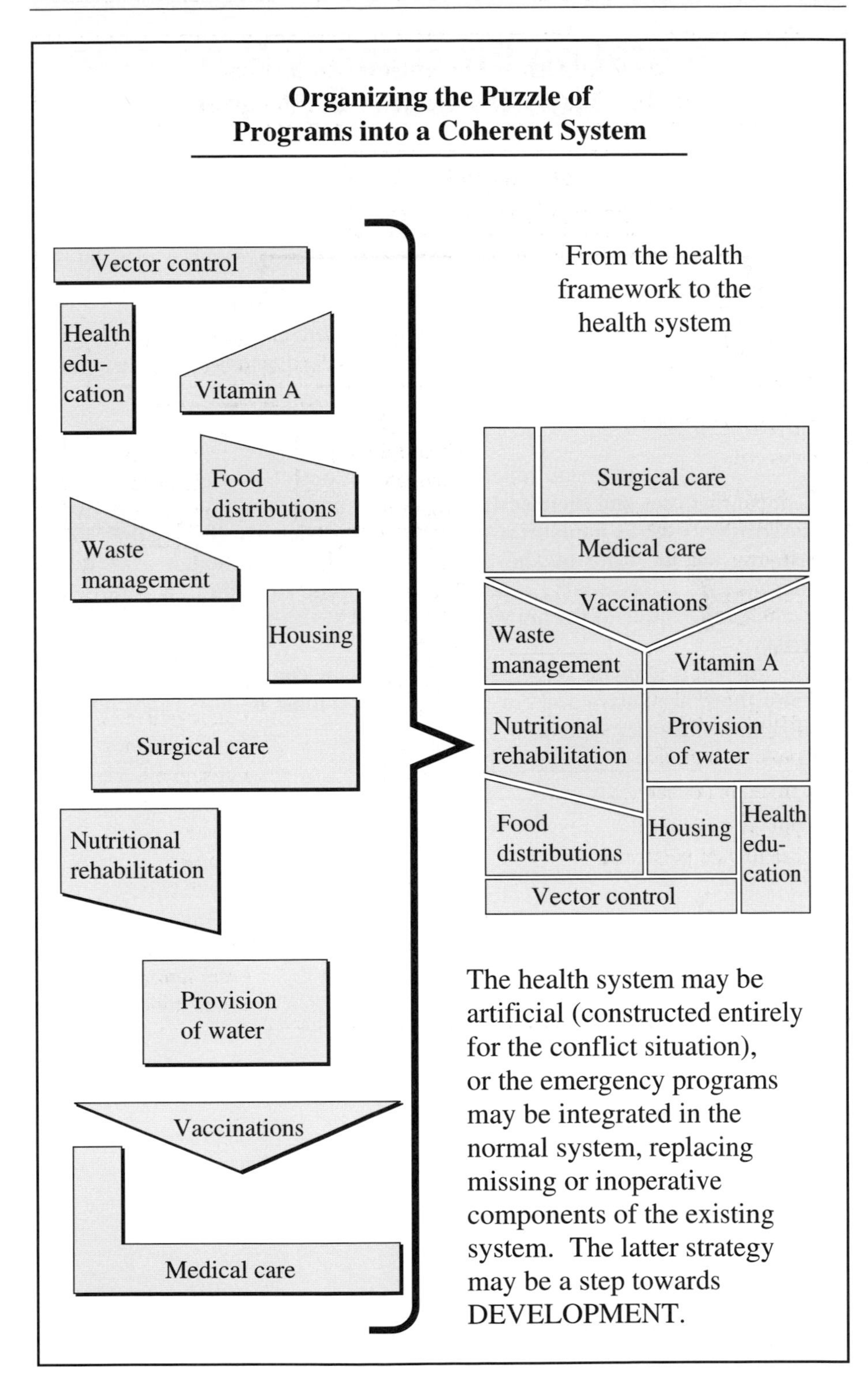
Organizing the Puzzle of
Programs into a Coherent System
Vector control
Health edu- cation
Vitamin A
Food distributions
Waste management
Housing
Surgical care
Nutritional rehabilitation
Provision of water
Vaccinations
Medical care
From the health framework to the health system
Surgical care
Medical care
Vaccinations
Waste management
Vitamin A
Nutritional rehabilitation
Provision of water
Food distributions
Housing
Health edu- cation
Vector control
The health system may be artificial (constructed entirely for the conflict situation), or the emergency programs may be integrated in the normal system, replacing missing or inoperative components of the existing system. The latter strategy may be a step towards DEVELOPMENT.

# V. Integrating Emergency Programs in a Health-Care System

Aid consisting in the provision of equipment, personnel, or logistic resources is integrated into the local health-care system. However, if the local system is unable to cope with the situation and external aid programs are necessary, they must somehow be integrated into a system, whether the local one or a parallel one created specifically for the emergency situation.[42]

The implementation of aid programs that are not integrated into some kind of comprehensive system is apt to result in ineffectiveness due to the absence of long-term follow-up and the lack of coherence between the different programs.

**Increasingly, humanitarian relief must take into account the capacities of the local facilities and their desire to manage crisis situations themselves. The strategy used by humanitarian agencies occasionally goes against this tendency for the sake of short-term effectiveness. Although a certain independence is necessary, especially in conflict situations, it does not preclude integration of the aid within the local health-care system — if one exists.**

**The important point to remember is that all measures taken to enhance health (both preventive and curative measures) must be integrated into a coherent health-care system.**

---

[42] This is often the case for populations living in large refugee camps, where the local system is unable to absorb the new population.

# Chapter 8

# DISASTERS AND DEVELOPMENT

***The inclusion of a chapter on development in a book about emergency situations may seem surprising, since the two subjects are apparently quite unrelated, even incompatible.***

***Emergency situations are often accused of draining financial and human resources that would have been better employed for development. Yet, some observers believe that disaster situations create propitious conditions, in the form of favorable socioeconomic changes, for new development programs.***

***The purpose of this chapter is to give health-care personnel working in emergency situations a better understanding of what development is, to define the ways their relief operation activity might endanger a development process, and, finally, to identify possible links between emergency operations and development activities.***

# I. The Conceptual Framework of Development

Is it realistic to try to define the concept of development?

"[...D]evelopment is a comprehensive economic, social, cultural and political process, which aims at the constant improvement of the well-being of the entire population and of all individuals on the basis of their active, free and meaningful participation in development and in the fair distribution of benefits resulting therefrom." [1]

Two important points should be mentioned in this respect.

## 1. The Concept of "Well-Being"

The concept of "well-being" does not have the same significance for all populations, depending on their cultural, social, ethnic, and religious characteristics (to name only a few). Consequently, every population, or at least every population group, must define its own development, based on its own conception of human rights.

1 Definition adopted by the United Nations General Assembly in its Declaration on the Right to Development, resolution 41/128, 4 December 1986.

*The concept of well-being* depends mostly on the socioeconomic context. For a Sahelian population, for example, well-being means guaranteed access to minimal food resources, while for a European population, it is the certainty of employment.

- What are essential rights?
- Which rights take priority?

The actual concept of human rights will be analyzed in Chapter 9 ("Protecting the Victims of Armed Conflicts"). A consensus should be reached, however, regarding the ultimate purpose of development; otherwise there is no point in trying to discuss the different possible approaches to it.

The title of this chapter, "Disasters and Development," is an invitation to link these two ideas and to perceive development from the very specific perspective of essential needs. Why not implement development plans that will insure the continuous coverage of these needs and prevent populations from falling victim to disasters at regular intervals? From this point of view, a developmental process can be defined as giving the largest possible number of people access to security, food, a healthy environment, and health.

Although essential needs are relatively well defined in relief operations,[2] this is not true of development projects. Moreover, the changes (improvements?) introduced by a development process will engender new needs. Thus, the ultimate purpose of development must be continually updated. After the provision of clean water comes the provision of hot water! Where should we stop?

## 2. Attaining that "Philosophical" Goal

To attain the goal of well-being, two approaches are possible: the economic approach and the social approach.

### 2.1 The Economic Approach

The economic approach gives priority to economic growth, which may be pursued in the agricultural sphere[3] or the industrial sphere.[4] The anticipated redistribution of wealth does not always occur, however. Inequality appears to have increased in Brazil,[5] and purchasing power in most African countries has

---

2 Although the socioeconomic context of the populations involved must be taken into account.

3 The goal is to develop agricultural production that can be exported.

4 This is the great hobbyhorse of economic development. In the sixties, countries such as Algeria and Brazil based their development on industry.

5 "The fruits of the economic miracle have benefited only a population of 30 to 40 million Brazilians who constitute the real domestic market. Thus, nearly two-thirds of Brazilians live in poverty and destitution, while 10%, the richest, hold nearly half of the national revenue." V. Prévot, , "Le Brésil: La croissance avant tout," in Sylvie Brunel, ed., *Tiers Mondes — Controverses et Réalités* (Ed. Economica, 1987), p. 217.

dwindled. Elsewhere, better results have been noted — in India and Taiwan, for example.

## 2.2 The Social Approach

The social approach assigns priority to social equality. Economic growth is merely a "necessary evil" to achieve social progress. The collapse of the socialist systems, however, showed the limitations of the latter. Almost all human beings are ready to participate in the redistribution of wealth — as long as it starts with them!

These two approaches should not be seen as opposites.[6] They are, in fact, two facets of a much more complex process that encompasses both of them:

"Development is possible only when the relevant sectors exist to permit the accumulation of capital, on one hand, and a substantial distribution of revenue, on the other [...D]evelopment strategy thus cannot consist in choosing between one sector and another; it is necessarily combinative."[7]

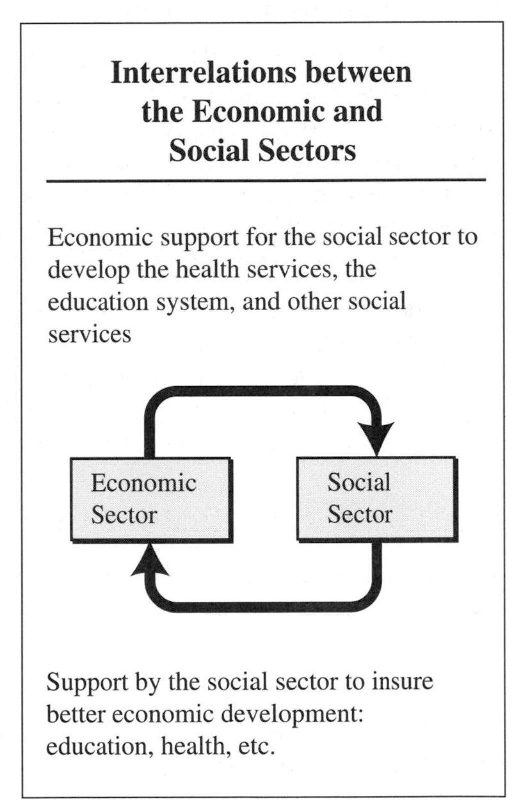


A UNDP study of 160 countries indicates that economic growth is a prerequisite for social development.[8] To put it plainly, countries are not going to spend money on social development until they have it to spend.

Exchanges between the economic and social sectors are bidirectional. On one hand, access to social services is not a gift from heaven. The cost of setting up facilities and training qualified health-care personnel must be covered by the national economy, unless international aid

---

6 "There is no conflict between growth and human development — though there may be a conflict between those who would allocate resources to the rich and those who would direct them to the poor." UNDP, *Human Development Report* (1991), p. 13.

7 M. Penouil, "Existe-t-il des modèles de développement?" in Brunel, ed., *Tiers Mondes*, pp. 208-209.

8 UNDP, *Human Development Report* (1991), p. 13.

takes over. On the other hand, a better national health status helps improve the performance of workers in the economic sector.

Although these examples certainly do not reflect the extreme complexity of the connections between the two sectors, they are explicit enough to show the necessity for a regulatory mechanism. In other words, who decides what form exchanges will take? This brings us to the political aspect of development.

## 3. Political Involvement

The broad socioeconomic policy lines formulated by governments are preponderant.[9] The redistribution of wealth may be limited to the economy when growth serves exclusively to finance more growth in this sector, without providing social benefits for those excluded from production. At the other extreme, resources drawn from the economic sector are immediately injected into the social sector, preventing the long-term economic investments that are the guarantee of continued growth over the long term.

The political sector must take into account a whole set of national factors (political classes, social organization, availability of natural resources, religion, existing level of development, necessity of long-term investments, etc.) in order to define a development policy that will help maintain a certain stability in the country. An uncoordinated approach to development — particularly a failure to respect the equilibrium between the social and economic systems — gives rise to a real danger of political instability.[10]

Two questions arise.

■ **Is political stability a factor in development?**
Situations of armed conflict by definition entail the breakdown of existing facilities, particularly the social services: education and health services are relegated to the background, far behind the services considered essential to the war effort. Under these conditions, development initiatives have practically no chance of implementation.

Although political stability is essential to development,[11] what it represents must still be defined: a wide democratic consensus on general policies, or a dictatorship which imposes its own "stability."

---

9 "No sustained improvement in human well-being is possible without growth. But it is even more wrong to suggest that high economic growth rates will automatically translate into a higher level of human development. They may, or they may not. It all depends on the policy choices the countries make." *Ibid.*, p. 14.

10 "Development changes the balance of power. Powers are brought down, new ones are created. Activities disappear, others are constituted. All these developments involve conflict." M. Penouil, *op. cit.*, p. 210.

11 "It is commonly acknowledged today that development requires political stability, which, in turn, is the guarantee of the continuity and steadiness of the governors' action." G. Hermet, "La Démocratie, luxe ou nécessité," in Brunel, ed., *Tiers Mondes*, p. 401.

At this point, pure economic and social reasoning must give way to the much larger realm of respect for human rights, and particularly for the right of peoples to choose their own form of political representation and socioeconomic development. Dictatorships, no matter what their orientation, do not lend themselves to a process of development, as witness numerous examples in Eastern Europe, Latin America, and Africa.[12]

- **Is development a factor in political stability?**

Development which favors a minority to the detriment of the majority generates conflict. It may also contribute to the emergence of new needs which cannot necessarily be satisfied and which will lead to a sense of inequality between social classes.

Paradoxically, through the very changes it induces, development creates instability to some degree; for that reason, development strategy must be readjusted to accommodate the socioeconomic changes and disruptions it occasions. In democratic countries, socioeconomic orientations evolve in tandem with political changes. Those changes, being the result of free elections, theoretically reflect the wishes of the community.

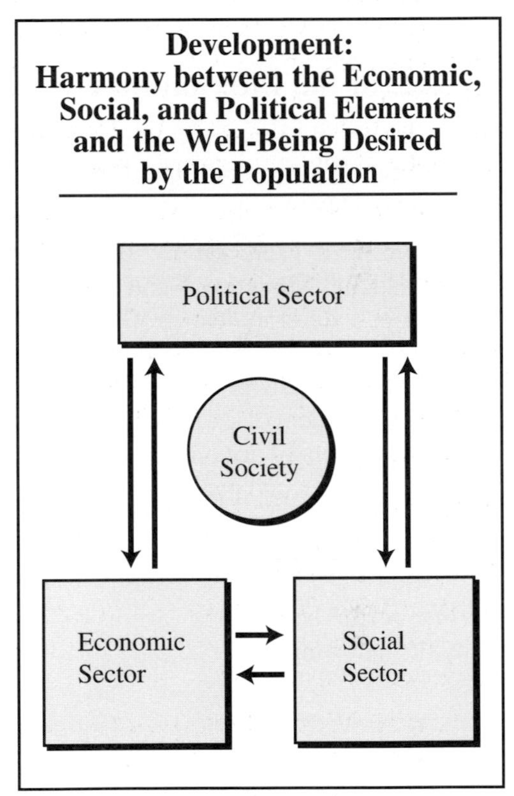


## 4. Role of the Geophysical Environment

The presence of mining resources, or abundant water, will help orient development towards heavy industry, or agriculture, or some other sector.

[12] "There may be a few exceptional regions where a strong power — one immediately thinks, military — permits a centralization so rigid that it is apt to paralyze any vague impulse towards agricultural progress — that is, change." J.P. Harroy, *Demain la famine, ou, La conspiration du silence* (Ed. Hayez-Bruxelles, 1979), p. 113.

## 5. Role of the Ecological Environment

The ecological environment is particularly important for agricultural development, since it concerns the balance between a population and its surroundings.[13] The aim here is not to judge between the advocates of high-tech agricultural development and those who promote development by traditional means; the truth undoubtedly lies somewhere between these two extremes, and differs for every location, depending on the nature of its soil, its climate, its cultural traditions, etc.

Any discussion of the balance between population and environment quite naturally raises the question of demographic growth and the strategy required to control it.[14]

## 6. Role of the International Environment

The definition and control of development policies are less and less the province of the national government. The dominant role of the international environment is reflected today in:

- the pressures exercised by the big international agencies, such as the International Monetary Fund and the World Bank, to oblige governments to adopt a development profile corresponding to the norms of developed countries. Usually, the changes imposed, termed "structural adjustments," reflect the interests of economic efficiency rather than social justice.[15]
- the reinforcement of the leadership of the northern nations, a leadership that is generally imposed not only by means of those countries' economic power and promotion of social progress, but also by their military power.[16]

## 7. The Global System

The interactions between the various systems making up a society can be summed up by the following chart:

---

[13] The concept of "carrying capacity."

[14] See P.J. Stewart, "The Ecology of Famine," in G. Ainsworth Harrison, *Famine* (Oxford Science Publications, 1988), p. 21.

[15] "UNICEF and the UNDP are in fact the only entities still defending nonconformist positions — the former by proposing in 1987 adjustment with a human face, and the latter by publishing its *Report on Human Development since 1990*." Jacques Berthelot, *Un système économique complexe qui profite d'abord au Nord, dans et hors l'ONU* (Editions Cordet-Panoramiques, 1994), p. 144.

[16] "The concept of sustainability is greatly endangered in a world that is one-fourth rich and three-fourths poor, that is half democratic and half authoritarian, where poor nations are being denied equal access to global economic opportunities, where the income disparity between the richest 20% and the poorest 20% of the world's population has doubled over the past three decades[....] The concept of one world and one planet simply cannot emerge from an unequal world. Nor can shared responsibility for the health of the global commons be created without some measure of shared global prosperity." UNDP, *Human Development Report* (1994), p. 21.

In this system, every possible interaction can be imagined, such as:

- the influence of the international economic system on the orientation and application of national economies;
- the impact of friction between civil society and the political system on the economic and social systems;
- the deterioration of the economic system caused by an ecological disaster, a deterioration which itself gives rise to social disturbances that may even affect the political system.

The interaction between these systems can be called development when changes in one or another of them contribute to a better overall equilibrium.

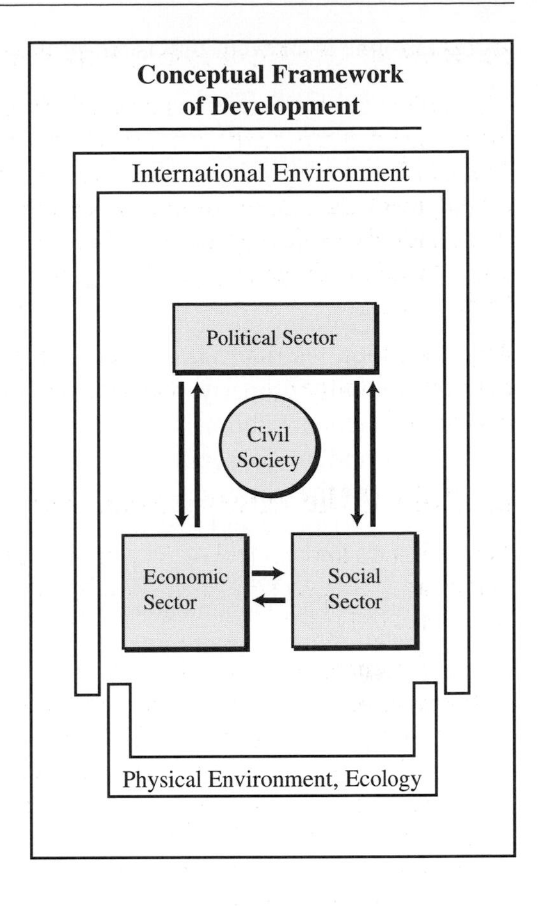


# II. The Conceptual Framework of Disaster

This section will define a simple framework to explain how disasters arise,[17] as well as the possible responses to them.

## 1. Definition of a Disaster

### 1.1 Terminology

*Disaster or Catastrophe*

"Disaster" and "catastrophe" are more or less interchangeable terms, although "disaster" is the most commonly used.

[17] The subject here is "natural" disasters, not those caused by conflicts.

"A catastrophe is an event that is harmful to the group that undergoes it." [18]

"A disaster is a crisis resulting from a failure in human interactions with the physical and social environment. Disaster situations outstrip the capacity of individuals and societies to cope with adversity." [19]

"A disaster is the convergence, at a given moment and in a given place, of two factors: risk and vulnerability." [20]

"A disaster can be defined as an event that occurs in most cases suddenly and unexpectedly, causing severe disturbances to people or objects affected by it, and resulting in loss of life and harm to the health of the population, the destruction or loss of community property, and/or severe damage to the environment. Such a situation causes a disruption in the normal pattern of life, generating misfortune, helplessness, and suffering, effects on the socioeconomic structure of a region or a country, and/or the modification of the environment, to such an extent that there is a need for assistance and for immediate outside intervention." [21]

- Three factors are essential in all these definitions:
  - the idea of a phenomenon or event which constitutes a trauma for a population or an environment;
  - the idea of a vulnerable point which will bear the brunt of the traumatizing event;
  - the idea of the failure of local resources to cope with the problems created by the phenomenon.

## *Risk*

The definition of risk must be associated with the idea of *probability*, which can be applied at two different levels: either to the phenomenon itself (the probability that a harmful event, such as an earthquake, flood, or conflict, will occur), or to that phenomenon's impact on the population and its environment. Although risk is commonly equated with the disaster itself, it really should be linked to the probability of a disaster's occurring.

The word "risk" is too general to be used without a "risk" of confusion, unless the sense in which it is employed is specified each time — no simple matter. If the word is used, its application must always be defined:

---

[18] R. Noto, P. Huguenard, and A. Larcan, *La médecine de catastrophe* (Ed. Masson, 1987), p. 11.

[19] HDI, *From Disaster Relief to Development*, Studies on Development, No. 1 (Geneva: Henry Dunant Institute, 1988), p. 170.

[20] G. Wilches-Chaux, "La vulnerabilidad global," in *Herramientas para la crisis: Desastres, ecologismo y formación profesional* (Popayan, Colombia: Servicio Nacional de Aprendizaje [SENA], Sept. 1989).

[21] Pan American Health Organization (PAHO), *Mitigation of Disasters in Health Facilities — General Issues*, Vol. I (1993), p. 1.

- risk of a natural or man-made phenomenon occurring (threat);
- risk of a disaster occurring (meaning the impact of a phenomenon on a population, which depends on the latter's vulnerability to the phenomenon).

### *Phenomena*

The phenomena that cause disasters may be classified by:

- *origin* — geophysical (volcanoes, for example), technological (chemical accidents), or human (conflict);
- *speed of onset* — abrupt (earthquake) or gradual (drought);
- *hierarchy*[22] — two levels of disaster should be distinguished: primary events without human intervention (earthquakes, volcanic eruptions, hurricanes, drought), and secondary events which are largely the consequence of the primary ones (floods, landslides, erosion).

### *Vulnerability*

Vulnerability has been given many definitions:

"A community's incapacity to absorb the effects of a given change in its environment." [23]

"Individuals and societies are vulnerable to disasters when they are in a weak position to handle the effects of a crisis. Three types of vulnerability may be distinguished: physical, organisational and psychological." [24]

"The concept of vulnerability has been widely used to denote a condition in which the physical and mental well-being required for a normal productive life is impaired and at constant risk. However, vulnerability in general usage includes any condition of exposure to hazards, risks and stresses. It can, for example, be that of an economy highly dependent on a few primary commodity exports, of a firm in a rapidly changing market, or of the illiterate in an increasingly literate environment.

The health-related vulnerability of individuals and communities is reflected in patterns of morbidity, mortality, and reproduction, and is the product of various forms of social and economic deprivation acting simultaneously." [25]

The essential points to remember from these definitions are that vulnerability:

---

[22] A. Lavell, "Desastres naturales y zonas de riesgo en Centroamérica: Condicionantes y opciones de prevención y mitigación," *CSUCA (Centro Superior Universitario de Centro América)* 4 (1991).

[23] G. Wilches-Chaux, "La vulnerabilidad global."

[24] HDI, *From Disaster Relief to Development,* p. 170.

[25] WHO, "Health Dimensions of Economic Reform," background document for the International Forum on Health: The Conditionality for Economic Development, Accra, Ghana, 4-6 December 1991 (Geneva: WHO, 1992), p. 11.

- is a multifaceted characteristic conditioned by individual, social, and structural factors, and that therefore any analysis must cover the entire chain of vulnerability, from the individual to the macroeconomic system;
- is on the whole linked to a community's degree of development;
- is characteristic of the most disadvantaged social strata (who lack information about the threat of a flood, live in precarious conditions, lack resources to cope with losses, etc.);
- is sometimes — or often — linked to the development process itself, which may create the conditions for a disaster (chemical and nuclear accidents, for example).

**Impact**

A disaster's impact is the "meeting" between a harmful phenomenon and a group of vulnerable factors. The impact may be on the population (number of displaced people, number of wounded, number of dead) or on the environment (extent of the destruction).[26]

A disaster's impact is variable; an earthquake may do no more than "shake the walls," or it may claim thousands of victims and cause massive destruction to the environment.

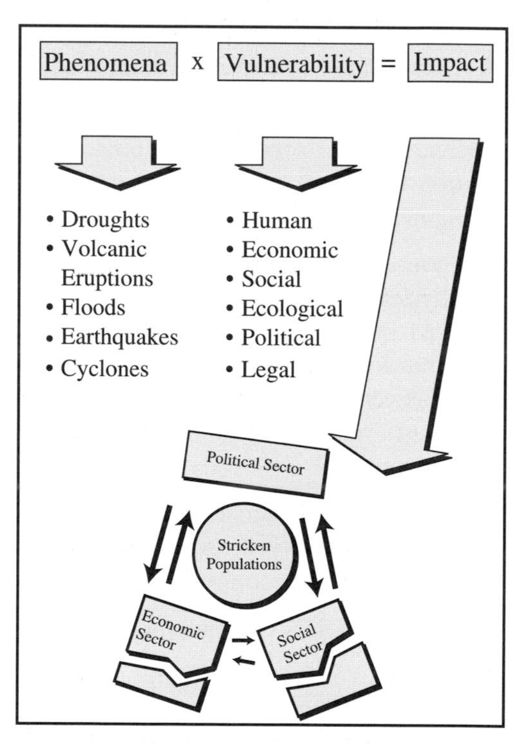


## 1.2 Defining a Disaster

The three concepts described above form the basis for a practical definition of a disaster situation, on which possible interventions at various levels can be grafted logically.

According to G. Wilches-Chaux, a disaster is defined by this formula:

**RISK x VULNERABILITY**
**=**
**DISASTER**

This definition, however, should be modified as follows: the word *risk* should be replaced by the word *phenomenon*, for the reasons given above, and the word *disaster* by the expression *impact of the phenomenon*; the

[26] Some authors tend to restrict the use of the word "impact" to the impact on people, and not on the environment. HDI, *From Disaster Relief to Development*, p. 173.

consequences of the phenomenon's impact may indeed be a disaster, but they may also consist merely in minor structural dysfunction, or else a temporary societal disorganization.

As an orientation guide to the complex tangle of factors leading to a disaster, the following "definition" may be helpful:

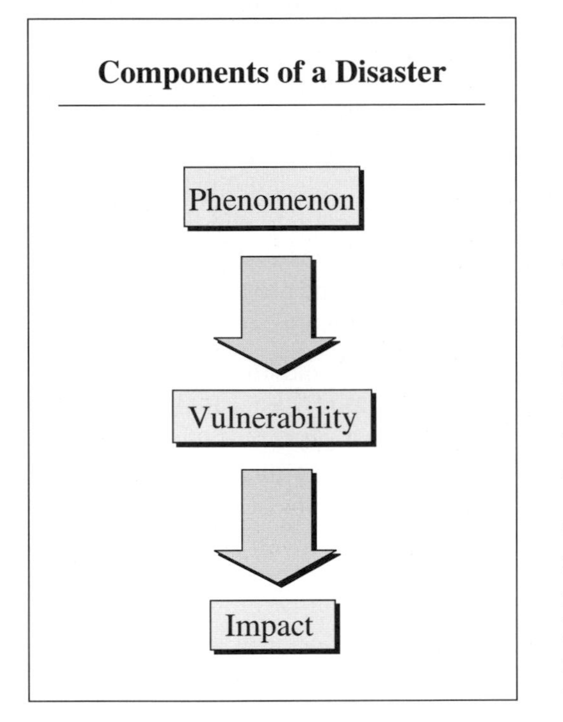


**An aggressive phenomenon is always on the lookout for vulnerability in order to create problems — either minor ones or major ones that create true disasters.**

This section will deal exclusively with disasters caused by natural and technological phenomena. Situations of armed conflict will be studied in Chapter 9 ("Protecting the Victims of Armed Conflicts").

Over the last thirty years, the number of victims claimed by natural phenomena and technological accidents has been growing steadily. There does not seem to have been a significant increase in the number and magnitude of natural phenomena such as volcanic eruptions and earthquakes; the number of vulnerable people, however, has increased considerably. This factor, then, merits a more particular study.

# 2. Importance of Vulnerability in the Mechanism of Disasters

## 2.1 Definition of Vulnerability

The study of the different types of vulnerability and its counterpart, the study of the ability to cope with adversity, is very fashionable. In disaster situations, the tendency is to restrict the notion of vulnerability to individuals or groups of individuals, such as children and pregnant women. Of course, the probability (or risk) that these groups will suffer the most has been demonstrated. Nonetheless, to link the emergency to development, the field of vulnerability must be expanded to cover areas that may be less familiar to health-care personnel working in emergencies, but which are fundamental to development.

Similarly, a disaster is often very restricted geographically. Accordingly, the local factors reinforcing the initial phenomenon's impact on the vulnerable groups must be sought out. These factors, however, are often linked to national and international structural defects. Although no effort will be made here to link the minutiae of local disturbances to the new world order, it should at least be understood that they are part of a vast and complex whole.

"Vulnerability manifested at the micro level has to be placed within these larger structures and systems, which extend beyond boundaries to the national, regional, and global level. The strategies to deal with vulnerability have therefore to act at several levels — the local level, of the community and the households within it, the national level (in terms of sectoral and macroeconomic policies), and the global level (in terms of international policies and programmes relating to aid, technical assistance, and economic relations between countries)." [27]

The publication of several works on the subject[28] and the United Nations' declaration of "The International Decade for Natural Disaster Reduction" have greatly helped to popularize the issue. They establish an important link between emergency relief and development activities. That is why this section focuses on the reduction of vulnerability as an example of development.

## 2.2 Types of Vulnerability

There are several kinds of vulnerability, as shown previously in the conceptual framework of development (section I-7).

### *Ecological Vulnerability*

Ecological vulnerability is usually a secondary effect of the combination of primary geophysical phenomena and a particular social behavior. Heavy rainfall in densely populated rural zones with a high degree of deforestation will give rise to disasters which develop slowly (erosion) or abruptly (landslides).

### *Economic Vulnerability*

The economic system is particularly vulnerable in developing countries. This vulnerability appears in many forms, which are intermixed with each other and with the other types of vulnerability. They can be distinguished as follows:

---

[27] WHO, "Health Dimensions of Economic Reform," p. 11.

[28] See, for example, G. Wilches-Chaux, "La vulnerabilidad global," and M. Anderson and P. Woodrow, *Rising from the Ashes* (1989).

*Individual and Family Economic Vulnerability*

Due to insufficient income, some rural populations are unable to survive a year of bad harvests. The absence of both food reserves and the financial means to buy the food they need makes them very vulnerable to climatic vagaries. In general, the mortality associated with disasters is inversely proportional to revenue.

*Local Economic Vulnerability*

Local economic vulnerability is a problem in geographical areas that are unfavorable to economic development. In the agricultural domain, for example, this may mean areas with traditionally poor soil, or soil that has become so as a result of deforestation and erosion.

In addition, economic difficulties have driven rural populations into the cities, where they are concentrated in unsafe areas (for example, the flooded regions in El Salvador in 1989). Development itself is a source of vulnerability. Agricultural policies that advocate single-crop farming leave farmers with nothing to fall back on in case of accidents, be they climatic, agronomic (crop diseases), or economic (price collapse).[29] In this case, the most vulnerable families will be those with a low production capacity due to the limited land available to them for cultivation.

*National Economic Vulnerability*

Inconsistent economic development policies, corruption, and city officials' lack of interest in rural areas are a few of the factors that help increase the vulnerability of populations at the end of the economic chain. Economic underdevelopment means that the installation of infrastructure essential to the economy cannot be financed. This plays a major role in disasters, in which the road network, means of communication (telephone), etc., are so important.

*International Economic Vulnerability*

Economic vulnerability follows the Dow Jones index. An international economic recession does not have much effect on the volume of international aid sent to countries in the grip of disaster. However, if there is no acute emergency, programs to prepare for or prevent disasters (dams for flood control, for example) are cut to the bone. As a result, all the groundwork done to reduce certain types of local and national vulnerability will be disrupted.

The international economy, by controlling the prices of raw materials and foodstuffs, directly influences the income of a large proportion of the rural populations of developing countries (*cf.* the collapse of cocoa prices).

[29] Examples are cocoa in Ivory Coast and peanuts in Senegal.

The examples are many. The role of humanitarian agencies working in emergency situations is usually limited to identifying family and local economic vulnerability, with no involvement in the resolution of national and international problems.

*Social Vulnerability*

The types of social vulnerability most relevant to disaster situations are human and institutional vulnerability.

*Human vulnerability*

- *Individual vulnerability* affects the classic vulnerable groups, who are found in disaster situations just as in normal situations.
- *Family vulnerability*: The concept of "every man for himself" in disaster situations must be seen in context:

"The stress of the threat or impact will intensify the bonds between members and often the family will respond as one unit — a system. This system has flexible boundaries, open to interaction with other systems in the recovery process, either systems of extended kin or organizations that provide necessary aid and resources." [30]

Although the family is a factor in stability, the converse is also true: family breakup is a factor in vulnerability.

- *Community vulnerability*: A community's degree of organization and social cohesion is a key factor in its mechanism of response to disaster. According to Wilches-Chaux,

"The level of social traumatism resulting from a disaster is inversely proportional to the affected community's level of organization. Societies which possess a complete network of formal or informal social organizations can absorb the consequences of a disaster much more easily.[31]

This cohesion depends on several elements, including education, culture (fatalism), and physical environment. Thus, in Ethiopia:

"To a peasantry living in acute destitution and imminent danger, survival considerations are always paramount, and every peasant learns the techniques of survival as part of his/her everyday experience. These techniques may be crude or ingenious depending on the frequency of disasters experienced by the peasantry, the perceptions of the people and the stock of accumulated knowledge having to do with production and survival, the resources (natural and social) of the community, and the social relations and communal values existing at a given time." [32]

---

[30] Beverley Raphael, *When Disaster Strikes* (London: Hutchinson, 1986), p. 170.
[31] G. Wilches-Chaux, "La vulnerabilidad global."
[32] D. Rahmato, "Peasant Survival Strategies in Ethiopia," *Disasters* 12, No. 4: 327.

### *Institutional vulnerability*

Within the concept of social vulnerability, a distinction should be made between relief organizations and health-care services.

- **Relief organizations**:[33]

In developing countries, local mutual-aid societies are organized to varying degrees, but they all depend on the country's economic resources, and the human resources to manage them. They lack the technological know-how required to deal with emergency situations, whether in the preparatory or implementational phases.[34]

- **Health services**:

The vulnerability of the health services can be analyzed at both the physical and organizational levels. On the physical level, these services may be vulnerable, for example, because of their proximity to disaster-prone areas, or because the facilities were not built to earthquake standards. On the administrative level, a lack of organization in large health facilities (hospitals) can only grow worse in situations involving a mass influx of patients.

### *Political Vulnerability*

Political instability makes countries particularly vulnerable to disasters. The presence of an armed conflict in Ethiopia potentiated the devastating effects of the 1984 drought, by delaying and then limiting access to the areas affected by the lack of water.

Populations may lack autonomy due to:

- the authoritarianism of a political regime which leaves little scope for individual and community initiatives; this type of "political culture" may remain very strong even during disaster situations;
- bureaucracy, often associated with authoritarianism, which tends to slow down and sometimes block the decisions that need to be made in an emergency;
- the absence of a contingency plan for disasters; the "disaster formula" defined earlier shows well the importance of prevention and preparation measures. To be carried out, however, such measures must first of all be integrated in a national disaster contingency program, and, second, be motivated by a real political will to implement them. These conditions are seldom met, owing to inadequate economic means and contradictory social priorities.

---

[33] Including the Red Cross and Red Crescent Societies.

[34] This problem is not unique to local relief organizations; many supposedly international organizations lack professionalism.

*Vulnerability of the Legal System*

The law, considered as a counterforce, may induce the authorities to meet their responsibilities in preventing disasters. The application of the law in this domain, however, still leaves much to be desired. The prevention of certain types of disaster is indeed a function of official measures: evacuating populations from stricken areas, putting certain zones off limits (for example, prohibiting agriculture on the sides of a volcano). Such measures are difficult to enforce, however, if the authorities have no viable alternatives to offer these populations.

## 3. Interactions Between the Different Types of Vulnerability

The number of different types of vulnerability, which encompass several levels of society, offers some idea of the complexity of the interactions between them. An example is population concentrations in areas with a strong probability of a major geophysical phenomenon (earthquake, volcanic eruption) occurring. Moving these populations elsewhere is practically unthinkable, not only for purely sociocultural reasons, but also — and especially — for economic reasons; this is true primarily of populations living close to volcanoes,[35] rivers, and deltas.[36]

This interaction is still more complex when disasters give rise to mass population displacements; they break up the social fabric, cut people off from their normal sources of food, expose them to a new microbiological environment, etc.

These factors interact at several levels and may create a real chain reaction. Thus, latent malnutrition (individual vulnerability) and agricultural underdevelopment (economic vulnerability) combine to create a nutritional disaster (exercising its impact on the groups that are already malnourished) in the wake of a drought (phenomenon).

The drought itself may be considered as the result (impact on agricultural regions) of a phenomenon (drop in rainfall) in areas already ecologically devastated by erosion, deforestation, the absence of irrigation works, etc. (economic vulnerability).

In the first case, the drought is considered as the phenomenon, and in the second case, as the disaster. This is a way of analyzing the different stages in the evolution of a disaster situation and of identifying all the factors that cause it. The ultimate consequence is the loss of human lives.

---

[35] With respect to volcanoes, the problem of vulnerability is, ironically, linked to economics. Volcanic regions are very fertile, with a particularly high agricultural potential. See G. Wilches-Chaux, "La vulnerabilidad global."

[36] It is estimated that in 1980 there were 1,800 dead and 32 million people otherwise affected by floods in India. The Swedish Red Cross affirms in this respect: "Prevention is better than cure."

An aggressive phenomenon is always on the lookout for vulnerability in order to create problems; the latter themselves become aggressive phenomena in turn, looking for other kinds of vulnerability.

This chain reaction eventually ends in the loss of human lives.

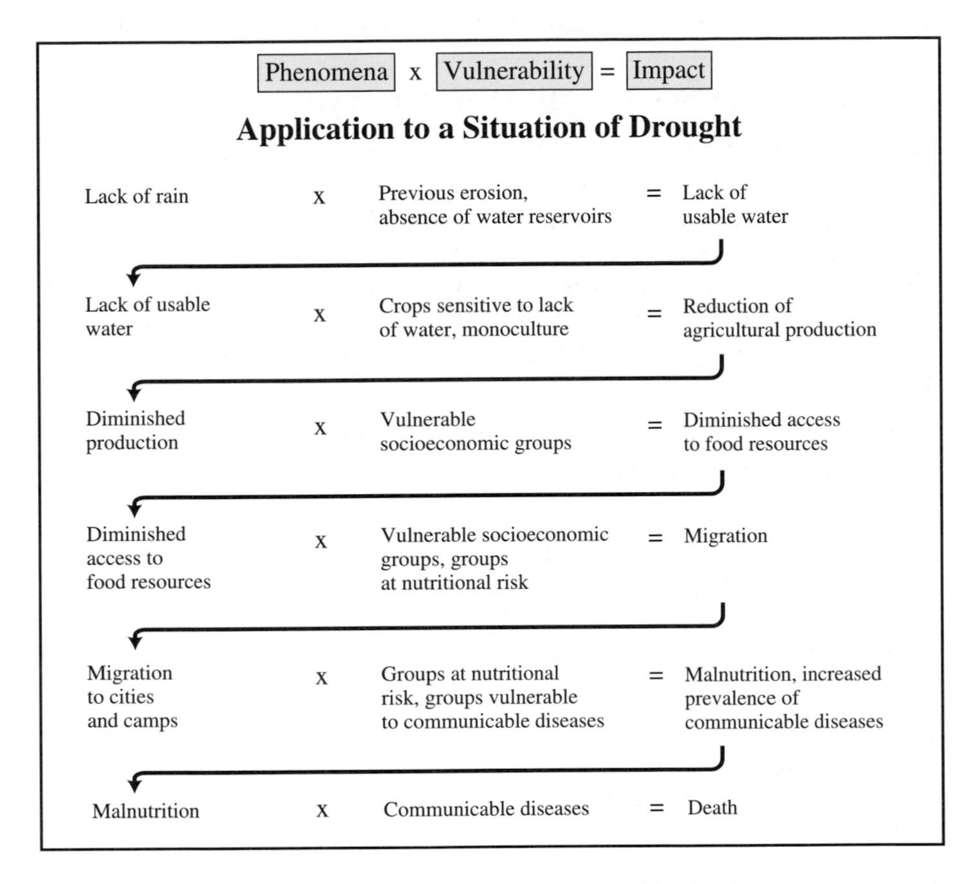


This chain can be shown more generally as a spiral (see chart).

## 4. Possible Responses

The responses possible in a disaster situation can be classified in terms of the formula discussed earlier:

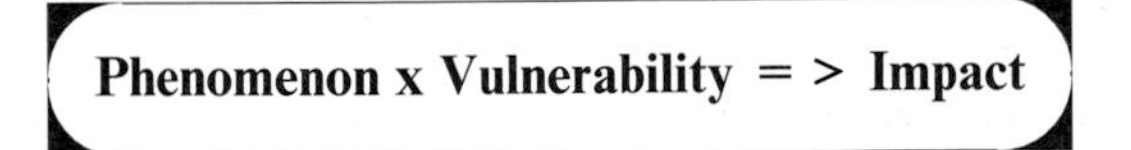

**Spiral of Disasters**

Ecological disaster
→ Agricultural disaster
→ Food disaster
→ Social disaster
→ Nutritional disaster
→ Human disaster

### 4.1 Responses to the Initial Phenomenon

Earthquakes, volcanic eruptions, and climatic disturbances (rain, cyclones) cannot be prevented, though cyclones and rain can be predicted, as can earthquakes (with considerably less accuracy, however). The effectiveness of early-warning systems depends on both the reliability of the prediction and the degree to which populations have been prepared to respond to instructions given in cases of alert.

### 4.2 Responses to the Impact

In the course of the preceding chapters, the strategies and techniques of assistance have been discussed in detail. It was shown that aid can be channeled directly to the victims, as in the case of food distribution, or towards services, as in the supply of drugs to local hospitals.

The rehabilitation of services consists in repairing the facilities that have been damaged in the course of the disaster so that they can function as they did before. They may be reconstructed as they were before the catastrophe, or, if possible, improvements may be incorporated which reflect the lessons learned from the unfortunate experience of the disaster. For example, following an earthquake, structures may be rebuilt in accordance with anti-seismic norms.

| **Phenomenon X** | **Vulnerability** | = | **Impact (0 ↓ Disaster)** |
|---|---|---|---|
| Prevention | Reduction | | Relief<br>Rehabilitation<br>Reconstruction |
| ↓ | ↓ | | ↓ |
| EWS<br>Education | Education<br><br>Construction according to earthquake standards<br>Dams against flooding, measures against erosion | | Contingency plan for disasters, emergency stores<br>Aid to victims<br>Rehabilitation of facilities |

These may be considered as true development activities, designed to make populations less vulnerable to harmful phenomena in future.

## 5. Intervention Strategy in the Wake of a Disaster

Aid to victims is an essential task, and one that local resources are best suited to perform. International relief must be considered as back-up support for local mutual-aid systems.

Rehabilitating the facilities damaged by the disaster must be part of the emergency strategy. In the short run, it is more efficient and less expensive to repair a water-supply system than to settle for distributing water from tanker trucks. The two measures can obviously be combined. Similarly, agricultural rehabilitation programs are essential to take over from food distribution programs.

Reconstruction cannot be undertaken without preliminary identification of the areas of vulnerability that gave way under the shock of the initial phenomenon. The reduction of vulnerability is the link permitting the transition from emergency programs *per se* (aid, rehabilitation) to a development program that will undertake the changes needed to reduce vulnerability.

# III. Link Between Emergency and Development: the Reduction of Vulnerability

*An aggressive phenomenon is always on the lookout for vulnerability in order to create problems; the latter become aggressive phenomena in turn, looking for other kinds of vulnerability.*

This theorem serves as a link between emergencies and development; the actual junction between the two is the *reduction of vulnerability*.[37] An emergency situation may reveal latent areas of vulnerability, which will be the starting point for thinking about the best way to prevent crises. The factors to be considered are represented in the following chart.

[37] "The reduction of human vulnerability to disasters and the strengthening of people's coping capacity are among the primary goals of development." HDI, *From Disaster Relief to Development*, p. 177.

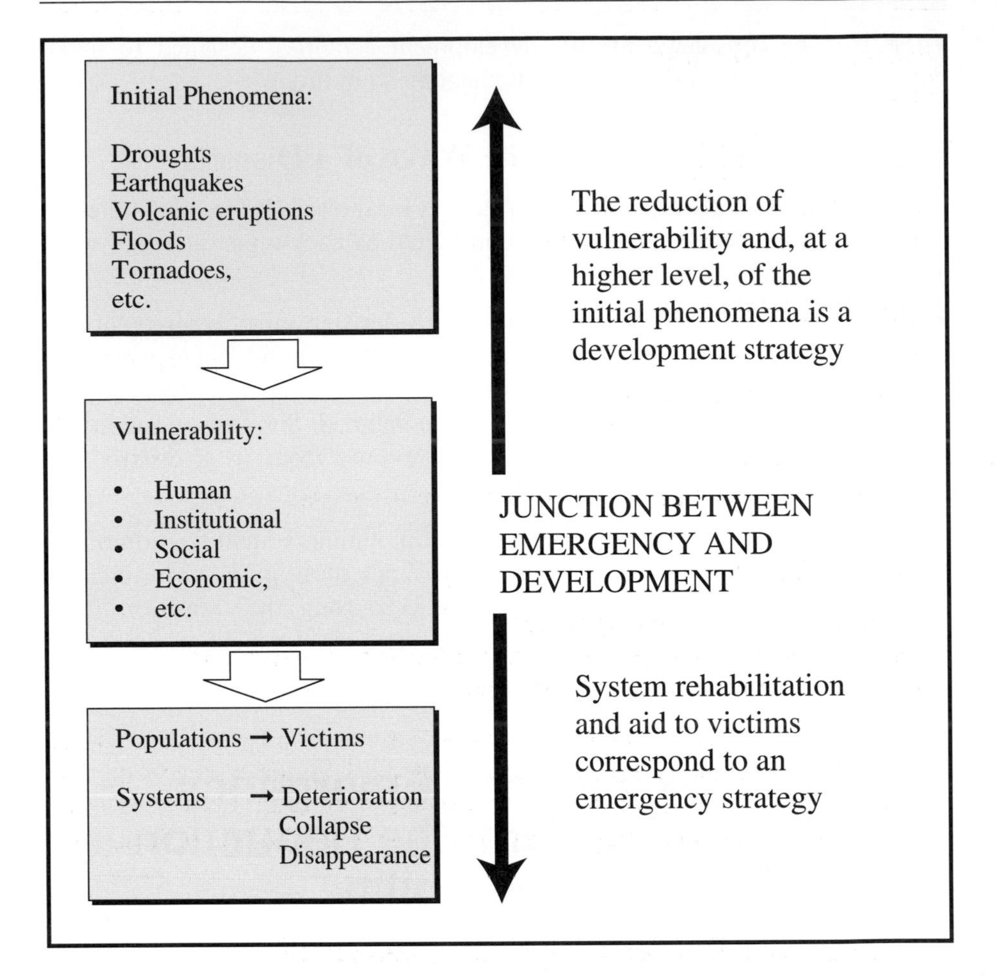


## 1. Identification of Vulnerability Within the Conceptual Framework of Development

The conceptual framework of development comprises all the types of vulnerability described earlier:

*Ecological vulnerability*

- Desertification
- Deforestation
- Pollution

*Physical vulnerability*

- Location of populations near dangerous areas

*Economic vulnerability*

- Poverty
- Insufficient income
- Single-crop farming
- Foreign debt
- International economic situation

*Social vulnerability*

- Illiteracy
- Inadequate health-care facilities
- Dysfunctional health services
- Cultural taboos
- Inadequacy of institutions responsible for disaster relief

*Political vulnerability*

- Centralized decision-making processes
- Lack of political will to prevent or soften the impact of disasters
- Lack of a contingency plan for disasters

All these kinds of vulnerability are part of the conceptual framework of development, and a damaging natural or technological phenomenon will upset or even block the functioning of the system, causing it to break down at its most vulnerable points. The more fragile the system's previous equilibrium, the greater this effect will be.[38]

## 2. The Choice Between Types of Vulnerability

The immediate vulnerability of a population living on the sides of a volcano is to be confronted with the risk of an eruption. This kind of vulnerability must be balanced against the vulnerability the population would have if it migrated to less fertile agricultural areas, or towards urban centers where finding employment would be problematic.

The choice depends largely on:

---

[38] "Comparing the 1972 earthquake in Managua, Nicaragua, with that in California in 1971 illustrates the point. The seismic activity level of the California earthquake was significantly higher, registering 6.8 on the Richter scale as compared to 5.6 in Managua. On the Mercalli scale (measuring the extent of physical damage over surface area) the California earthquake caused major damage (IX-XI level damage) over 100 square kilometres, whereas Managua registered a lower level of damage to a smaller area. The population directly affected by the earthquake in California was 13 times that of the earthquake in Managua. But in Managua around 5,000 people died; in California just 60. Clearly, levels of economic development and disaster preparedness have a profound impact upon the suffering caused by natural events." International Federation of Red Cross and Red Crescent Societies, *World Disasters Report* (1993), p. 34.

- the capacity of individuals to cope with this sort of change (education, change of work, etc.);
- the capacities of the community threatened with necessary cultural change;
- the capacities of the economic system, which may or may not permit such changes;
- the political will to assist the threatened community in its transition from one way of life to another.

### 3. The Relationship Between the Reduction of Vulnerability and the Increase of Existing Capabilities in the Framework of a Development Process

For humanitarian agencies, the link between emergencies and development is clearly the reduction of vulnerability.[39] Any contribution to a balanced, lasting development process must originate in what is available locally. Of course, the development of these local capacities may call for external technological inputs, foreign expertise, or external financial support; but it should not consist in importing a model of development defined in another context where the social, economic, and political parameters are completely different. Development activities therefore must be redefined to fit the context for which they are planned. Moreover, the threatened community itself must be responsible for identifying the measures that should be taken to improve the situation over the long term, and for implementing them. Finally, the common denominator of most kinds of vulnerability is human vulnerability: a deficient deductive level, absence of professional qualifications, socioeconomic habits that harm the environment. Increasing capacities in these areas offers the best chance of influencing the structural vulnerability of the economic and social systems.

Looking at the disaster situations most frequently encountered, we will identify the main types of vulnerability and the capacities required to counter them, concentrating on those linked to structure rather than circumstances.

## IV. Applications

This section will cover drought, earthquakes, floods, and volcanic eruptions. The following table gives an idea of their respective impacts on the communities affected by them.[40]

---

39 "Few non-governmental agencies concerned with disasters can afford to get involved in expensive, traditional prevention activities such as building levees. Nor can agencies, except perhaps the large UN bodies, expect to get involved in the 'top-down' national preparedness and mitigation strategies, but there are numerous opportunities for working with the potential victims to make their environment less prone and themselves less vulnerable." Anders Wikjman and Lloyd Timberlake, *Natural Disasters: Acts of God or Acts of Man?* (Earthscan, 1984), p. 127.

40 International Federation of Red Cross and Red Crescent Societies, *World Disasters Report*, p. 103.

Impact on Communities: Total Number of People Affected, 1967-1991

| | *Number of People Affected* | *Number of People Injured* | *Number of People Killed* |
|---|---|---|---|
| Droughts | 1,426,239,250 | 18 | 1,333,728 |
| Earthquakes | 42,943,009 | 741,420 | 646,307 |
| Volcanic Eruptions | 1,938,270 | 6,868 | 27,642 |
| Floods | 1,057,193,110 | 266,336 | 304,870 |

# 1. Droughts

Droughts are an ideal example for a study of vulnerability, as they are numerous and involve a complex interaction of factors.

## 1.1 Interaction of Phenomenon and Vulnerability

### *Vertical Chain of Reaction*

Changes in rainfall, whether a decrease compared to the usual level or a anarchical distribution of rainfall over the year, may result in a lack of usable water for agriculture, due to preexisting erosion[41] and the absence of any reservoir system. The final result is an ecological disaster.

This disaster, in turn, will endanger those crops sensitive to lack of water, reducing agricultural production[42] and thereby giving rise to an agricultural disaster. The drop in agricultural yield will affect the economically vulnerable groups,[43] who will have trouble obtaining food.

These problems will be all the more serious if the society in which they occur has a vulnerable social structure (dysfunction of traditional mechanisms of mutual aid, families broken up by war, a displaced population which is not socially

[41] An absence of vegetation encourages water to run off on the soil surface directly to rivers and streams, without seeping down to the water table. This erosion may be the result of deforestation, itself related to overpopulation.

[42] Those regions that practice intensive single-crop farming, which generally involves high water consumption, are particularly vulnerable.

[43] These are the groups whose means of economic compensation are limited, mainly because of latent underdevelopment: no monetary reserves, no food stocks from one year to the next, etc.

homogeneous, etc.). Families are then no longer able to provide for their minimum food needs, moving from shortages to disaster.

At first, a food disaster[44] will affect the most vulnerable groups in a family, or the classic groups "at nutritional risk": children under the age of five years,[45] pregnant and lactating women, the elderly, the handicapped, and the sick. For these people, the food disaster will be reflected in a nutritional disaster. If the lack of food continues, the entire population will be affected.

In developing countries, which do not possess the resources, the institutions, or the infrastructure required to assist such populations, the disaster will result in a high mortality rate. The mortality rate of the Ethiopian refugees who arrived in eastern Sudan in 1985 has been estimated as 18 to 45 times higher — depending on population group — than that of the local population.[46]

### *Horizontal Ramifications*

The linear cause-effect progression that characterizes a disaster has horizontal ramifications as well. Society is not a homogeneous entity; factors such as education, experience of previous crises, and the general level of development influence social cohesion and help to explain the different behaviors observable within a single society facing a crisis. The more extended the ramifications, the more complex the analysis of causes will be, involving all aspects of life: economic, social, cultural, and political.

## 1.2 Measures to Reduce Vulnerability and/or Increase Capacities

Attacking the problem from the end of the chain would mean dealing only with the nutritional consequences of a crisis caused much further back — that is, by a situation of underdevelopment. Since the goal of this chapter is to establish the link between emergencies and development, we must look at the *end* of an emergency situation and analyze how the experience of crisis can induce changes in both victims and authorities which will prevent, or at least mitigate, future crises.

The following measures could be taken for a rural population stricken by drought.

---

[44] Characterized by the loss of access to food resources.

[45] MSF studies indicate that children of two and three years old are most affected.

[46] It should be noted that drought was one of the factors that led the Ethiopians to migrate; but another was political instability. Michael Toole and Ronald Waldam, "Prevention of Excess Mortality in Refugee and Displaced Populations in Developing Countries," *Journal of the American Medical Association* 263, No. 24 (27 June 1990): 3297.

### *Climate*

The only possible measures against the climatic phenomenon itself is surveillance by an early-warning system (EWS).[47]

### *Ecological Disaster*

All measures tending to increase the availability of water should be promoted. These include:

- water storage systems
  - improvement of natural reservoirs
  - creation of artificial reservoirs
- reduction of deforestation
  - exploitation of alternative sources of energy
- reforestation
  - development of tree nurseries
- reduction of erosion
  - modification of livestock-raising practices
  - development of soil conservation techniques

### *Economic Disaster*

The aim here must be to reduce the population's dependence on a single source of food supply. This can be done by:

- encouraging saving;
- developing markets;
- diversifying the means of subsistence — for example, by the introduction of cottage industries.

### *Agricultural Disaster*

Steps must be taken to strengthen the agricultural system and to make it less vulnerable to the vagaries of the climate. In addition to the measures already mentioned in connection with water-supply management and the reduction of erosion, these steps could include:

- crop diversification;
- the institution of cooperatives for the sale of seeds and exchanges of equipment;
- dissemination of know-how (new farming techniques);

[47] EWSs are studied in Chapter 6 ("Epidemiology").

- improved methods of raising livestock;
- increase of arable land;
- access to local markets to sell produce and purchase equipment.

These measures are essentially technical. Undoubtedly, some of them will involve changes in farming systems and farmer organization — changes that will not be possible unless the necessary political adjustments are made. Moreover, this technical approach may prove counterproductive if it is implemented without the consent of the populations concerned and regardless of their traditions and their motivation for change. The farming system may be based on ancestral tradition; and although technically it may be prejudicial to agricultural yield, it may help maintain the fabric of the social system, thereby helping the population to survive serious crises. Preventing an agricultural disaster is not exclusively a matter of technical expertise; sociocultural and political factors must also be taken into account.

### *Food Disaster*

Steps can be taken to preserve access to food resources in cases of threatened or actual shortages. These steps include:

- maintenance of the social structure;
- respect for the traditional mechanisms of mutual aid;[48]
- development of household food-storage techniques to reduce food loss due to the inroads of rats and insects;
- development of local aid organizations — for example, National Red Cross (or Red Crescent) Societies — which will be ready to lend their help when traditional means are or threaten to become inadequate.

### *Nutritional Disaster*

Here the means of prevention are more limited:

- health education to prevent nutritional mistakes that may compound the problem of food shortage;
- access to health-care services — good immunization coverage will prevent a measles epidemic, for example, from striking down children already weakened by malnutrition;
- access to potable water.

[48] "In the most typical case, a peasant may travel to a neighbouring or distant country which is untouched or only lightly affected by drought and famine to borrow food from a relative, a friend, or someone with whom such an arrangement can be made." D. Rahmato, "Peasant Survival Strategies in Ethiopia," *Disasters* 12, No. 4: 331.

The earlier intervention in the chain of vulnerability takes place, the greater the chances that serious food and nutritional crises can be avoided. This raises the whole problem of humanitarian strategy in the field of famine relief.

In the first place, although the onset of serious food crises can be predicted, usually it is not until the media become interested that the authorities concerned — local, national, and international — go into action. The second difficulty is that sending food aid in a crisis does not solve the underlying problem. Its roots often lie in preexisting underdevelopment; the current crisis, latching onto it, only emphasizes economic, sociocultural, and political structural inadequacies.

The benevolent approach of food aid which has predominated up to now should be completely revised in favor of a preventive approach designed to correct structural inadequacies.[49] At a certain point, it becomes difficult to tell whether the activities undertaken — development if they attack the root of the problem, emergency relief if they attack the consequences — derive from one strategy or the other. Food aid to a population whose food resources, according to predictions, will not meet their normal needs within six months, is still an emergency measure; agricultural aid in the form of distribution of seeds, tools, and draft animals, in contrast, is a rehabilitation measure. Finally, improving the management of the water used for agriculture and changing farming techniques come under the heading of development rather than rehabilitation.

To classify different activities objectively according to whether they constitute emergency aid, rehabilitation, or development, the following criteria are used:

- Who decides?
- Who implements?
- Who pays?
- Are structures modified?
- Is there progress towards self-sufficiency?

# 2. Earthquakes

## 2.1 Interaction of Phenomenon and Vulnerability

Many studies have shown that in an earthquake, it is the most disadvantaged populations who suffer the greatest loss of life. The explanation can be found in an analysis of vulnerability, particularly its social aspects:

- housing, where construction does not accord with earthquake standards;[50]

---

[49] In this respect, development activities are eminently political.

[50] "Ignorance and poverty increase the vulnerability of marginal groups because their housing is inadequate or built using faulty construction techniques, and, above all, because their settlements are located in high-risk areas and the infrastructure is overburdened." PAHO, *Health Conditions in the Americas,* Vol. I (PAHO, 1990), p. 203.

- health-care facilities themselves fall prey to destruction in an earthquake;
- health-care facilities are ill-prepared to receive large numbers of casualties;
- restricted access to health-care facilities.

### 2.2 Measures to Reduce Vulnerability

Measures to reduce vulnerability are also generally designed to reduce underdevelopment. They include the implementation of standards, particularly construction standards. Another important step is reorganizing the health-care services:

"Disasters hinder development by destroying the infrastructure and by using up the health services' scanty resources for emergencies or rehabilitation. However, they also provide an opportunity to genuinely reform and improve the health system, because they encourage such changes as better distribution of services or a shift from large hospitals to comprehensive and decentralized health services. Such measures were adopted in Mexico City during the reconstruction of the hospitals destroyed by the earthquake."[51]

## 3. Floods

Here again, the connection with underdevelopment is obvious: populations concentrated in fertile but high-risk areas, absence of dams or dikes to hold back flood waters, flimsy housing which will not stand up to flooding.

Environmental vulnerability could conceivably be reduced, through reforestation and the construction of dams and water reservoirs. Such projects are realistic only if the community agrees they are justified and is willing to maintain them in the long term.

## 4. Volcanoes

The vulnerability associated with volcanoes is not limited to actual eruptions, which certainly entail human losses but whose consequences in the long term are not as great as those engendered by the constitution of pyroclastic deposits (lahar).[52] These may upset the hydrological balance in the region. To these effects must be added the destruction of infrastructure such as bridges, which are swept away by the flood of pyroclastic deposits. In the long run, the number of people affected by this imbalance is much greater than the number of victims directly affected by the initial volcanic eruption.

---

[51] *Ibid.*

[52] Deposits created by the cinders and other particles emitted by volcanoes and concentrated in declivities (such as river beds) by rain, upon contact with which they solidify.

Measures to reduce vulnerability focus on:

- the initial phenomenon — prediction through early-warning mechanisms;
- the community — information on dangers, education about the steps to be taken in case of an alert;
- buildings — construction of new buildings (hospitals, schools) outside the danger zones;
- the environment — protection of low-lying regions by constructing dams to channel the flow of pyroclastic deposits;

# V. The Difficult Transition from Emergency Programs to Development Programs

## 1. Autonomous Emergency Programs: an Artificial Paradise

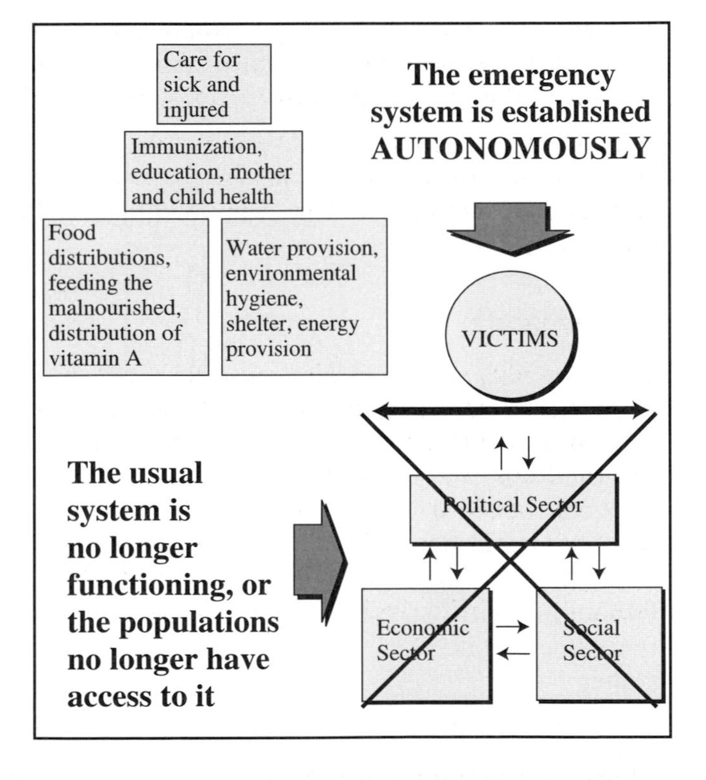


The initial phase of disaster situations presents the risk that emergency programs will be instituted that are totally unconnected with the existing systems. Obviously, in certain situations, when populations have been displaced and are no longer integrated in any development framework (no more economic system, no more social service infrastructure, no more political system), it will be necessary to set up a completely artificial environment, in which food distributions replace agricultural production, water is distributed by tank trucks, and medical care is provided free by benevolent agencies.

The dangers of this approach are evident:

- the authorities normally in charge of the local systems relinquish responsibility;
- the victims become chronic aid recipients who will gradually lose any sense of being autonomous within a system of their own. Everybody is happy — both the humanitarian agencies, who are able to demonstrate their efficiency, and the victims, who little by little will come to consider the emergency system as a normal way of meeting their essential needs.

Emergency interventions are often necessary, of course, and no criticism of them is intended here; but if the emergency should necessitate the establishment of an artificial system that takes the place of the usual systems, then the emergency strategy absolutely must reflect a long-term perspective aiming at the eventual restoration of the original systems.

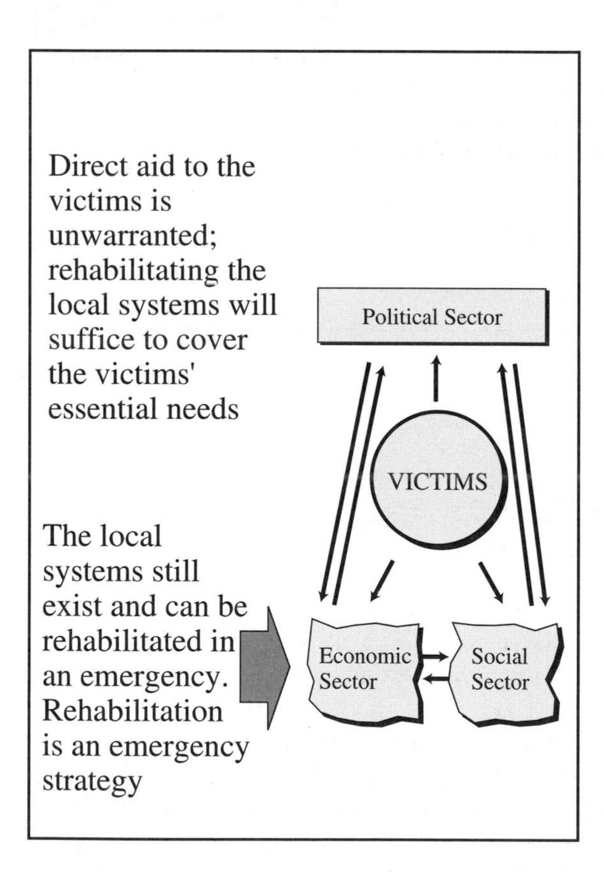


## 2. Rehabilitation as a Form of Emergency Intervention

If the link between the victims and the local systems still exists, and the dysfunction of the latter is linked to material supply problems or a temporary lack of personnel, as may be the case for hospitals and water supply stations, for example, then an intervention to rehabilitate the local systems will be enough to solve the problem. Rehabilitation comes under the heading of emergency strategy.

## 3. Combining Direct Aid and Rehabilitation Programs

When the problems involved require major rehabilitation interventions, it will be necessary to combine emergency interventions in the form of direct aid to the victims (food distribution, medical care) with rehabilitation programs that will take over as soon as the local systems have been restored to their former operational level. These two kinds of programs are part of a well-planned emergency strategy, in which the medium-term solution is anticipated from the beginning of the intervention.

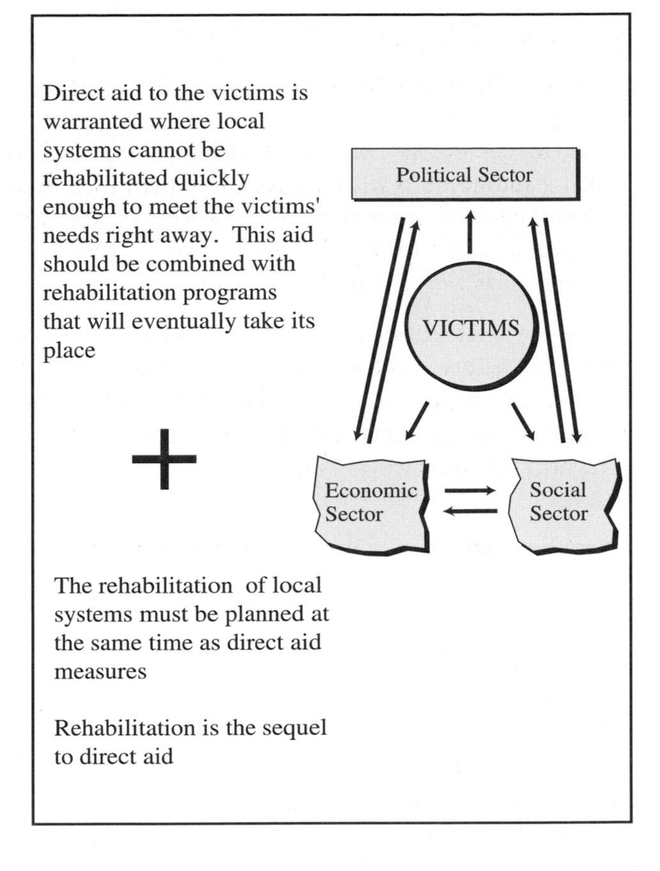


## 4. Distinction Between Rehabilitating and Developing Local Systems

Rehabilitation consists in restoring local systems. Clearly, if those systems suffer from major deficiencies which make them particularly vulnerable, the question may arise whether rehabilitating them is appropriate, or whether perhaps they should be structurally modified to make them more effective. In this case, real development programs must be envisaged, comprising two lines of action. One will involve examining system vulnerability, determining corrective measures, and applying them; the other will seek to develop existing local capacities and give the local personnel responsibility for implementing all stages of the programs. Overall, development programs should help raise people's standard of living and make them less vulnerable to disasters.

The number of natural disasters continues to increase as years go by, as does their impact on the socioeconomic sector,[53] leading to an ever-widening gap between the needs of the vulnerable groups and the local capacity to meet them. The reasons for this growing gap should be sought in the deteriorating economic situation of many developing countries, the degeneration of the environment, migration to the cities, increased technological risks, and the burden of demographic growth, which forces entire populations to move into high-risk areas.

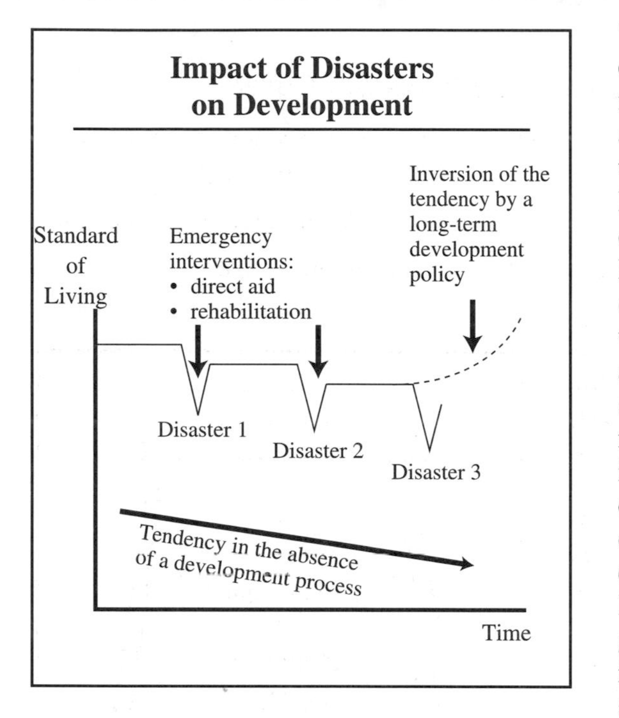


"Probably the most significant cause of the rise in the number and impact of disasters is population growth, which is forcing people to live in more marginal and dangerous places — low-lying land liable to flooding or areas close to active volcanoes. And as more and more of the planet is settled, earthquakes are more likely to strike inhabited areas. Population increases and industrial development also lead to environmental degradation. Deforestation and overgrazing, for example, have increased the number and severity of droughts and floods.

[...]

Disasters in developing countries are an integral part of their poverty cycle. Poverty causes disasters. And disasters exacerbate poverty. Only sustainable human development — which increases the security of human beings and of the planet we inhabit — can reduce the frequency and impact of natural disasters."[54]

---

53 "The number of disasters which strike continues to grow. In recent years, the number of persons affected by these disasters has been increasing at the rate of 6 per cent per year, which corresponds to three times the annual population growth. Along with ever-mounting economic losses, the inevitable result is a serious negative impact on sustainable development." Final document issued by the United Nations World Conference on Natural Disaster Reduction, Yokohama, Japan, 23-27 May 1994.

54 UNDP, *Human Development Report* (1994), p. 29.

This slide towards levels of greater and greater vulnerability can be arrested only through the institution of coherent policies that envisage not only measures to cope with the immediate effects of disasters, but also the necessity for long-term action focusing on the underlying factors that make certain populations particularly vulnerable to disasters.

# VI. Harmonizing Development Policies

## 1. Development Policies at the National Level

Development policies that are centered mainly on the economic sector are no longer sacrosanct, and provision for social needs is becoming a priority:

"The 1980s: Economic restructuring is considered the premise of development.

The 1990s: Reforming social policies has become an imperative." [55]

Although the importance of the social sector is now realized, the task of actually doing something about it is hindered by both lack of economic means and an increase in social needs. This is true not only in the developing countries, but also in the developed countries where the era of the welfare state is coming to an end.

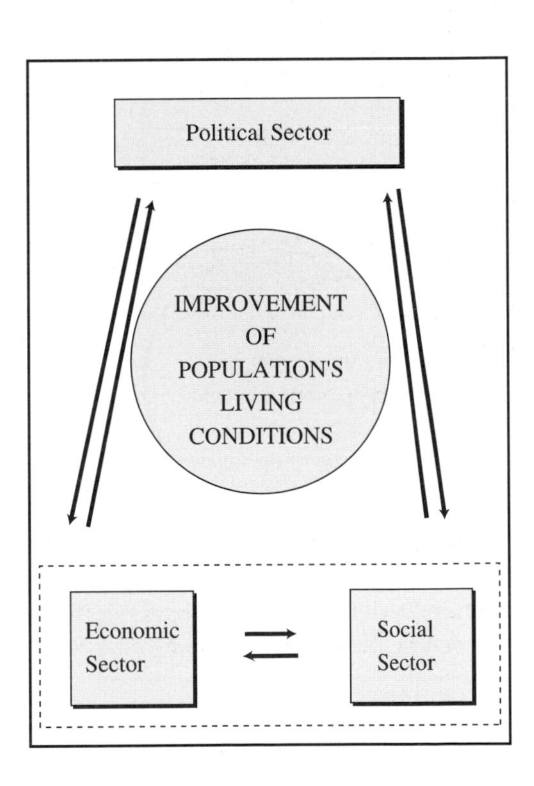


This chapter would not be complete without an analysis of the relations between the political system and the population it represents or is supposed to represent. Political systems play a role in:

- defining social and economic policies. Today the debate between liberalism and a Marxist approach no longer has any currency.

[55] International Development Research Centre (IDRC), *Explore* (Jan. 1994).

- the strategies for applying these policies — consensus, imposition by force, equity, centralization or decentralization.

The exercise of power must be analyzed in terms of the relations existing between the government, the parliament, the judiciary, the forces that maintain order, the army, and the social groups. The expression of a nation's values varies according to ethnic differences, socioeconomic level, and ideologies. However, there should be a consensus between a population and its political system regarding reciprocal rights and obligations. For example, the population has:

- the right to express itself;
- the right to access to health services;
- the right to decent housing;
- the right to education;
- the right to independent justice;
- the duty to respect the rules established to maintain order.

The State, on the other hand, has:

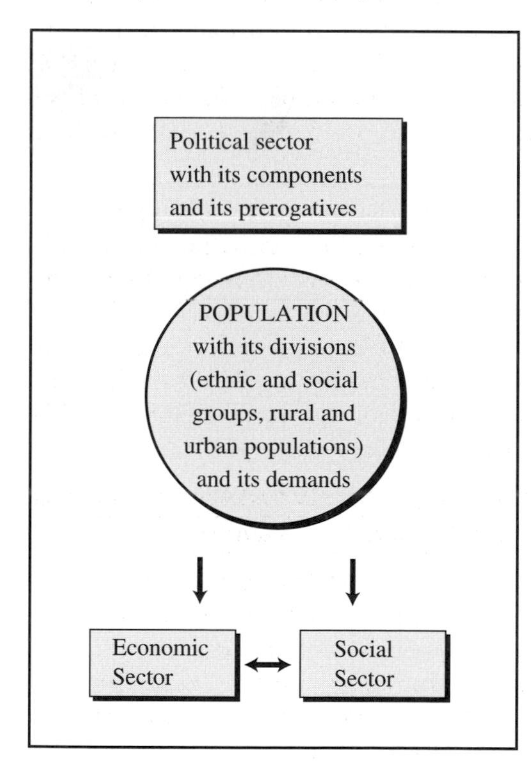


- the right to levy taxes;
- the right to maintain order;
- the duty to maintain the country's territorial integrity.

The promotion of harmonious development must take into account all these factors, which often pit individuals against governments, governmental authorities against one another, or individuals against one another.

The contract that ties individuals to the established power defines the "rights of citizens." In lawful States, the norms and procedures for their application which govern relations between individuals (private law) or relations between individuals and the public authorities (public law) are established by democratic rules — that is, those decreed by "the people." Depending on whether the election system is majority rule or proportional representation, the will of the "people" will be more or less faithfully represented. The majority system, however, favors the emergence of one party to the detriment of the others:

"Such a system amplifies the score of the majority party, for the latter can carry the majority of the seats with 51% of the ballots cast (and thus fewer than half of the registered voters). This party could then apply its program without difficulty; but is it fair play to eliminate from power 49% of the voters?" [56]

Although the 51/49 ratio is still better than that achieved under dictatorial regimes, in which a tiny percentage of individuals imposes their law on the entire society, it well illustrates the limits of democracy. In this respect, however, major progress has been made: "The 1980s were in many ways a decade of democratic transition — as many military dictators ceded power to civilian administrations and one-party States opened themselves up to multiparty elections." [57]

# 2. Development in an International Perspective

## 2.1 The Predominance of the Economic Factor

The world's economic systems are becoming increasingly interdependent, and a country's economic development cannot be conceived without due consideration of the international economic environment. In the economic sector, the multinational companies control two-thirds of world trade. The income of the African coffee-grower, for example, depends directly on the prices set by these companies.

A number of international organizations try to encourage the development of national economic systems while instilling respect for international economic rules. These organizations include the IMF (International Monetary Fund), the WTO (World Trade Organization) which replaces the GATT (General Agreement on Tariffs and Trade), the IBRD (International Bank for Reconstruction and Development) — commonly called the World Bank — the EBRD (European Bank for Reconstruction and Development), and UNCTAD (United Nations Conference for Trade and Development).

**Is the ultimate goal of trade liberalization to promote the well-being of all human beings or the socioeconomic interests of the wealthiest countries?**

International relations are based essentially on political and economic interests. Thus, donor countries expect commercial benefits from the aid they provide to the developing countries, in the form of opportunities to buy primary goods at rock-bottom prices, to sell equipment, or to supply factories ready for use. "National self-interest — military, political or commercial — is sometimes thought to be an inevitable consideration for the donor country. It is often said that aid is merely an instrument for achieving foreign policy objectives." [58]

[56] Odon Vallet, *L'Etat et le Politique,* Collections Dominos (Flammarion), p. 50.
[57] UNDP, *Human Development Report* (1994), p. 32.
[58] UNDP, *Human Development Report* (1991), p. 75.

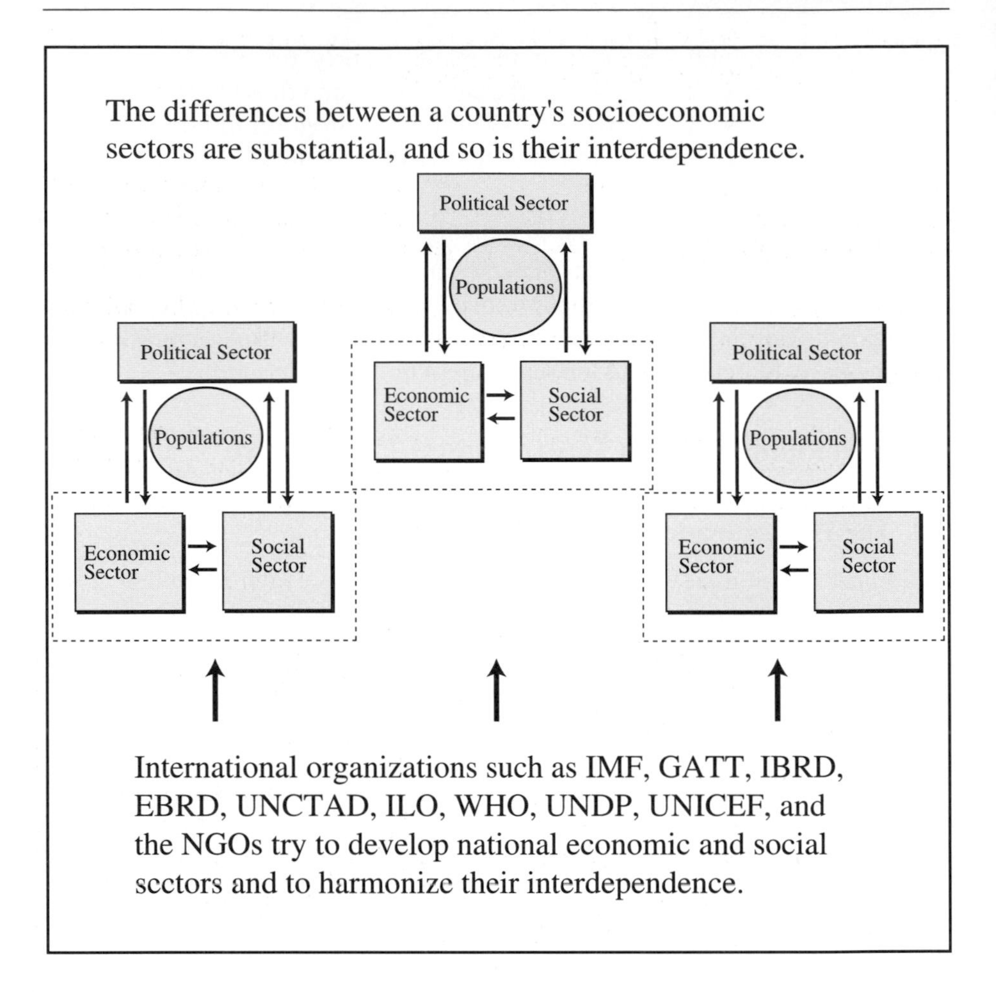


## 2.2 The Emergence of the Social Sector

Nevertheless, the social sector has not been abandoned. Certain international agencies influence national policies, such as WHO (founded in 1946) in the health field, the ILO (International Labor Organization, founded in 1919) in the realm of labor law, and UNESCO (United Nations Educational, Scientific, and Cultural Organization, founded in 1945) in the education field.

These sectors are obviously interdependent, and organizations which by definition are oriented exclusively towards the economic sector, such as the IMF, have realized the importance of the social factor:

"Up until the end of the eighties, the Fund considered that social policies and income distribution were the prerogative of sovereign, independent governments, and that its own statutes did not give it a mandate in this area. It underlined its 'political neutrality' in this respect, pointing out that the battle against poverty depended on economic stability.

(...)

From the end of the eighties, however, the battle against poverty became a more important objective for the Monetary Fund, given the accumulation of examples of stabilization programs that had had a harmful effect on the poorest groups."[59]

However, the remedies advocated to reduce poverty are usually palliative measures (subsidies to consumers, social services, etc.) rather than long-term social development objectives.

In its 1990 annual report, the UNDP proposed that the performances of countries no longer be evaluated by that "ineluctable" yardstick of gross national

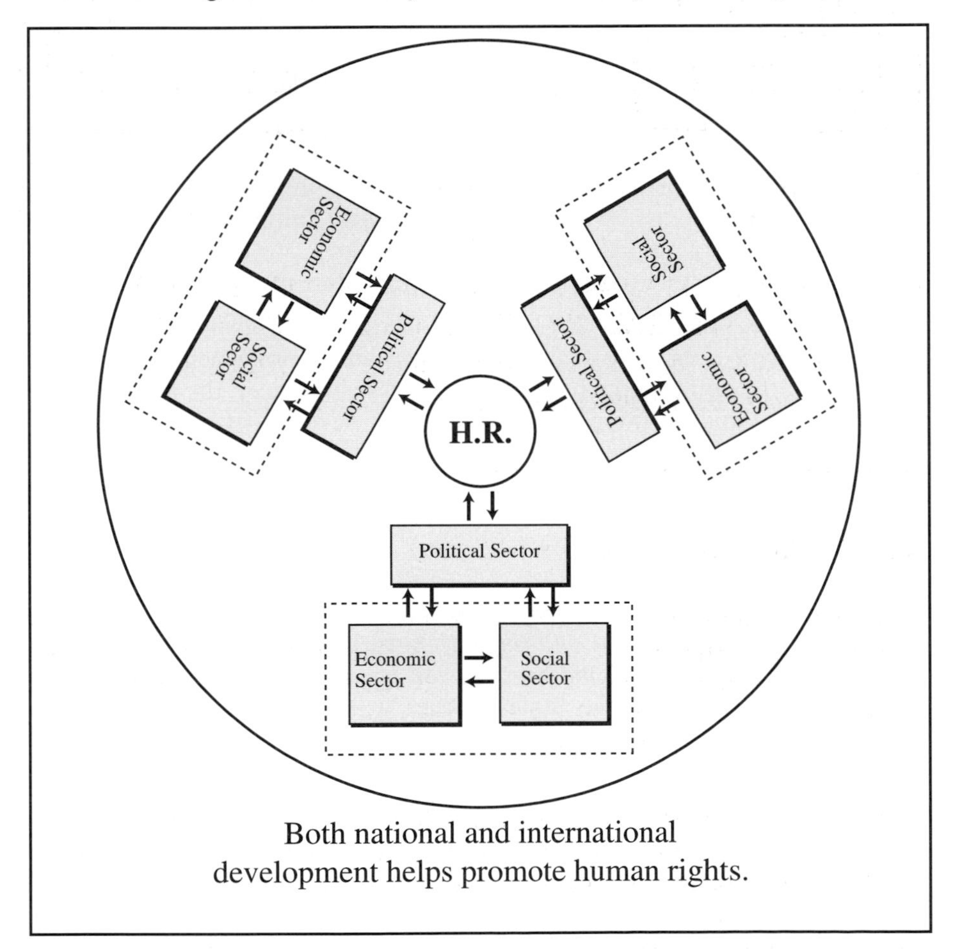


Both national and international development helps promote human rights.

[59] Patrick Lenain, *Le FMI* (Collection Repères, 1993), p. 60.

product (GNP) per inhabitant, but by an indicator of human development, to be constituted by a set of parameters centered on three main factors: life expectancy, education, and living conditions. Canada was in first place according to the indicator of human development, whereas it would fall to eleventh place on the GNP scale. Developing the performance of socioeconomic systems is no longer a goal in itself, but a means of improving the living conditions of all populations. The human being is now the center of development policies.

## 2.3 International Human-Rights Law as an Intervention Strategy for Development

The United Nations Organization has been very active in this domain; its strategy is defined in the following articles.

*Article 2 of the Declaration on the Right to Development*:

"1. The human person is the central subject of development and should be the active participant and beneficiary of the right to development.

2. All human beings have a responsibility for development, individually and collectively, taking into account the need for full respect for their human rights and fundamental freedoms as well as their duties to the community, which alone can ensure the free and complete fulfilment of the human being, and they should therefore promote and protect an appropriate political social and economic order for development.

3. States have the right and duty to formulate appropriate national development policies that aim at the constant improvement of the well-being of the entire population and of all individuals, on the basis of their active, free and meaningful participation in development and in the fair distribution of the benefits resulting therefrom." [60]

*Article 11 of the International Covenant on Economic, Social and Cultural Rights* was adopted by the UN General Assembly on 16 December 1966 (emphasis added):

"1. The States Parties to the present Covenant recognize the right of everyone to an *adequate standard of living* for himself and his family, including adequate *food, clothing and housing*, and to the continuous improvement of living conditions. The States Parties will take appropriate steps to ensure the realization of this right, recognizing to this effect the essential importance of international co-operation based on free consent.

2. The States Parties to the present Covenant, recognizing the fundamental right of everyone to be *free from hunger*, shall take, individually and through international co-operation, the measures, including specific programmes, which are needed:

[60] General Assembly Resolution 41/128 of 4 Dec. 1986.

(a) To improve methods of production, conservation and distribution of food by making full use of technical and scientific knowledge, by disseminating knowledge of the principles of nutrition and by developing or reforming agrarian systems in such a way as to achieve the most efficient development and utilization of natural resources;

(b) Taking into account the problems of both food-importing and food-exporting countries, to ensure an equitable distribution of world food supplies in relation to need." [61]

*Articles 2 and 3 of the Declaration on Social Progress and Development* (1969):

**"Article 2**

Social progress and development shall be founded on respect for the dignity and value of the human person and shall ensure the promotion of human rights and social justice [...]

**Article 3**

The following are considered primary conditions of social progress and development:

(a) National independence based on the right of peoples to self-determination;
(b) The principle of non-interference in the internal affairs of States;
(c) Respect for the sovereignty and territorial integrity of States;
(d) Permanent sovereignty of each nation over its natural wealth and resources;
(e) The right and responsibility of each State and, as far as they are concerned, each nation and people to determine freely its own objectives of social development, to set its own priorities and to decide in conformity with the principles of the Charter of the United Nations the means and methods of their achievement without any external interference;
(f) Peaceful coexistence, peace, friendly relations and co-operation among States irrespective of differences in their social, economic or political systems."

*Article 1 of the Covenant on Civil and Political Rights* was adopted by the UN General Assembly on 16 December 1966: "All *peoples* have the right of self-determination. By virtue of that right they freely determine their political status and freely pursue their economic, social and cultural development" (emphasis added).

## 2.4 Disasters and Human-Rights Law

The connection between disasters and human rights is clear. The sight of injured people, malnourished children, populations uprooted from their homes in the

[61] Resolution 2200 A (XXI).

wake of catastrophe, usually unleashes an international reaction based on the prime human right: the right to life. Emergency relief is the best way of insuring survival and the restoration of living conditions to what they were before the disaster. Unfortunately, these conditions are usually precarious, constantly in danger of tipping over into emergency again. Emergency situations have the merit of pinpointing the most vulnerable population groups, who will not escape the poverty cycle without the help of a serious development policy.

Whether at the level of emergency disaster relief or during the development process that follows, States must develop legal instruments that clearly establish the responsibilities of the national and international authorities concerned.

## *National Legislation*

Prevention plans have been prepared in many countries. National legislation establishes the responsibilities of various organizations involved in disaster prevention and relief. In Jamaica, for example, a body known as the Office of Disaster Preparedness and Emergency Management (ODPEM) is empowered to raise funds itself for its interventions.

In many countries, however, the institution of disaster prevention programs meets with numerous obstacles. The lack of financial means limits the implementation of prophylactic measures that do not have an immediately perceivable impact. Social, ethnic, and religious discrimination contributes to an increase in the vulnerability of the poorest members of society. Consequently, taking disasters into account in national development programs may seem paradoxical insofar as poverty and inequality are becoming increasingly manifest.

## *International Legislation*

UN General Assembly resolution 43/131 of 8 December 1988 underlines the importance of humanitarian aid and emphasizes the role of the States; in it, the General Assembly:

"1. *Reaffirms* the importance of humanitarian assistance for the victims of natural disasters and similar emergency situations;

2. *Reaffirms* also the sovereignty of affected States and their primary role in the initiation, organization, co-ordination and implementation of humanitarian assistance within their respective territories;

3. *Stresses* the important contribution made in providing humanitarian assistance by intergovernmental and non-governmental organizations working with strictly humanitarian motives;

4. *Invites* all States in need of such assistance to facilitate the work of these organizations in implementing humanitarian assistance, in particular the

supply of food, medicines and health care, for which access to victims is essential [...]."

The importance of preventing disasters was underlined by General Assembly resolution 44/236 (1989) proclaiming the next decade as the "International Decade for Natural Disaster Reduction," the main goals of which were to analyze national vulnerability and to participate in drawing up a prevention plan.

The International Decade has served as a basis for changing national mentalities, allowing leaders to draw support from international recommendations in order to change their approach to disaster situations:

"The advent of the International Decade for Natural Disaster Reduction (IDNDR) changed that, providing practitioners at the national level with the international credentials they lacked. Gradually, the Decade has weeded out those practitioners — amateurs and professionals — who have failed to master new methods and techniques, or who cling to the old way of equating disaster prevention and mitigation with stockpiling equipment, blankets, and old clothing." [62]

The need to integrate disaster prevention in a global policy based on human development is regularly emphasized in international seminars, such as the round table organized in Berlin on the subject of "Disaster Mitigation and Prevention Policies for Sustainable Development" (25-28 January 1994), which concluded in its final declaration: "National and international agencies responsible for development planning should play the leading role in the promotion and implementation of developmental activities aiming to reduce vulnerability to disasters."

These two basic principles — the integration of disaster prevention in a global development policy and the States' primary responsibility in both devising prevention programs and managing response — have challenged the role of international humanitarian agencies, which had a tendency to monopolize disaster interventions without concerning themselves with local response capacities or possibilities of prevention, the starting point for any development process. Countries in Latin America and Asia have demonstrated their ability to confront their responsibilities in both disaster response and disaster prevention; whereas others, notably in Africa, are inexorably plunging deeper into the downward spiral of poverty.

[62] PAHO, *A World Safe from Natural Disasters* (1994), p. 3.

**Emergency practitioners must be able to integrate disaster prevention programs into the wider perspective of the major problems facing humanity at the dawn of the 21st century:**

- **anarchical management of natural resources**
- **economic development based exclusively on mercenary considerations**
- **uncontrolled population growth**
- **lack of social equality**
- **mass population migrations**
- **increase in the number of disasters due to increased vulnerability and the augmentation of risks entailed by anarchical development**

**Unless it resolves these fundamental imbalances, humanity will witness a growing increase in the number and extent of conflicts.**

# Chapter 9

# PROTECTING THE VICTIMS OF ARMED CONFLICTS

***Protecting the victims of armed conflicts is a field in which humanitarian aid is both much in demand and particularly difficult to implement. The context of this protection is defined by the following sequence, the three main elements of which will be briefly described:***
- ***the conditions permitting peace;***
- ***the factors that cause peaceful situations to develop into war;***
- ***the factors that favor a return to peace.***

# I. Definition of the General Framework

## 1. Peace

Peace may be defined as the result of a perfect balance between the systems within a country, allowing all the people of a nation to benefit from the full enjoyment of their rights. On the international level, the same kind of balance is necessary for peace between nations.

This approach, based on an idyllic view of the world, is probably utopian. In reality, relations between human groups are based on power struggles, in which the adversaries often resort to force.

"Inquiry into the nature of peace and how to build it can be framed in two ways. From the systemic perspective, it can be conceptualized as a world system where the probability of war, especially war among major states, goes way down. From an interaction perspective, it can be conceptualized as a great reduction in the probability that political actors will resort to violence to achieve their ends." [1]

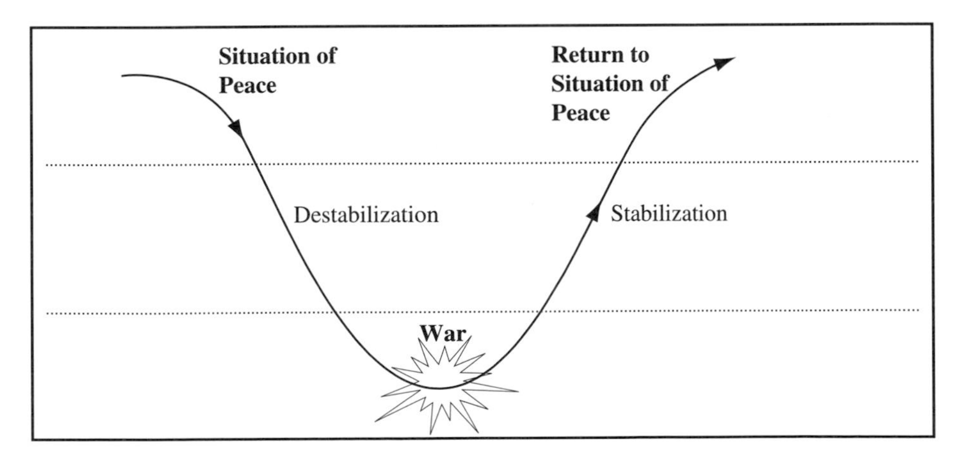


[1] John A. Vasquez, *The War Puzzle*, Cambridge Studies in International Relations, 27 (Cambridge University Press, 1993), p. 264.

For the International Red Cross and Red Crescent Movement,
"peace is not simply the absence of war, but rather a dynamic process of co-operation among all States and peoples; co-operation founded on freedom, independence, national sovereignty, equality, respect of human rights, and a fair and equitable distribution of resources to meet the needs of peoples."[2]

The conditions permitting the maintenance of peace were examined in the previous chapter. There is, on the national level, the connection established between peace and the promotion of human rights, and, on the international level, the necessary inter-State cooperation aimed at promoting the development of the most disadvantaged nations. Peace and development are linked: development is essential to reduce the risks of armed conflict, while peace is a prerequisite for development.

Also noted was the importance of the challenges humanity will face during the next decades. If these challenges are not met, they are liable to increase the risk of armed conflicts between nations.

## 2. Armed Conflicts

Armed conflicts do not occur unexpectedly. Behind the immediate factors that trigger them, analysis reveals other, deeper causes, such as territorial demands, socioeconomic inequality, economic interests, the defense of political ideologies, burgeoning nationalism, the struggles of ethnic minorities, racism, and arms proliferation.

### 2.1 Prevention of Armed Conflicts: Intervention at the Source

Development in the broad sense — that is, the promotion of human rights — helps prevent conflicts by reducing socioeconomic inequalities, abolishing discrimination, and permitting political expression for all citizens. Decreased military spending and disarmament can also help promote development, if the resources initially earmarked for arms are correctly used to benefit the most impoverished.

The United Nations' peacekeeping efforts are essential. The UN organizations work to promote human rights in the world. Moreover, when differences arise between States, the UN plays an arbitrating role, asking the adversaries to seek a peaceful solution:

"The parties to any dispute, the continuance of which is likely to endanger the maintenance of international peace and security, shall, first of all, seek a solution

[2] "What the Red Cross and Red Crescent Movement Does and Wants to Do for Peace," *International Review of the Red Cross* 750 (Nov./Dec. 1984): 327.

by negotiation, enquiry, mediation, conciliation, arbitration, judicial settlement, resort to regional agencies or arrangements, or other peaceful means of their own choice."[3]

Article 2(4) of Chapter 1 of the United Nations Charter prohibits the use of force between States. The Security Council, however, can ask the member States to take coercive measures (Art. 39), using armed force (Art. 42) or other means (Arts. 40, 41).

## 2.2 International Humanitarian Law

Along with efforts to promote the political resolution of conflicts, intervention is necessary to minimize the effects of such conflicts. The desire to limit the consequences of war does not imply acceptance of the principle of war; it reflects, rather, a pragmatic approach, based on the realization that in spite of efforts to maintain peace, war exists.

International humanitarian law is "a set of rules aimed at limiting violence and protecting the fundamental rights of the individual in time of armed conflict."[4] To do this, international humanitarian law strives to regulate the conduct of hostilities and to guarantee the protection of non-combatants.

### *Conduct of Hostilities*

Rules have been laid down to regulate the methods and means of combat. These rules are primarily those constituting the law of The Hague. This body of law restricts or prohibits the use of certain means of warfare during a conflict, and includes:

- The Declaration of St. Petersburg (1868), which outlawed the use of certain types of projectiles in time of war.
- The Declaration Concerning Expanding Bullets, prohibiting the use of bullets that expand or flatten easily in the human body (1899).
- The Geneva Protocol for the Prohibition of the Use of Asphyxiating, Poisonous or Other Gases, and of Bacteriological Methods of Warfare (1925).
- The Convention on the Prohibition of the Development, Production and Stockpiling of Bacteriological (Biological) and Toxin Weapons and on their Destruction (1972).
- The Convention on the Prohibition of Military or Any Other Hostile Use of Environmental Modification Techniques (1976).
- The Protocol on Non-Detectable Fragments (1980).
- The Protocol on Prohibitions or Restrictions on the Use of Mines, Booby-Traps and Other Devices (1980).

---

[3] United Nations Charter, Ch. VI, Art. 33, Par. 1 (1945).
[4] *Human Rights and the ICRC: International Humanitarian Law* (Geneva: ICRC, 1993), p. 3.

- The Protocol on Blinding Laser Weapons (1995).

The last three instruments are part of the 1980 United Nations Convention on Prohibitions or Restrictions on the Use of Certain Conventional Weapons which May Be Deemed to Be Excessively Injurious or to Have Indiscriminate Effects. The Additional Protocols of 1977 contain many rules concerning means and methods of warfare — for example, Articles 35, 36, and 37 of Protocol I.

In war situations, health-care personnel are confronted with the consequences of the use of arms (surgeons, for example, see the results of anti-personnel mines), and those of the military tactics employed (public health personnel and displaced populations). Operating from the perspective of prevention, health-care personnel are naturally concerned in particular by the possibilities of limiting the means of warfare. The role of health-care personnel is, of course, to tend those wounded by mines, but also to address the issue on another level, respect for the international humanitarian law that prohibits the indiscriminate use of mines.[5] Similarly, health-care workers know the dramatic effects that population movements have on health. Their role is therefore to educate all those who bear some of the responsibility for such decisions and their consequences.

At another level of prevention, the health-care personnel also have a responsibility to warn against the development of new weapons. The perfection of laser weapons that cause permanent blindness in those hit, and the possibility of producing such weapons on a large scale directly concern the professional conscience of health-care workers; it is their duty to draw attention to the dramatic effects the use of these weapons is likely to have.

### *Protection of Non-Combatants*

Individuals are extremely vulnerable in situations of armed conflict.

"There are few situations in which the individual encounters greater dangers than in war. And it is in a situation of war that the individual is also the most vulnerable."[6]

---

[5] "The ICRC is firmly of the opinion that the only effective measure is to ban the use and production of anti-personnel landmines. [It is] also of the opinion that there should be strict controls on the use and design of anti-vehicle mines which in practice have led to casualties among both local civilian and humanitarian workers, including ICRC delegates, who need to use the roads to reach the victims. The ICRC notes with satisfaction that several States have joined the call for a ban on anti-personnel mines and earnestly hopes that others will do so before the Review Conference itself." Statement by the International Committee of the Red Cross (24 Oct. 1994), at the 49th session of the United Nations General Assembly, First Committee Agenda Item 66: Convention on Prohibitions or Restrictions on the Use of Certain Conventional Weapons which May Be Deemed to be Excessively Injurious or to Have Indiscriminate Effects.

[6] Cornelio Sommaruga, "Le CICR et la protection des droits de l'homme," talk given at the inaugural meeting of the 23rd teaching session of the International Institute of Human Rights, Strasbourg, 6 July 1992.

Civilian populations suffer in particular in situations of armed conflict; forced displacement, extortion, and assault are all frequent violations of international humanitarian law. The situation of prisoners, wounded, and shipwreck survivors is often particularly precarious. Nor should the impact of armed conflict on local systems be forgotten:

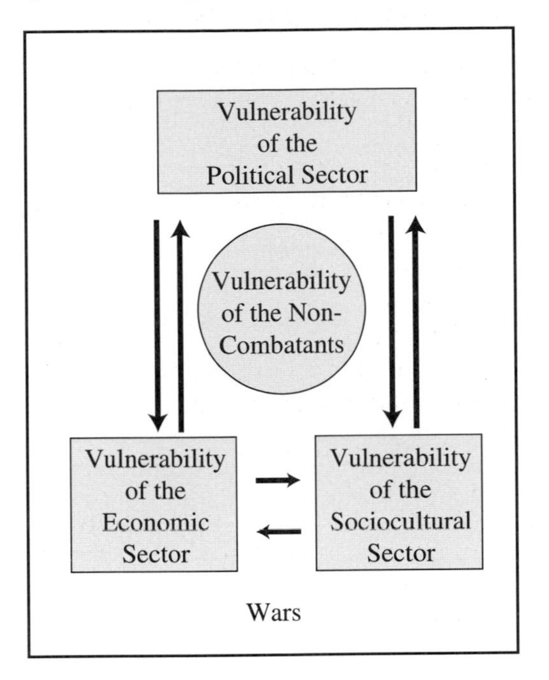


- disruptions of the economic system; in some rural areas, landmines restrict access to agricultural land.
- destruction of social infrastructures such as hospitals, water-supply services, etc.
- impairment of the social fabric, including disruption of normal mechanisms of mutual aid.
- destabilization of political structures, leading to a loss of control over the main functions of the State: police, justice, armies.

All these disruptions affect non-combatants — especially since many countries have underlying structural deficiencies to begin with, which are aggravated by armed conflict. The protection of essential services is linked to the protection of individuals.

**The protection of non-combatants is based essentially on the 1949 Geneva Conventions and their two Additional Protocols of 1977.**

Henry Dunant's account of the Battle of Solferino led to the adoption in 1864 of the first Convention for the Amelioration of the Condition of the Wounded in Armies in the Field. In 1868, the draft of the Convention for the Amelioration of the Condition of Wounded, Sick and Shipwrecked Members of Armed Forces at Sea was adopted by an international conference in Geneva, but it was not until 1899 that the draft convention was ratified by the States at the first international peace conference, in The Hague.

World War I (1914-1918) exposed the gaps in prisoner-of-war protection:
"[...] by sending delegates in the camps, it was able not only to bring the comfort of a friendly visit to prisoners of war, but also to make an impartial judgment of the treatment accorded to them and to persuade the Detaining Powers to make improvements which were called for by the tenets of the Red Cross. Once the war was ended, the International Committee of the Red Cross [...] lost no time in

seeking to profit from experience gained during the war to improve the conditions of prisoners of war by giving them a regular statute."[7]

The Geneva Convention Relative to the Treatment of Prisoners of War was adopted on 27 July 1929, by the Diplomatic Conference of Geneva.

The world war of 1939-1945 claimed many victims among the civilian population (deportations, bombings, summary executions), who belonged to a category of persons unprotected by any convention. Back in 1934, the ICRC had prepared a draft convention concerning the protection of civilian populations in wartime, which was to be submitted to a diplomatic conference scheduled for the beginning of 1940. However, the conference was prevented by the outbreak of World War II. Thus, it was not until 1949 that the fourth Geneva Convention Relative to the Protection of Civilian Persons in Time of War was adopted, by a diplomatic conference held in Geneva from April 21 to August 12. At the same time the conference adopted the revisions proposed for the first three conventions. Together, these four documents make up the Geneva Conventions of 12 August 1949.

The Diplomatic Conference of 1974-1977 on the Reaffirmation and Development of International Humanitarian Law Applicable in Armed Conflicts ended on 8 June 1977 with the adoption of two Protocols additional to the Geneva Conventions: "Supplemented in this way, borrowing copiously from the Hague law — which itself had been in great need of updating since 1907 — the Geneva Conventions henceforth constitute an impressive monument of 600 articles of which almost 150 are new."[8]

Finally, customary law is also cited for the protection of war victims. This law is not written, but reflects accepted practice.

## 3. Return to Peace

Peace may be reestablished in various ways. The test of strength between the two parties to the conflict may end in the victory of one of them. Negotiations between the two, with or without an intermediary, may resolve the situation. Peace may be reestablished by these negotiations or by the pressure of international diplomacy. Finally, it may result from outside intervention by one or several countries acting under the mandate or with the authorization of the UN Security Council. In such a case, the armed forces under the control of the UN act in accordance with Article 42 of the UN Charter.

---

[7] Jean Pictet, ed., *Commentary, Geneva Convention Relative to the Treatment of Prisoners of War*, Vol. 3 (ICRC, 1960), p. 4.

[8] ICRC, *Commentary on the Additional Protocols of 8 June 1977 to the Geneva Conventions of 12 August 1949* (Geneva: Martinus Nijhoff Publishers, 1987), p. XXXIV.

The UN also plays a predominant role in peacekeeping operations, by installing observers, deploying armed forces, or else establishing civilian personnel in the areas concerned.

A return to lasting peace depends not only on the cessation of hostilities, but especially on a recognition of the causes that led to the conflict. In non-international conflicts, the solution is usually political, and the UN plays a primary role: it provides for immediate measures ranging from the provision of aid to the holding of free elections, to the placement of a country under administrative supervision. In the longer term, maintenance of a lasting peace will involve socioeconomic change. This falls in with the options proposed in the preceding chapter involving the link between development and human-rights promotion. The need to link emergency interventions to a long-term strategy based on development is a major preoccupation of humanitarian agencies:

"More and more, the international actors, including the United Nations, the donor organizations, the NGOs, and the humanitarian groups, are preoccupied by peacemaking, the maintenance of peace, and the rehabilitation of war-torn

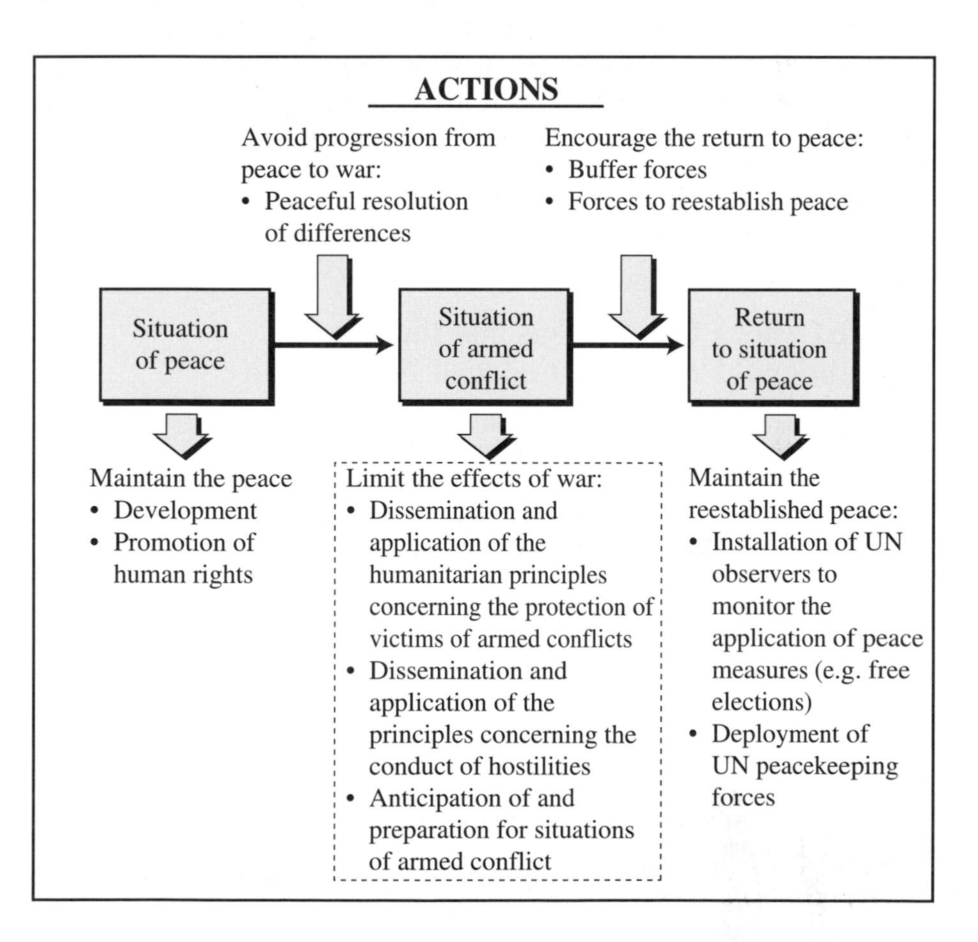

societies. Their particular responsibility is to facilitate reconstruction and development in the long term."[9]

The purpose of war is to destroy, while that of development is to build. The reestablishment of peace after an armed conflict is an essential condition for undertaking development activities.

The UN's role is primordial in reestablishing and maintaining peace, and also in promoting development. International humanitarian law contributes to the restoration of peace in that it helps maintain a humanitarian oasis during the conflict:

"The first and most obvious contribution of international humanitarian law to peace is the maintenance of relations based on law between States and other Parties in a situation where force otherwise predominates. This accepted discipline in the use of force is essential for the re-establishment of peace."[10]

# II. Specific Points of International Humanitarian Law Useful for Health-Care Personnel

This section will examine those points of the Geneva Conventions and their two Additional Protocols which are essential to health-care personnel if they are to understand the legal framework in which they operate.

## 1. The Geneva Conventions and their Two Additional Protocols: Fields of Application

The four Geneva Conventions and Additional Protocol I are applicable in international armed conflicts. Additional Protocol II applies to non-international armed conflicts. It should be noted, however, that Article 3, common to all four Conventions, also concerns non-international armed conflicts. Article 3 is a miniature convention in itself, with three very important characteristics:

- it is the only reference to non-international armed conflicts in the Conventions;
- it contains a summary of the main basic guarantees;

---

[9] IDRC, *Explore* (Jan. 1994), p. 7.

[10] Yves Sandoz, "The Red Cross and Peace: Realities and Limits," *The Journal of Peace Research* 24, No. 3 (Sept. 1987): 292.

- since it does not change the legal status of the parties to the conflict, its application cannot turn the conflict into an international armed conflict.[11]

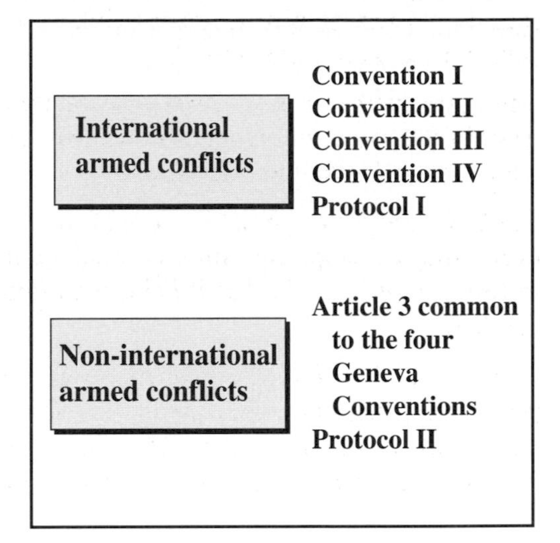


Despite this last provision, the text was adopted only after long negotiations with the States which saw it as interference in their internal affairs.[12]

International humanitarian law applies in situations of armed conflict, and emphasizes both the belligerents' duties towards

> **"Article 3**
>
> In the case of armed conflict not of an international character occurring in the territory of one of the High Contracting Parties, each Party to the conflict shall be bound to apply, as a minimum, the following provisions:
>
> (1) Persons taking no active part in the hostilities, including members of armed forces who have laid down their arms and those placed *hors de combat* by sickness, wounds, detention, or any other cause, shall in all circumstances be treated humanely, without any adverse distinction founded on race, colour, religion or faith, sex, birth or wealth, or any other similar criteria.
>
> To this end, the following acts are and shall remain prohibited at any time and in any place whatsoever with respect to the above-mentioned persons:
>
> (a) violence to life and person, in particular murder of all kinds, mutilation, cruel treatment and torture;
> (b) taking of hostages;
> (c) outrages upon personal dignity, in particular, humiliating and degrading treatment;
> (d) the passing of sentences and the carrying out of executions without previous judgment pronounced by a regularly constituted court affording all the judicial guarantees which are recognized as indispensable by civilized peoples.
>
> (2) The wounded and sick shall be collected and cared for.
>
> An impartial humanitarian body, such as the International Committee of the Red Cross, may offer its services to the Parties to the conflict.
>
> The Parties to the conflict should further endeavour to bring into force, by means of special agreements, all or part of the other provisions of the present Convention.
>
> The application of the preceding provisions shall not affect the legal status of the Parties to the conflict."

[11] L.C. Green, *The Contemporary Law of Armed Conflict* (Melland Schill Monographs in International Law, 1993), p. 42.

[12] See Jean Pictet, ed., *Commentary, Geneva Convention Relative to the Protection of Civilian Persons in Time of War* (ICRC, 1958), p. 32.

non-combatants and the manner in which hostilities are to be conducted. The application of international humanitarian law must come to terms with military necessity: "The law of war can only be, in fact, a law of compromise between military necessity and humanitarian requirements."[13] This pragmatism, however, must not be interpreted as surrender to the armed forces present. The neutrality and impartiality of the humanitarian agencies allow them to negotiate with the authorities in charge of the military operations so that humanitarian requirements are respected to the extent necessary to protect the victims of the conflict.

The creation of a humanitarian "space" in situations of armed conflict will gain wider acceptance if humanitarian organizations are indeed seen by the parties to the conflict to be neutral and impartial.

## 2. Distinction Between International Humanitarian Law and International Human Rights Law

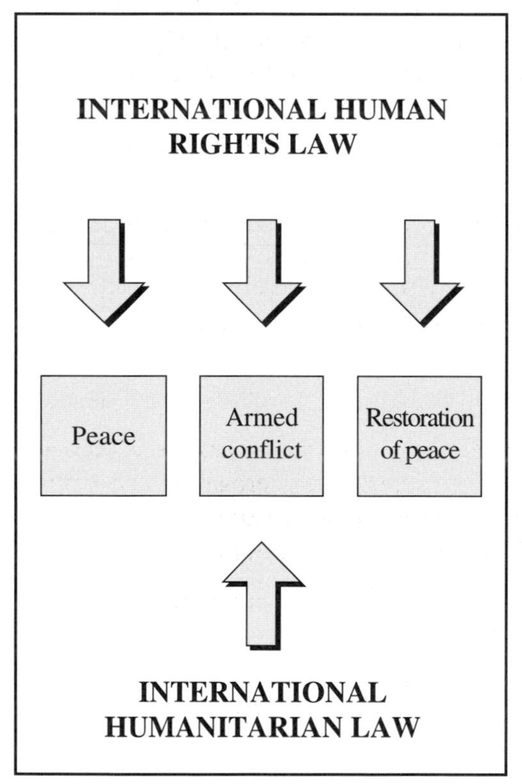


### 2.1 Fields of Application

International humanitarian law applies to situations of armed conflict, whereas international human rights law is applicable to all circumstances. Nonetheless, although international human rights law is, like international humanitarian law, applicable in situations of armed conflict, various factors tend to weaken its impact on them. As a result, international humanitarian law is dominant in this field.

International humanitarian law is a body of rules that the parties to a conflict must respect. These rules concern the parties' treatment of non-combatants (wounded, shipwrecked, prisoners of war, political prisoners, civilian populations), and also the parties' attitude towards the established systems (respect for the environment,

---

13 Maurice Torelli, *Le droit international humanitaire* (Presses Universitaires de France, 1985), p. 12.

respect for goods essential to the population's survival, respect for cultural sites, etc.). For example, Protocol II additional to the four Geneva Conventions provides that: "All the wounded, sick and shipwrecked, whether or not they have taken part in the armed conflict, shall be respected and protected." [14] Further on, it specifies:

"Starvation of civilians as a method of combat is prohibited. It is therefore prohibited to attack, destroy, remove or render useless, for that purpose, objects indispensable to the survival of the civilian population, such as foodstuffs, agricultural areas for the production of foodstuffs, crops, livestock, drinking water installations and supplies and irrigation works." [15]

These rules are particularly important for health-care personnel in their efforts to protect and assist war victims.

International human rights law directly concerns individuals and applies mostly to the individual's relations with the State. Human rights can be divided into three categories:

- those involving individual liberties — the right to freedom of expression, the right to freedom of movement, the right to respect for family life, etc.;
- those implying certain services provided by the State — the right to education, the right to health care, etc.
- those concerning the community as a whole — the right to development, the right to peace, etc.

"[W]e immediately see a difference in the manner in which humanitarian law and human rights treaties are worded. The former indicates how a party to a conflict is to behave in relation to people at its mercy, whereas human rights law concentrates on the rights of the recipients of a certain treatment." [16]

## 2.2 Derogations

The authorities are obliged to respect the provisions of international humanitarian law and ensure that they are applied. No derogation is possible. The rights they protect are inalienable — for example, prisoners of war cannot renounce their rights (Art. 7 of the Third Geneva Convention).

This is not true, however, of human rights law, from which the authorities can derogate in exceptional circumstances:

"In time of public emergency which threatens the life of the nation and the existence of which is officially proclaimed, the States Parties to the present

[14] Protocol II additional to the four Geneva Conventions of 12 August 1949, Art. 7, Par. 1.
[15] Protocol II additional to the four Geneva Conventions of 12 August 1949, Art. 14.
[16] Louise Doswald-Beck and Sylvain Vité, "International Humanitarian Law and Human Rights Law," *International Review of the Red Cross* (March/April 1993): 101.

Covenant may take measures derogating from their obligations under the present Covenant to the extent strictly required by the exigencies of the situation, provided that such measures are not inconsistent with their other obligations under international law and do not involve discrimination solely on the ground of race, colour, sex, language, religion or social origin." [17]

Nevertheless, the rights constituting the "hard core" of human rights cannot be put aside. These are the intangible rights — for example, the right to life, the right not to be subjected to torture or to inhuman or degrading punishment or treatment, and the right not to be enslaved.

### 2.3 Precision of Legal Rules

A contradiction may be seen between the impossibility of derogating from the rules of international humanitarian law and the obligation to make allowance for "military necessity." In fact, the provisions of international humanitarian law precisely define the limits of "military necessity": "Unlike human rights law, which is set out as a series of general rights which all persons have, humanitarian law takes the form of detailed rules which the parties to the conflict are bound to follow." [18]

### 2.4 Universality

The concept of universality was extensively debated during the Vienna Conference on Human Rights in 1993. Human rights laws are legal provisions which derive from moral values, the perception of which may vary from one culture to the next. Even the principle of the universality of human rights is not totally accepted, and the legal instruments adopted to protect human rights have not been universally ratified. In contrast, the treaties of humanitarian law have been ratified by most States.

### 2.5 Implementation

The rules governing the implementation of the two branches of international law are different. The United Nations has several mechanisms for the implementation of human rights law (for example, the Human Rights Commission); for humanitarian law, the ICRC plays a vital role.

## 3. The Application of International Humanitarian Law

The rules of international humanitarian law are sufficiently explicit to guarantee the protection of non-combatants. Yet reality has shown their application to be

[17] Art. 4 of the International Covenant on Civil and Political Rights (1966).
[18] ICRC, *Human Rights and the ICRC: International Humanitarian Law*, p. 5.

difficult, for several reasons. One reason is that States refuse or fail to apply international humanitarian law, although their responsibility to do so is clearly established in Article 1 which is duplicated in all four Geneva Conventions and Additional Protocol I: "The High Contracting Parties undertake to respect and to ensure respect for the present Convention [this Protocol] in all circumstances."

Another reason is that humanitarian agencies' access to victims may be restricted or forbidden, for various motives: refusal to recognize the existence of a conflict, a desire to prevent humanitarian organizations from witnessing violations of international humanitarian law, and, finally, security problems, especially in situations where the collapse of State infrastructures leads to a loss of control over armed groups.

In international armed conflicts, the ICRC is entitled to use a right of initiative specified in the Geneva Conventions (Art. 9, Conventions I, II, and III; Art. 10, Convention IV). In non-international armed conflicts, the ICRC's right of initiative is based on Article 3, common to all four Conventions. Article 4, paragraph 2, of the ICRC Statutes also invokes this right of initiative: "The ICRC may take any humanitarian initiative which comes within its role as a specifically neutral and independent institution and intermediary, and may consider any question requiring examination by such an institution." [19]

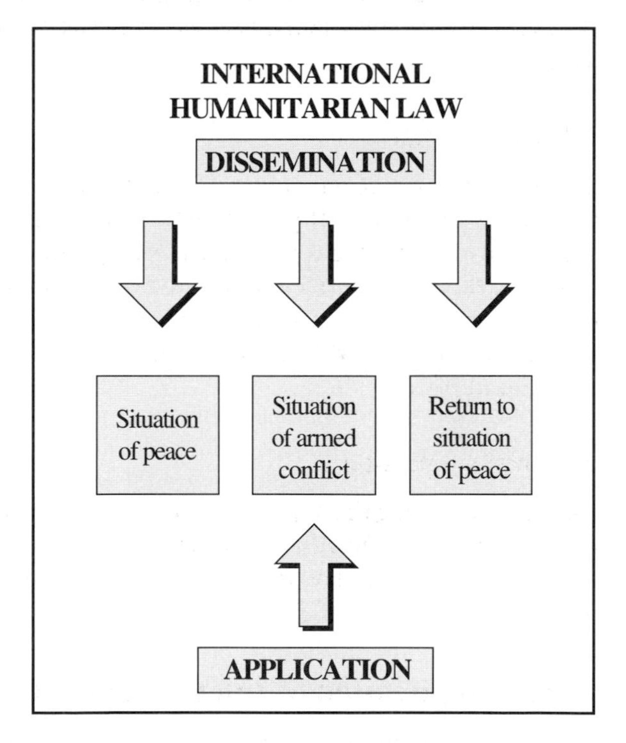


## 4. Dissemination of International Humanitarian Law

To be respected, international humanitarian law must be known. The dissemination of humanitarian rules is therefore essential if international humanitarian law is to be applied with maximum effectiveness and violations

[19] Statutes of the International Committee of the Red Cross, adopted in June, 1973, revised on 6 Dec. 1973, 1 May 1974, 14 Sept. 1977, 29 April 1982, and 20 Jan. 1988.

are to be avoided. During an armed conflict, efforts to publicize humanitarian law must be redoubled. The ICRC plays an essential role in this respect, but responsibility for dissemination lies chiefly with the States.

## 5. The Right to Assistance

The right to assistance is guaranteed by the Geneva Conventions (in particular Arts. 3, 23, 55 and 59) and Additional Protocols I (in particular Arts. 69 and 70) and II (Art. 18). The responsibility for organizing relief is clearly explained in the commentary on the Additional Protocols of 1977.[20] The authorities in charge have the primary role:

"The whole of the provision is based on the principle that States are primarily responsible for organizing relief. Relief societies such as the Red Cross and Red Crescent organizations are called upon to play an auxiliary role by assisting the authorities in their task."[21]

External assistance enters the picture if the authorities are unable to meet their obligations: "Such external aid is complementary; it is only provided when the responsible authorities can no longer meet the basic necessities of the civilian population whose survival is in jeopardy."[22]

It is important that health-care personnel understand this division of responsibility well. Thus, the decision to set up a surgical hospital to care for war-wounded should be based not merely on the presence of war-wounded, but on an analysis of the correlation between local surgical facilities and the care required by the wounded. Only if the local hospitals are unable to provide the necessary care can external intervention be contemplated.

## 6. Health-Care Personnel

Health-care personnel make an obvious contribution in favor of the victims of armed conflicts: care for the wounded and sick, prevention of disease, and improvement of living conditions are all areas in which they use their skills. However, their responsibilities go far beyond mere medical care. In certain cases, the presence of medical teams helps promote the safety of the victims, who without them would be subject to acts contrary to international humanitarian law — extortion, forced displacement, abduction, rape, etc. Of course, during an armed conflict, the authorities may also take advantage of the presence of medical personnel to project a favorable picture of the situation to the rest of the

---

[20] *Commentary on the Additional Protocols*, p. XXXIV.
[21] *Ibid.*, Protocol II, Art. 18, p. 1477.
[22] *Ibid.*, Protocol II, Art. 18, p. 1479.

world. To prevent this kind of abuse, health-care personnel must consider the victims' need for protection in all senses of the word, in addition to their health needs.

Many elements must be considered if the health-care personnel are to perform their tasks well. Access to the victims is the first condition. It is sometimes difficult to achieve for political and security reasons. Once access is obtained, protection of medical personnel, facilities, and convoys is essential. The correct use of the red cross emblem provides that protection.

## The Emblems of the Red Cross and the Red Crescent

In peacetime, the emblems of the red cross and the red crescent are used in the following situations:

- to denote membership in the International Red Cross and Red Crescent Movement (ICRC, Federation, National Societies);
- exceptionally and with express authorization, to mark ambulances and aid posts offering free care.

In times of conflict, the emblem is the visible manifestation of the protection accorded by the Geneva Conventions. It tells the combatants that certain people, medical units, or means of transport are protected by the Geneva Conventions and their Additional Protocols. In an armed conflict, the *protective* use of the emblem is authorized for the following:

- medical corps of the armed forces;
- staff and supplies of National Societies integrated in the medical corps of the armed forces;
- civilian hospitals;
- civilian medical units;
- other voluntary aid societies, with express authorization and on condition that their personnel be subject to military laws and regulations.

According to Article 44, paragraph 3, of the first Geneva Convention of 1949, the ICRC and the Federation, as "international organizations," enjoy privileged status and are authorized to use the emblem at all times.

Thus, the emblem is clearly subject to a very restrictive regimen, in order to maintain its protective function in the case of armed conflict. Each State has its own legislation concerning the use of the emblem, and the obligation to prevent or punish any improper use.

## General Protection of Medical Missions

The general protection of medical missions is covered by Article 16 of Protocol I and Article 10 of Protocol II. The latter states as follows:

"1. Under no circumstances shall any person be punished for having carried out medical activities compatible with medical ethics, regardless of the person benefiting therefrom.
2. Persons engaged in medical activities shall neither be compelled to perform acts or to carry out work contrary to, nor be compelled to refrain from acts required by, the rules of medical ethics or other rules designed for the benefit of the wounded and sick, or this Protocol.
3. The professional obligations of persons engaged in medical activities regarding information which they may acquire concerning the wounded and sick under their care shall, subject to national law, be respected.
4. Subject to national law, no person engaged in medical activities may be penalized in any way for refusing or failing to give information concerning the wounded and sick who are, or who have been, under his care."

Several points should be mentioned here:

- Medical activities must conform to the rules of ethics.
- Medical personnel are bound to observe discretion, meaning both respect for medical confidentiality as such and an obligation not to inform on patients.
- Medical personnel act within the framework of national legislation,[23] although the principle of respecting national legislation may conflict with the principle of not informing.
- The prohibition on punishing someone performing a medical function for the mere fact of keeping quiet about the wounded and sick under his or her care is relative, since this measure depends on the national legislation.
- The protection of health-care personnel is intended to reinforce the protection of the wounded and sick.

It should be noted that the rights protecting health-care personnel are inalienable:
"Members of medical personnel may in no circumstances, renounce any of the rights conferred on them by international humanitarian law [...] This categorical injunction is intended to prevent pressure being exerted on medical personnel to make them renounce their rights, and to preclude justification of a breach being claimed on the grounds that the victim had given its consent."[24]

## The Duties of Health-Care Personnel

Although health-care personnel enjoy some degree of protection so that they can assist the victims of armed conflicts, they also have a certain number of obligations:

- to respect the principles of medical ethics;

23 "It refers here not only to the law in force at the start of the conflict, but also to any new legislation introduced and brought into force by a State after the start of the conflict. The legal situation, the result of a compromise, has its shortcomings in that it might endanger the special protection to which the wounded and sick should be entitled." *Ibid.,* Protocol II, Art. 10, p. 1428.

24 Dr. Alma Baccino-Astrada, *Manual on the Rights and Duties of Medical Personnel in Armed Conflicts* (Geneva: ICRC/League, 1982), pp. 67-68.

- to provide care to all victims on the basis of need, without discrimination of any kind — total neutrality;
- not to bear arms, with the exception of light weapons for self-defense;
- to identify themselves as medical personnel.

## 7. Protection of Medical Facilities[25]

The Geneva Conventions (Art. 19ff I, Art. 22ff II and Art. 18ff IV) and the Additional Protocols (Art. 8ff/I and 7ff/II) provide for the protection of medical facilities and means of transport. Article 11 of Protocol II stipulates:

"1. Medical units and transports shall be respected and protected at all times and shall not be the object of attack.
2. The protection to which medical units and transports are entitled shall not cease unless they are used to commit hostile acts, outside their humanitarian function. Protection may, however, cease only after a warning has been given setting, whenever appropriate, a reasonable time-limit, and after such warning has remained unheeded."

According to the *Commentary on the Additional Protocols*,
"the term 'medical units' is a generic term covering both permanent units, which stay where they are (hospitals, laboratories, equipment depots, etc.), and mobile medical units, which may be moved as required (field hospitals, first aid posts, ambulances, etc.). The term 'medical transports' means any land vehicle (cars, trucks, trains, etc.), ship, craft or aircraft assigned to transporting the wounded, sick, and shipwrecked, medical and religious personnel, and medical equipment."[26]

Since protection ceases if the medical units and means of transport are used for hostile acts, the health-care personnel must apply the rules very strictly.

## 8. Monitoring the Observance of International Humanitarian Law and the Mechanisms of Sanction in Case of Violation

The best way of monitoring the application of international humanitarian law is to be present in the field, out where the victims are. This is the ICRC's *modus operandi*. Proximity to the victims allows observers to verify on the spot whether or not the rules of international humanitarian law are actually being respected. In this respect, access to the victims is a major concern for the ICRC.

The record on the application of international humanitarian law has so far been depressing: an increasing number of conflicts, in the course of which populations are attacked indiscriminately and refused the right to humanitarian relief.

---

[25] See also Baccino-Astrada, *ibid.*
[26] *Commentary on the Additional Protocols*, Protocol II, Art. 11, p. 1433.

Those States which are not parties to the conflict also have a certain responsibility when it comes to violations of international humanitarian law. Article 1 common to the Geneva Conventions[27] requires of them that they make an effort to ensure respect for the law in all circumstances by taking the appropriate practical measures:

- a delegate can make oral representations to the local authorities;
- a detailed report can be submitted to the government concerned;
- a memorandum can be sent to all the governments signatory to the Geneva Conventions.

The ICRC employs the last option only with the greatest caution, to preserve its effect and keep it from being seen as a political stand.

Generally speaking, the ICRC does not make its observations public. Indeed, its role is not to denounce violations of international humanitarian law, but rather to help the parties to a conflict to apply the law. This being said, the ICRC reserves the right to take a public stand if its requests are not met and if doing so is in the interest of the victims.

These measures may seem weak in relation to the seriousness of certain violations, especially because the latter show a tendency to increase. The ICRC must maneuver between two risks: being accused of doing nothing, if it does not take a public stand; or being accused of taking a political position, if it denounces the situation publicly.

# III. Applications

## 1. Protection of Civilian Populations

Civilian populations are doubly affected by armed conflicts — directly, by the attacks on them, and indirectly, by the deterioration of the essential services on which their survival depends: agriculture, medical services, water supply services. Moreover, civilian populations are often forcibly displaced and their fundamental rights are violated (summary executions, abductions, etc.).

The use of legal instruments can have a decisive impact on the intervention strategy used in the field of health. Numerous studies have shown, for example, that during massive population movements, the mortality rate may be up to 15 times higher than normal.[28] Knowing these facts, health workers can warn

[27] "The High Contracting Parties undertake to respect and to ensure respect for the present Convention in all circumstances" (Art. 1, common to all the Conventions).

[28] "Centers for Disease Control, Famine-Affected, Refugee, and Displaced Populations: Recommendations for Public Health Issues," *Morbidity and Mortality Weekly Report* 41, No. RR-13 (24 July 1992).

authorities about the risks of population displacement, and back up their arguments with the legal instruments cited below.

**The Protection of Civilian Populations against Forced Displacement**

Protocol II, Article 17, provides:

"1. The displacement of the civilian population shall not be ordered for reasons related to the conflict unless the security of the civilians involved or imperative military reasons so demand. Should such displacements have to be carried out, all possible measures shall be taken in order that the civilian population may be received under satisfactory conditions of shelter, hygiene, health, safety and nutrition.

2. Civilians shall not be compelled to leave their own territory for reasons connected with the conflict."

According to Article 85, line 4a, of Protocol I, the following acts are considered grave breaches:

"the transfer by the Occupying Power of parts of its own civilian population into the territory it occupies, or the deportation or transfer of all or parts of the population of the occupied territory within or outside this territory, in violation of Article 49 of the Fourth Convention."

Keeping civilian populations in their normal environment depends on such factors as security conditions and the scope of "military necessity." Finally, if the civilian population remains on its home ground, its means of subsistence must be protected. Here again, health-care personnel can turn to legal instruments.

**Protection of Means of Subsistence**

Article 14 of Protocol II guarantees the protection of goods indispensable to survival:

"Starvation of civilians as a method of combat is prohibited. It is therefore prohibited to attack, destroy, remove or render useless, for that purpose, objects indispensable to the survival of the civilian population, such as foodstuffs, agricultural areas for the production of foodstuffs, crops, livestock, drinking water installations and supplies and irrigation works."

This article is clear. However, a point brought out by the *Commentary on the Additional Protocols of 8 June 1977 to the Geneva Conventions of 12 August 1949* merits reflection; it refers to failures to take the necessary measures to supply a population with goods indispensable for survival.[29] Such an omission could become a sort of combat method by abstention, which is contrary to the spirit of the article. It remains to be determined whether the omission is due to a deliberate

---

[29] *Commentary on the Additional Protocols of 8 June 1977 to the Geneva Conventions of 12 August 1949,* p. XXXIV.

desire to starve the civilian populations, or whether it is a result of a material inability to implement the measures required. Protocol I includes similar provisions (Art. 54).

The constitution of neutral zones may also be contemplated as an intervention strategy to guarantee the protection of the means of subsistence, the health-care services, and the civilian populations as such.

**The Concept of Neutral Zones**

"The idea here is to shelter civilian populations from hostilities, mainly by creating hospital or neutralized zones and by forbidding attacks on hospitals and civilian medical transport, which are permitted to use the protective emblem for this purpose."[30]

Civilian populations, however, often have no choice. As the ICRC has pointed out,[31] in a conflict civilians are often caught between two evils. If they stay in their homes, they are exposed to the dangers of war (bombing, landmines, attacks, famine) and are apt to find themselves without means or medical care. If they flee, they are still at the mercy of the combatants, as potential hostages risking arrest, summary execution, or "disappearance." Such population movements, spontaneous at first, are apt to become forced, where the armed forces seek to isolate insurgents.

People displaced within their own country are protected by Article 3 and Protocol II.

## 2. Population Displacements

The protection of refugee populations poses specific problems. The fact that civilians are obliged to seek refuge elsewhere, within their own or in a foreign country, is the direct consequence of a violation of international humanitarian law, which has failed to protect them in their home environment: "Violation of humanitarian law, actual or feared, is the cause of most movements of displaced persons or refugees in situations of armed conflict."[32]

The term "refugee" refers to a person who has sought refuge in another country, i.e. who has crossed an international border. An internally displaced person is still within the borders of his or her country. Although both categories of people often have very similar needs, their legal protection is quite different and requires separate examination.

---

[30] Y. Sandoz, "La notion de protection dans le droit international humanitaire et au sein du Mouvement de la Croix-Rouge," in Swinarski, ed., *Etudes et essais sur le droit international humanitaire*, p. 978.

[31] "Personnes déplacées et droit international humanitaire," ICRC declaration to Human Rights Commission, 48th session, ICRC (19 Feb. 1992).

[32] Declaration by the Executive Committee of the Programme of the UN High Commissioner for Refugees, 42nd session, ICRC, 9 Oct. 1991.

## 2.1 Refugee Populations

### Definition of the Term "Refugee"

The term "refugee" was defined by the 1951 UN Convention Relating to the Status of Refugees and the Protocol of 1967:
"[a person who]...owing to well-founded fear of being persecuted for reasons of race, religion, nationality, membership of a particular social group or political opinion, is outside the country of his nationality and is unable or, owing to such fear, is unwilling to avail himself of the protection of that country; or who, not having a nationality and being outside the country of his former habitual residence, is unable or, owing to such fear, is unwilling to return to it."[33]

Many refugees flee their countries not because of personal persecution, but because of war at home. They are refugees from violence, who make up the mass population movements that are particularly common in Africa. The Organization of African Unity (OAU) Convention Governing Specific Aspects of the Problem of Refugees in Africa confirms this expansion of the traditional definition:
"The term 'refugee' shall also apply to every person who, owing to external aggression, occupation, foreign domination or events seriously disturbing public order in either part or the whole of his country of origin or nationality, is compelled to leave his place of habitual residence in order to seek refuge in another place outside his country of origin or nationality."[34]

### The Principle of "Non-Refoulement"

"No Contracting State shall expel or return ('refouler') a refugee in any manner whatsoever to the frontiers of territories where his life or freedom would be threatened on account of his race, religion, nationality, membership of a particular social group or political opinion."[35]

This principle is also laid down in the United Nations Declaration on Territorial Asylum (1967), the OAU Convention Governing Specific Aspects of the Problem of Refugees in Africa (1969), and the American Convention on Human Rights (1969).

### Protection in the Host Country

The 1951 Convention concerns the rights of refugees within the host country with respect to legal status, employment, education, housing, etc. Article 2 of that convention stipulates that refugees are bound to conform to the laws and regulations of the host country.

---

33 Article 1(A)2 of the 1951 Convention Relating to the Status of Refugees, amended by Article I(2) of the Protocol of 1967.

34 Convention Governing Specific Aspects of the Problem of Refugees in Africa, OAU, Article I(2)-1969.

35 Convention Relating to the Status of Refugees (1951), Article 33(1).

One of the goals of UNHCR is to ascertain that refugees are being treated in accordance with internationally recognized standards.

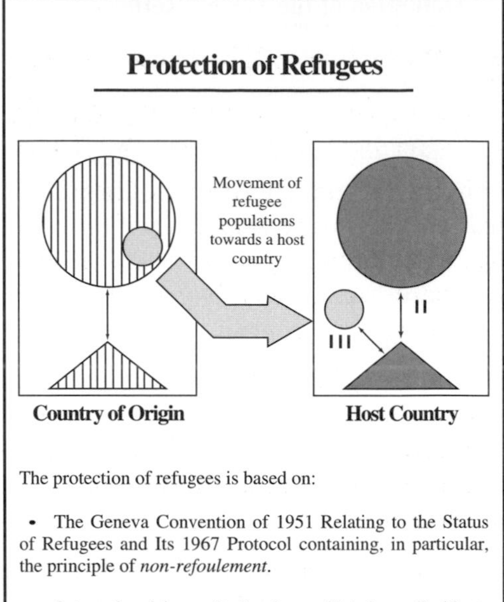


## Long-Term Solutions

Three solutions can be envisioned in the long term:

- repatriation to the country of origin;
- settlement in the host country;
- resettlement in a third country.

Repatriation to the country of origin is the most sensible solution, since it restores refugees to their own sociocultural environment. Repatriation must be voluntary, and it is essential that protective measures be taken, including an assurance that the security conditions that caused the refugees to flee in the first place have been resolved, a guarantee that essential needs can be met as soon as the refugees return home (housing, food, etc.), and, finally, measures to afford refugees some possibility of finding a job again.

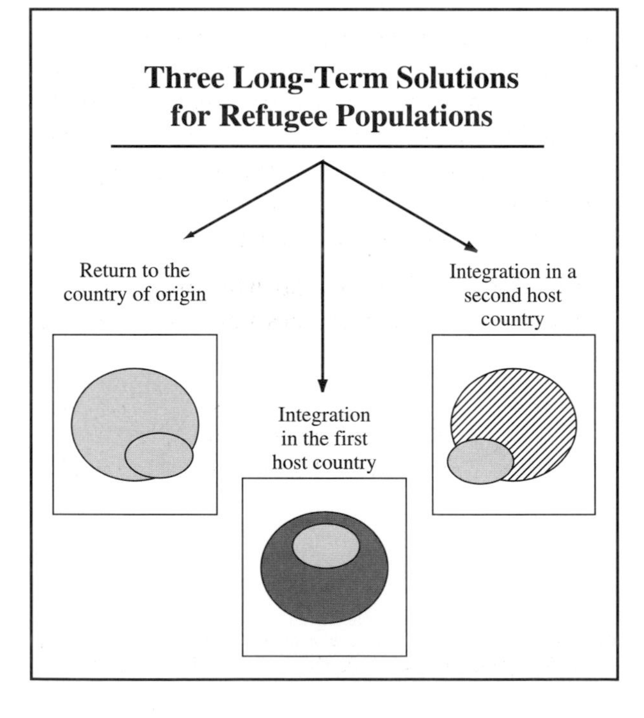


Settling the refugees in the first host country is also an option, if the security conditions of the country of origin remain uncertain and the host country agrees to integrate the refugees into the local population.

Moving them to a third country can be contemplated when the first two solutions are not possible.

## 2.2 Protection of Displaced Persons in their Own Countries

A slightly different problem involves displaced people still living in their own countries, though not in their own homes:

"[W]hen civilians are forced to leave their homes owing to serious violations of international humanitarian law, they are still *a fortiori* protected by this law. This protection may come from the law applicable either to international or to internal conflicts, as both types of conflict may result in displacements of people within their own country."[36]

Civilians may be forced to leave their homes for many reasons, the chief of which is undoubtedly armed conflict. Armed conflicts can give rise to two types of displacement: either the civilians are moved by force by the authorities or an armed opposition group, or they flee because of the general spread of violence, for example as a consequence of shelling or famine.

In both cases, the displaced persons are protected by humanitarian law. Since most displacements take place during internal armed conflicts, it is the law on internal conflicts that applies: Article 3 common to the Geneva Conventions and Additional Protocol II. In some cases, however, the displacements take place during international conflicts, in which case humanitarian law in its entirety applies.

Humanitarian law protects internally displaced persons as members of the civilian population, which benefits from comprehensive immunity against the effects of the hostilities. Protocol II prohibits attacks against civilians. It is also prohibited to destroy objects indispensable to the survival of the civilian population. And as we have already seen, forced displacements are expressly prohibited (Art. 17, Protocol II). In general, civilians are to be treated humanely. The internally displaced are also entitled to receive assistance.

Displaced persons are often very vulnerable, in particular when they are in the power of an authority which is not in a position or does not wish to assume responsibility for their protection.

The number of displaced persons has risen sharply in recent years. They now number more than refugees. There is every reason for the international community to show concern for their plight, but not at the expense of other

[36] Jean-Philippe Lavoyer, "Refugees and Internally Displaced Persons: International Law and the Role of the ICRC," *International Review of the Red Cross* 305 (March-April 1995): p. 171.

categories of victims whose need for protection and assistance is often just as great.

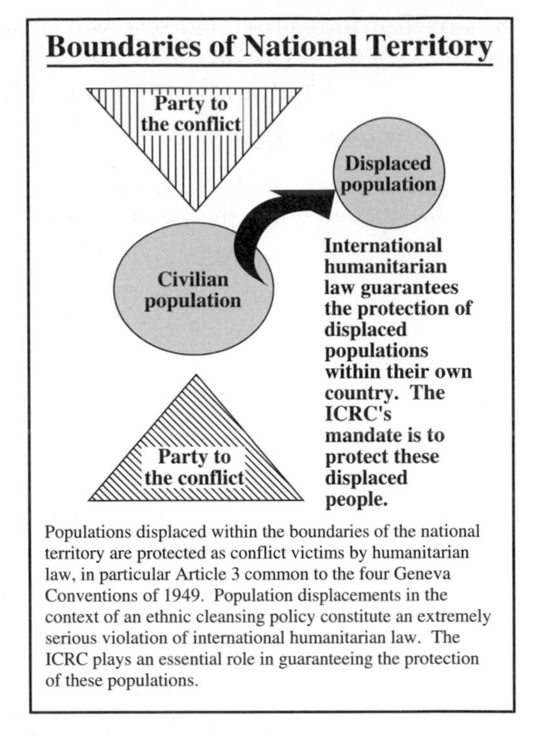


Populations displaced within the boundaries of the national territory are protected as conflict victims by humanitarian law, in particular Article 3 common to the four Geneva Conventions of 1949. Population displacements in the context of an ethnic cleansing policy constitute an extremely serious violation of international humanitarian law. The ICRC plays an essential role in guaranteeing the protection of these populations.

## 2.3 Prevention of Population Displacements

In this context, the word "prevention" means the possibilities of guarding against a situation where a population will be obliged to flee its usual place of abode for reasons of security. International humanitarian law contains the necessary provisions to protect civilian populations, and compliance with it should save them from having to flee during an armed conflict. Prevention at this level, then, means insuring that international humanitarian law is applied.[37]

---

[37] "Human dignity is generally very severely affected by the fact of having to leave one's home on account of events associated with armed hostilities or other forms of violence, because of the utter dependence in which the displaced persons find themselves. States should therefore adhere to a policy designed to *prevent displacement*. For this, much greater importance will have to be attached to respect for humanitarian law." "The ICRC and Internally Displaced Persons," *International Review of the Red Cross* 305 (March-April 1995): 183.

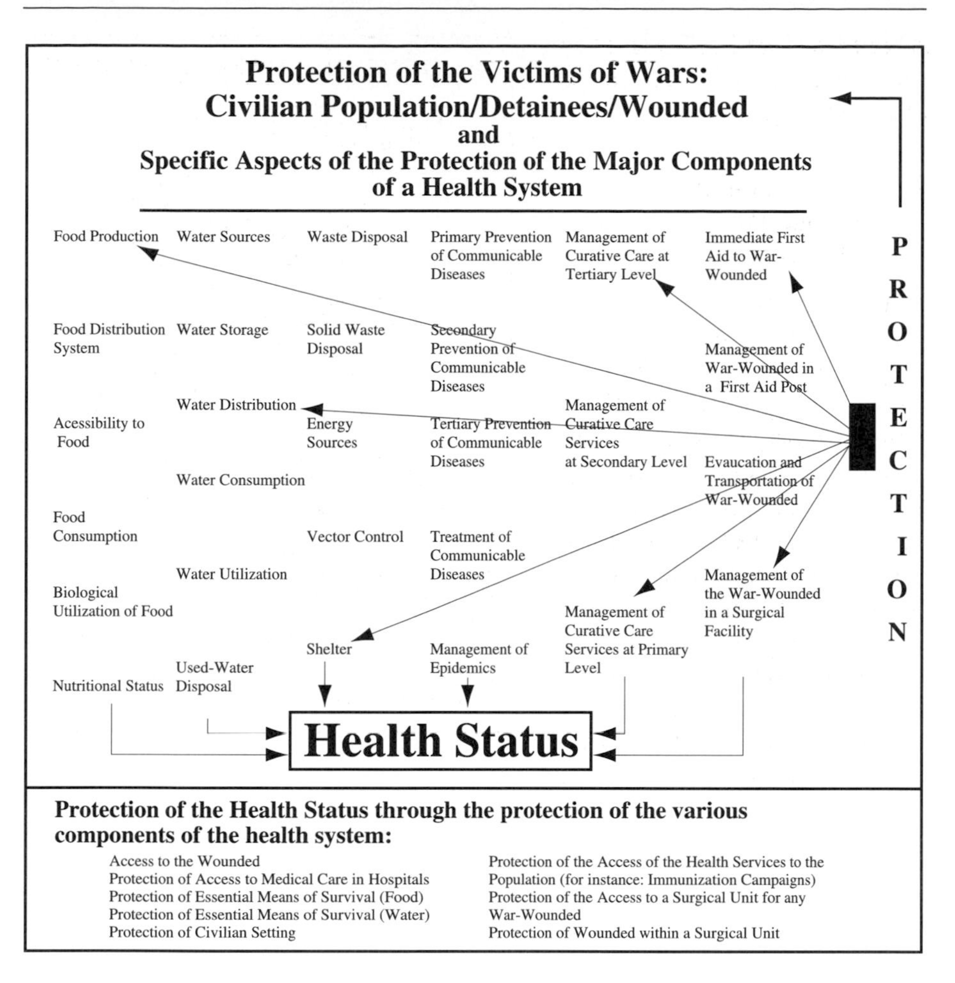


**Cooperation between legal experts and health-care personnel must be reinforced.**

- **Their proximity to the victims gives health-care personnel the opportunity to experience at first hand the problems involved in protecting them. To derive the maximum benefit from this advantage, health-care personnel should be better acquainted with the application of international humanitarian law.**
- **Legal experts, in turn, might study the use of epidemiological tools, which are very useful for inquiries into violations of international humanitarian law.**

**The convergence of these two kinds of skills should improve humanitarian interventions on behalf of the victims of armed conflicts.**

## Chapter 10

# INTRODUCTION TO HUMANITARIAN ETHICS

***The amateurism of the early eighties gave way to the gradual development of a more professional approach, and humanitarian interventions are now conducted according to principles that are accepted by all the major humanitarian organizations. Thus, the fundamental principles of the Red Cross and the Red Crescent provide the basis for a definition of the humanitarian ethic. Some of these principles have been adopted in United Nations resolutions:***

- Humanity
- Impartiality
- Neutrality
- Independence
- Voluntary service
- Unity
- Universality

***"The work of the International Red Cross and Red Crescent Movement is guided by seven Fundamental Principles, which were adopted by governments too at the International Conference of the Red Cross held in Vienna in 1965. The Movement notes with great satisfaction that three of these principles, namely humanity, impartiality and neutrality, were mentioned in General Assembly resolution 46/182 and thus recognized as the cornerstone of all humanitarian endeavour."***[1]

# I. Moral Code of Humanitarian Organizations Regarding Victims

This chapter defines a code of conduct based on experience. The worker in the field must be able to define a practical code of conduct to serve as a guide in the management of his or her activities. To that end, this chapter will review the planning cycle described in Chapter 1, and identify the ethical problems that may arise at each step.

[1] Cornelio Sommaruga, President of the ICRC, "Strengthening of the Coordination of Humanitarian Emergency Assistance of the United Nations Organization," Statement before the UN General Assembly (New York, 20 Nov. 1992), published in *International Review of the Red Cross* 202 (Jan./Feb. 1993): 52.

The planning cycle can be summed up in three main stages:

- initial assessment, to determine the problems arising in a given situation and to establish priorities.
- program design for high-priority problems, to define objectives, select activities, and mobilize the resources needed to implement health-care programs.
- evaluation of outcome, including the use of resources, the benefits from the activities, and the impact on the victims' health.

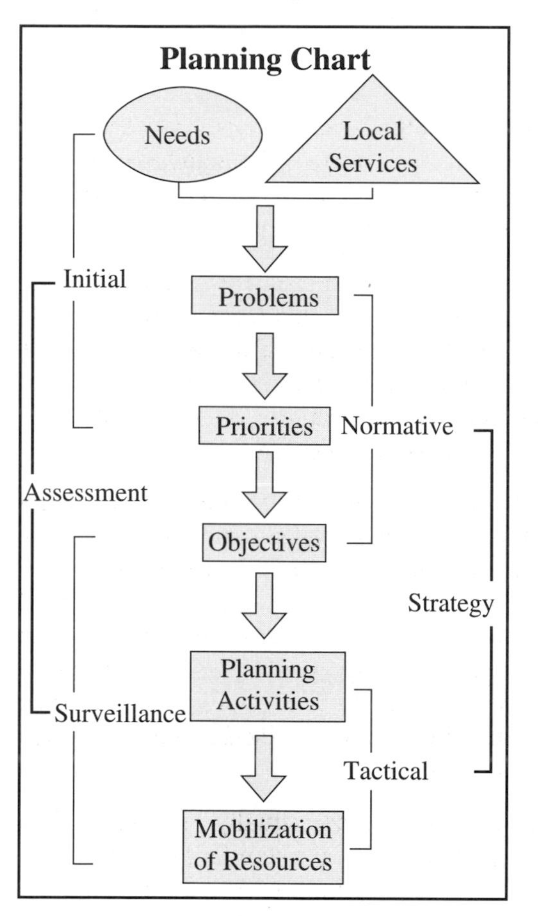


# 1. Ethics and the Decision to Intervene

## 1.1 Restrictions on Initial Assessments

The mere arrival of an assessment team in a disaster area arouses hopes of assistance in the victims. The consensus among humanitarian agencies today is that initial assessments must be carried out before any humanitarian intervention programs can be planned. On one hand, the victims must understand that intervention will be contemplated only if the problems identified correspond to the mandate of the agency implementing the assessment; on the other, agencies must be able to respond if urgent problems have been observed in the course of the assessment. An ethical problem arises when agencies carry out surveys without having the intention or the means of intervening later should it be necessary.

If the problems observed are not urgent, new assessments will be proposed and carried out at regular intervals, to see how the situation develops. This approach is acceptable only if it is shown that the problems identified can wait, and there is no risk that they will worsen quickly. A preemptive intervention can prevent certain problems associated with emergencies.

For international humanitarian agencies, the purpose of the initial assessment is to determine whether any problems necessitate outside assistance. Such problems are defined as being the result of an imbalance, actual or potential, between the victims' needs and the capacity of local resources to cope with them.

Ethical issues arise on two levels: the needs of the victims, and the potential of local services.

## 1.2 Victims' Needs

### *The Concept of Vital Needs*

In a situation of armed conflict, all the humanitarian organizations agree that the main focus should be on vital needs — that is, those needs that must be met first if the victims are to survive: access to food, access to health-care services, access to water, etc.

In developing countries, a population's normal needs are in fact limited to vital needs, so the humanitarian agencies hardly need to deliberate over what should be done. In a different sociocultural context, where essential needs are covered by local services, the demands of the victims and the authorities concern non-vital needs which are normally met. A humanitarian intervention, then, will restore the balance that existed before the crisis. There is no ethical problem here.

However, if levels of intervention are compared by country, the question arises whether this extension of "needs" into the non-essential realm does not lead to a double standard, since interventions to help populations in developing countries will be limited to vital needs, while those for developed countries will be expanded to other domains. Is it possible to limit the concept of impartiality to a given context, and to adjust the aid given to victims of a particular country to its usual standard of living? Or should the concept of impartiality be carried to a much more global level? If the latter, perhaps all victims of conflicts should be treated alike, whatever the previous sociocultural level.

Everyone knows that different emergencies are not equally "interesting" to donors. Given this fact, it may be tempting to define the standard in a particular situation on the basis of the resources provided by the international community. This idea is unacceptable, however, for it merely reinforces the tendency of certain humanitarian agencies to intervene only in dramatic situations, to the detriment of situations that are more catastrophic but offer no political or media interest.

The preceding chapters of this book defined the ethical bottom line for intervention. Determining the upper limit is more difficult. To do it, the framework of our analysis must be expanded to include protection needs and a comparison of the specific needs of all the groups of victims in a given situation.

*The Comprehensiveness of Needs*

The concept of "vital needs" is often limited to material needs, if not physiological needs pure and simple. This view tends to restrict humanitarian interventions to the provision of material aid, when often the victims' need of protection is even greater.

In a situation where essential material needs are covered, the humanitarian agencies may be tempted to cover non-vital needs in order to maintain their presence and thereby provide a certain degree of protection to victims being subjected to repeated violations of their rights. Similarly, a non-urgent intervention to help a particular group sometimes permits access to another group of victims whose essential needs may not be covered.

## 1.3 Local Services

As mentioned in Chapter 9, international humanitarian law assigns the responsibility for meeting victims' needs to the national authorities. In practice, application of this principle can pose serious problems.

### Do All the Victims Have Access to Essential Services?

If discrimination exists (based on political affiliation, ethnic origin, etc.), all humanitarian agencies will condemn it to one extent or another, but the practical problem remains: what should be done for the victims?

The main factor in deciding if intervention is justified is whether the needs not being met because of discrimination are vital or not. After all, if the victims face a vital risk, it is ethically difficult to do nothing but censure the authorities responsible for the discrimination. Intervention in this case must be accompanied by negotiations with the authorities to try to change their attitude.

### Is the Quality of the Local Services Satisfactory?

The local authorities may judge the services offered to the victims to be of good quality, whereas outside observers would consider them inadequate. A distinction should be made between services that are inadequate because the personnel lack the resources necessary to do their work properly, and services that are inadequate because the local personnel has no interest in the victims. In the first case, humanitarian agencies can remedy the observed deficit; in the second case, it is difficult to do anything about lack of motivation in workers who themselves may be struggling to survive.

## 1.4 Decision-Making

In practice, deciding whether or not to intervene is not as simple as might be supposed from the basic concept, which is to intervene if local services are not able to cover the victims' vital needs. To facilitate the decision-making process, situations can be classified according to various combinations of two basic criteria: whether the victims' needs are vital and the potential of the local services. The following diagram reflects the different types of situation.

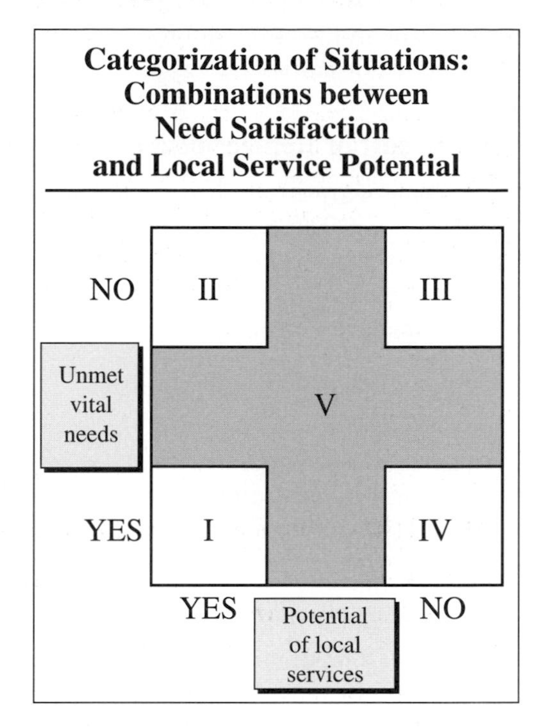


I. Assessment reveals vital needs that are not being met, although the local services have the potential to take care of the victims. Is this inconsistency due to discrimination, lack of organization, or a refusal to accept the responsibilities imposed by international humanitarian law?

II. Assessment does not reveal any vital needs that are not being met. Further inquiry is indicated to make sure that the authorities are also insuring the protection of the victims (security, preservation of the family unit, etc.).

III. Vital needs are covered, but local services are inadequate; this inadequacy may affect only non-vital needs. In this case, the question arises as to whether international relief should be provided for the non-vital needs. The decision will be based on a consideration of the previous socioeconomic level and the protection needs of different groups of victims. If the latter's safety is not guaranteed, the presence of humanitarian agencies may be desirable, even by means of aid programs that do not cover vital needs.

IV. Vital needs are not met and the local services are not able to cope with the situation. In this case, international aid is necessary.

V. Situations in the middle zone are more difficult to define. It may be impossible to discover whether vital needs are being covered, or it may be difficult to establish whether local services are available to the victims.

This matrix is not designed to make decisions automatic, but rather to facilitate them by pinpointing a certain number of parameters within each category.

## 2. Ethics and Intervention Strategy

The term "normative strategy" is used to describe the selection of priorities and goals for an intervention, while the word "tactics" refers to the order in which the activities of an intervention program will be carried out. The ethical problems involved in normative strategy are outlined below.

### 2.1 Support or Replacement of Local Services?

The victims of armed conflicts require services able to cover their essential needs: health-care services, systems to supply food and water, housing, and guarantees of security. Over the last decade, certain non-governmental organizations have tried to assume the responsibility themselves for the institution and provision of services for such victims.

#### Is This Approach Justified?

The primary responsibility for the care of a population falls on the local authorities. Only if they fail to meet it should the humanitarian agencies step in to remind them of their duties towards the victims and, if necessary, to take the practical measures required.

The ICRC's position in this respect is clear:

"The aspect of the ICRC's relief policy which is visible to the outside world is the provision of food or medicines to keep individuals or populations alive, alleviate their suffering and avoid their future being compromised by the effects of illness, injury or malnutrition. However, this is merely the most conspicuous feature of a much broader policy. First and foremost, the ICRC endeavours to ensure that the *de jure* or *de facto* authorities allow the population access to the essential resources and services needed for its survival and for the community to function properly and, where necessary, that they provide whatever assistance is required."[2]

Here, ethics are the basis for the criteria the humanitarian agencies will use in deciding to implement a replacement strategy. Such a strategy is unavoidable when there is no local facility to take care of the victims, and might involve, for example, building a hospital to treat war-wounded in a region with no hospitals at all. It is difficult to determine criteria when facilities exist but do not function in a satisfactory manner, or, worse, when the services furnished are below the standards that would be considered normal in a particular context.

Humanitarian agencies give themselves the "right" to take over the facilities in question in order to improve their performance, reorganizing their management, investing in them, etc. In this case, the question of the facility's autonomy or

[2] Marion Harroff-Tavel, "Action Taken by the International Committee of the Red Cross in Situations of Internal Violence," *International Review of the Red Cross* 294 (May/June 1993): 214.

dependence vis-à-vis the authorities normally responsible arises. Without real control over the facility's operation, relief organizations cannot expect rapid change; the aid they provide will go to produce services which will always be below the norm. At the other end of the spectrum, however, a total appropriation of the facility amounts to a strategy of dependence.

In short, humanitarian agencies must respect what already exists, but, at the same time, they must know how to take its place if necessary. Any attempt of this sort should, of course, be subject to careful reflection. Besides the colonialist overtones of this approach, its long-term effects must be considered — for example, the risk that the local authorities will abdicate their responsibility.

The criteria for replacement might be the following:

- discriminatory access to services;
- practices dangerous for victims;
- external presence necessitated by insecurity;
- urgency of an effective intervention.

The replacement strategy also solves another problem — that of neutrality, when there is a risk that one party to the conflict will consider humanitarian aid to the facilities of the other party as evidence that the humanitarian intervention is not neutral.

Despite its advantages, replacement strategy must be limited to those situations where the local facilities do not meet the criteria of neutrality and efficiency called for by an emergency situation.

Thus, to insure coverage of a population's need for hospital care, for example, a humanitarian agency could:

- reestablish access to health facilities that are inaccessible to certain groups of victims;
- assist local health-care facilities by furnishing the equipment necessary for proper functioning;
- build a hospital independent of the local health system.

**What should the policy be concerning a medical facility that has the human but not the material resources needed to treat patients, and which refuses to treat people from a particular ethnic group?**

There are four options:

- Assist the facility, since the aid supplied will be used to treat at least part of the population — although this amounts to accepting discrimination.
- Negotiate until the facility agrees to accept all patients without discrimination, then assist it — realizing, however, that if the facility refuses, the population will be deprived of necessary care.
- Assist the facility in spite of everything, and negotiate to obtain access for all. Although a means of pressuring the authorities will thereby be lost, the aid will

help at least part of the population. The relief agency offers access to care to one population group, but without accepting the discrimination against the other group. The threshold of tolerance remains to be defined, as well as an acceptable time limit for concluding the negotiations.
- Accept the discrimination and find another solution for the excluded group—for example, providing a new facility for it.

**What should be the policy concerning a civilian population whose vital needs are not covered and who are suffering from extortion by an armed group?**

There are three possibilities:
- Withhold assistance in order to protest the treatment meted out to the civilian population. This amounts to delivering a death sentence against the civilians, who will lack food, medical care, and other necessities, so that in fact it is the victims and not those responsible for the extortion who are penalized.
- Intervene without comment. This may improve the material situation of the civilian population (unless material aid is diverted by the armed group), but will not improve the victims' security.
- Assist the populations concerned and exert pressure on the leaders of the armed group or the regional authorities. This is the most sensible approach, but presents the risk of hardening the authorities' stance vis-à-vis the humanitarian organizations, which may ultimately be denied access to the victims.[3]

These two examples show how difficult it is to find a way of satisfying the victims' immediate needs while still maintaining ethical principles.

## 2.2 Strategy and Violations of International Humanitarian Law

Confronted with violations of international humanitarian law, humanitarian agencies have a choice of two strategies which, although apparently contradictory, are in fact complementary. One involves appealing to international public opinion, while the other employs discretion in bilateral negotiations with the responsible authorities.

The strategy of denouncing violations of international humanitarian law is meant to alert governments and the international community in general to the difficulties humanitarian agencies face in the normal performance of their work. The danger of this strategy, as mentioned above, is that it can harden the attitudes of the authorities responsible for blocking access to the victims; this may affect other vulnerable groups who already benefit from the presence of humanitarian agencies.

[3] In other words, they may be expelled for interfering in the internal affairs of the State.

The strategy of discretion consists in betting on the success of bilateral negotiations with the authorities responsible for the violations of international humanitarian law to persuade them to change their attitude towards the victims.

Humanitarian agencies must choose between these two strategies. The ICRC has opted for discretion, whereas other organizations, such as Amnesty International, have chosen public denunciation. The two approaches are complementary, but in general each organization adheres to the line it has adopted.

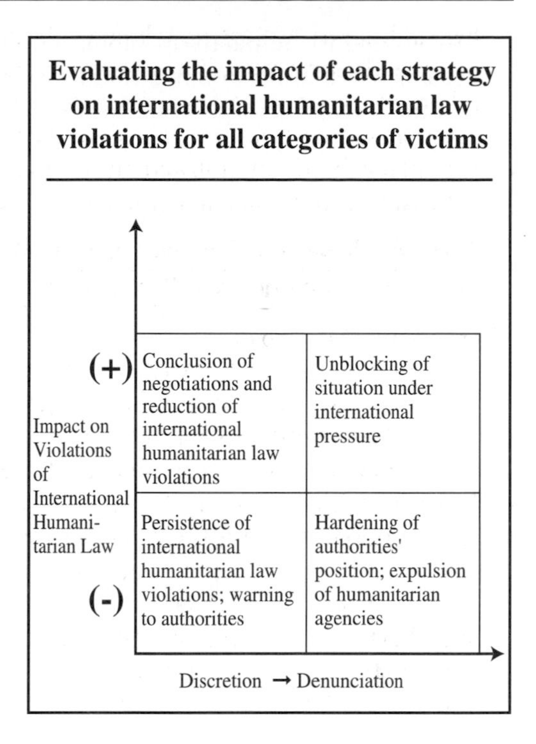


### The Limits of Denunciation and Discretion

The option of discretion has its limits. Accordingly, when negotiations lead nowhere and international humanitarian law is repeatedly violated, it is reasonable to change strategy. The switch to denunciation should be made only after careful deliberation. The ICRC reserves the option of appealing to the international community when it believes that all other forms of action have proven to be in vain. As it stressed in a declaration before the Commission on Human Rights, it calls upon both the parties to a conflict and the international community to make every effort to put an end to unacceptable practices of every kind, including, of course, the detention of thousands of civilians in dangerous conditions.[4]

## 2.3 Humanitarian Strategy and the Interests of the Parties to the Conflict

Usually, the victims have not chosen their camp. However, the parties to the conflict frequently choose their victims. This poses several problems.

- **The Policy Concerning Hostage Populations**

Is it wise, for example, to assist populations that the local political or military authorities are trying to keep in their homes, when security conditions are

[4] ICRC, Declaration to the Commission on Human Rights, first extraordinary session, 13-14 Aug. 1992.

dangerous and the populations should be evacuated? Logically, efforts should not be made to maintain populations in their normal environment if they are in danger there; instead, they should be helped to seek refuge elsewhere. The ethical problem becomes complex, however, when the insecurity is a policy intentionally pursued by one of the parties to the conflict precisely in order to force the population to leave home. In a situation of this kind, it is reasonable to help these residents to remain where they are, if that is what they want. However, humanitarian agencies face an ethical dilemma in the case of populations that want to leave. If they help them leave, they are lending themselves to the purge policy of one of the parties to the conflict; if they try to keep them in their homes, they are exposing them to danger.

- **Impartiality of Humanitarian Aid**

The concept of impartiality is often misunderstood by the parties to a conflict. Assisting victims in the territory of the enemy is considered as support for the enemy's war effort rather than a humanitarian act.

- **Proportionality of Needs**

From the ethical point of view, humanitarian relief should be adapted to needs. This means that in a situation involving victims on both sides, but with more needs on one side than the other, more aid will be given where the need is greater. The authorities concerned may see this disparity as unjust if, for example, they have the "misfortune" to have fewer victims or needs in the territory they control, or if they are better organized than the enemy to supply the needs — partially or totally — of the victims who depend on them. Thus, the authorities who discharge their obligations properly may feel penalized in comparison with the enemy, whose victims, abandoned, will be taken care of by the humanitarian organizations. This is why, in order to attract humanitarian aid, authorities often inflate or even invent statistics concerning the number of victims, or else claim that the local facilities are unable to meet the needs of the population.

What should be done? Stick to the principle of proportionality? Help each side equally? Assist according to need and publish "good conduct" reports for the party that meets its responsibilities? There should be no deviation from the true meaning of the principle of proportionality, which is to grant humanitarian aid *proportionally to the needs* of the victims.

## 2.4 Strategy and Prevention

All problems have causes; relief teams must be aware of possible ways of preventing those causes.

### Technical Prevention of the Immediate Causes of Medical Problems

The principle of preventing medical problems (instead of waiting for them to appear and then treating them) is now accepted by all the major humanitarian agencies. Accordingly, it can be hoped that there will be fewer and fewer of the following:

- nutrition rehabilitation centers operating without the support of food distributions;
- clinics treating diarrhea while the staff gives no thought to monitoring water quality;
- displaced-person camps which do not provide immunization against measles.

These practices can be considered as professional lapses, insofar as rules exist and the failure to comply with them (except in extreme cases where constraints make compliance impossible) is usually due to ignorance.

### The Political Approach to Preventing Health Problems

The concrete example of injuries caused by anti-personnel mines illustrates this level of intervention. In many conflicts, notably in Afghanistan and Cambodia, the danger caused by mines persists long after the hostilities end, and it is civilians who continue to suffer the consequences.

"Those who look after people injured by anti-personnel mines and who, day after day, witness the suffering caused by these pernicious weapons, those who produce artificial limbs to help maimed children as they try to cope with their disability, all ask themselves what can be done to put an end to this terrible scourge."[5]

The role of medical personnel is above all to care for these wounded; but they also have a moral obligation to ask how such injuries can be prevented.

### How Can Such Injuries Be Prevented?

The prospects for preventing the manufacture and sale of anti-personnel mines appear doubtful, unless the international media put pressure on the governments involved in mine manufacture to cease production completely. However, prevention efforts can also focus on the way mines are made, although this may sound bizarre at first. Yet these weapons could, in fact, be fitted with devices causing them to self-destruct automatically a certain length of time after they are put in the ground. Finally, with respect to the use of mines, the goal is to prohibit, or — more realistically — to limit their use, by means of precise rules.

These three levels are linked. Prohibition of the use of mines goes together with intervention in mine production and trade. Intervention at these levels, however, is political.

---

[5] Rémi Russbach, "Anti-personnel Mines: A Disgrace for Humanity," *International Review of the Red Cross* 202 (Jan.-Feb. 1993): 57.

Health-care personnel working in the framework of humanitarian operations are not, of course, responsible for seeking political solutions to this problem. But it is clearly incumbent on them to point out, indeed, to denounce, the consequences of mine use to the political, military, and diplomatic authorities, and to sensitize the media to the problem.

#### Preventing Population Migrations

In situations of armed conflict, respect for the rules of international humanitarian law will prevent entire populations from having to flee their homeland. These refugees from violence flee, not because they are personally persecuted, but because of the dangers of the conflict itself: indiscriminate bombing, arbitrary displacement, confiscation of essential goods, etc.

## 2.5 Strategy and Selection of Intervention Programs

In planning a program for a given situation, humanitarian agencies may be tempted to make choices not on the basis of the victims' most urgent problems, but according to their media and/or political impact. Thus, a humanitarian organization may be tempted to select "good" programs — that is, programs that do not involve complicated logistics, that present little risk of political involvement, and that make a big splash in the media.

The most typical example is probably the choice between nutrition rehabilitation programs and food distribution programs. In situations where there is no food, it must be kept in mind that setting up a nutrition rehabilitation program unsupported by food distributions will not contribute to a general improvement in the victims' living conditions. Moreover, this strategy may relieve the international community of any sense of responsibility, through the involvement of the media. For the media, the fact that the malnourished are being treated is enough to show the outside world that something is being done and, consequently, that the problem is in the process of being solved.

In making choices, then, health-care personnel must be able to examine the issue in ethical terms, balancing the choices made on the basis of the victims' needs against those reflecting the humanitarian agencies' interests.

## 2.6 Emergency Strategy and Development

The concept of preventing problems at their source indirectly poses the issue of integrating a developmental dynamic into emergency operations. It is often unrealistic to try to link an emergency operation with development in situations of armed conflict; peace is essential to development.

"When conflicts break out, mutually reinforcing efforts at peacemaking and peace-keeping come into play. Once these have achieved their objectives, only sustained, cooperative work to deal with underlying economic, social, cultural and humanitarian problems can place an achieved peace on a durable foundation."[6]

For humanitarian agencies working exclusively in conflict situations, the problem is not to plan development activities that can be carried out once peace has been restored, but rather to incorporate a long-term alternative in the emergency strategy from the very beginning. The agencies specializing in emergency relief are reluctant to do this for several reasons:

- lack of expertise in this field;[7]
- lack of financial means once the emergency is over;[8]
- lack of personnel to meet both urgent demands and long-term demands.

Despite these obstacles, however, every emergency aid program must include some reference to a long-term solution — even if it consists in nothing more than delegating the responsibility to specialized agencies.

The solutions commonly proposed are not truly long-term solutions, since they usually consist in rehabilitation programs designed to restore facilities to their former state. This is not genuine development, since no radical changes are made in the techniques used or in individual behavior, nor are the established systems challenged.

For a rural population with no food resources, the priority is, of course, food distribution. However, from the moment preparation begins for a food aid operation, thought should be given to alternative measures that will eventually replace the food distributions. One possibility might be, for example, providing the population with seeds and tools so that they can return to their usual agricultural activities and achieve a certain self-sufficiency.

The search for a long-term solution is related to humanitarian ethics.

## 3. Ethics and Program Development

Programs are developed in several stages:

- determination of objectives;
- planning of activities;
- mobilization of resources.

---

6 Boutros Boutros-Ghali, *An Agenda for Peace* (United Nations, 1992), p. 33.

7 Health problems are similar in both "normal" and emergency situations. However, the strategy for solving them is fundamentally different in the two cases.

8 Emergency situations are a great financial drain owing to their media impact on the international community during the acute phase of the crisis. Once the peak has passed, the media and, consequently, donor governments lose interest and turn to other crises. It then becomes very difficult to cover the needs of populations who will require continued assistance to institute long-term solutions allowing them, if not to avoid new crises, at least to mitigate their effects.

## 3.1 Ethics and the Determination of Objectives

Determining objectives consists in defining the limits of an intervention program: nature of the action, number of people targeted, anticipated duration, and expected outcome. Although this method is very "technocratic," it provides the framework for a number of questions which delineate the ethical issues.

### *Selecting the Program's Target Population*

**Access restricted to certain population groups**

Selecting the target population may pose problems. What should be done, for example, if access is limited to certain geographical areas? The options are:

- to meet the needs of the populations living in these areas;
- to wait and put pressure on the authorities in order to gain access to all the victims;
- to combine the two approaches.

**Civilian populations are mixed in with armed groups**

Humanitarian aid is not intended to supply the needs of armed groups. Yet in practice, especially in situations of guerrilla warfare, civilians and soldiers are often intermingled. In certain cases, civilian populations are actually hostages of the armed groups. What, then, should be the policy of the humanitarian agencies?

In theory, assistance must be exclusively reserved for non-combatants whose vital needs are not covered. In practice, it is difficult to separate the civilians from the armed groups. Aid can be planned according to the number of civilians targeted. Some of the aid will probably go to armed groups, and the civilians' vital needs may not be covered. If the armed group is included in the intervention program, the aid providers are deliberately contributing to the war effort.

One way of getting around this problem is to minimize the aid's attraction for combatants; for example, relief workers could replace food distributions with meal distributions, as was done in Somalia.

**Displaced and resident populations**

In interventions to benefit displaced populations, a problem inevitably arises concerning the line to take with the resident population, who are usually no better off than the victims.

Taking exclusive responsibility for displaced populations in such situations is apt to be misunderstood by the local authorities, especially since access to the displaced populations depends largely on their good will. However, this political aspect should not mask the ethical problem. And, although there is no question of "buying" access to the victims by including the resident populations in an extensive assistance program, the two points of view can, nevertheless, be reconciled. On one hand, humanitarian organizations cannot take care of an entire region; on the other, local authorities may argue that their people suffer from the same problems, but have not had the "luck" to be affected by the conflict.

It may be possible to:

- direct aid to the displaced populations in such a way that there will be positive fallout for the resident population;
- select groups at risk, not only to help them, but also (and especially) to show the local authorities that the needs of their own people are also being taken into account.

It is possible to go much further in instituting development programs for resident populations, since they are unlikely to have to move on to a new environment.

*Duration of the Intervention*

The duration of a humanitarian intervention cannot be anticipated on the basis of political and military factors. This acknowledged fact should not, however, obscure the real issue: planners should not, in any case, set an arbitrary time limit for a program, but rather decide in advance on criteria for terminating the intervention. One essential criterion is the victims' ability to provide for their own vital needs. A lack of financial resources or the loss of media coverage cannot be used as pretexts to stop a humanitarian intervention.

Another ethical problem arises when organizations embark on programs without having the resources necessary to keep them operational for an adequate period. The necessity of cutting off aid is all the more dramatic if vital needs are involved.

When the policies of the authorities involved are contrary to the victims' interests, humanitarian agencies may legitimately wonder whether they should conclude their operation before the appointed time. Before deciding, they must consider both the impact withdrawal will have on the authorities' attitude and the consequences for the health of the victims.

## 3.2 Ethics and Activity Planning

An intervention program is made up of a set of activities which must obey certain ethical rules.

**Each activity must contribute to the general objective of the program of which it is a part**

In the very specific example of a program to control tuberculosis, a certain number of activities can be identified, such as:

- immunization with BCG;
- screening for patients presenting positive sputum;
- treating the cases identified.

Immunization with BCG can be done separately from the other two activities. The limits of this proceeding are known and accepted. In contrast, screening for positive TB cases without preparing to treat them is a step that merits careful thought. If no treatment is to be provided, the necessity for screening is questionable. Even worse, in cases of tuberculosis, is to begin a program but stop it for lack of funds before patients have completed their treatment. Not only does the disease continue its course, but this practice is likely to increase resistance to antibiotics.

#### Emergency Activities and Respect for Local Norms

Another problem is what to do when the humanitarian organization is certain that the local norms do not match those generally recognized as effective. In the case of tuberculosis, for example, the commonly recommended treatment regimen for emergencies is short (6 months); this is acknowledged to be both more effective and less costly[9] than long treatments (12-18 months). Yet in many developing countries, the national policy is to use the long treatment for tubercular patients. Under these circumstances, what should be done for a refugee or displaced person presenting TB with positive sputum? The options are:

- Ignore the national policy and treat the patient in the most effective way. This, however, introduces a double standard favoring the victims of the conflict or disaster.
- Treat the refugees or displaced people according to international standards, while at the same time promoting these norms on the national level.
- Apply the national policy, knowing that the unstable political situation makes follow-up of patients over an extended period uncertain, and that this type of treatment is ineffective and contrary to medical ethics.

The *second solution* is the only one that reconciles medical ethics with the promotion of development activities for the country.

### 3.3 Ethics and the Mobilization of Resources

#### Resources and Respect for Local Customs

The examples of what not to do, such as distributing corn in Asia or pork in Moslem countries, are notorious. Local eating habits must be respected.

#### Cost of Emergency Interventions

The volume and cost of the resources mobilized for emergency situations are often disproportionate to the resources normally available in the countries

---

9 If the cost/benefit analysis takes into account not only the cost of the drugs, but also social and economic costs.

concerned. Some observers have seen this as an ethical problem, comparing the impact of emergency interventions with the results that development agencies could have achieved with the financial manna of emergency aid.

The cost of emergency interventions can be attributed to two basic factors: the use of resources from outside the country, and the necessity of mobilizing resources quickly. Why are humanitarian interventions always urgent? Emergencies rarely erupt all at once. Early signs can often be detected in advance. Accordingly, it should be possible to predict the emergency and:

- pre-position food stocks in advance, using ordinary means of transport rather than the expensive options;
- lay in stocks of drugs in areas at risk.

Anticipating emergencies would reduce costs and permit an immediate response to victims' needs. From a practical standpoint, of course, this approach raises certain logistical problems (storage of food and drugs for an indefinite length of time) and political problems (acceptance by the authorities of a prediction of war).

### Use of Resources from Outside the Country

The use of resources from outside the country is often necessary. In every case, the consequences of deciding to use outside resources must be carefully weighed. For example, the food resources required for a relief operation may be purchased in the trouble zone itself; or in the country, but outside the trouble zone; or in neighboring countries; or, finally, they may be imported from Europe, the US, or other surplus countries. Merely ascertaining whether food is available locally is not sufficient; a whole group of factors must be analyzed.

- *Buying locally*

Buying locally offers several advantages: costs are lower (food, transport, maintenance, etc.), the food is more quickly available (short transport time, no customs duty), and it is better suited to local dietary habits. All these factors make local purchasing very attractive.

However, it should be remembered that local buying may unbalance a shaky local market, and that local merchants will refuse to sell their food stocks in order to push prices up.

- *Buying in neighboring countries*

The risks involved in buying supplies in the bordering regions or countries are the same as for buying locally, though they are less certain and less extensive.

- *Importing from Western countries*

Importing food from Western countries presents major disadvantages in terms of delivery time and cost (even if it is not the aid agency that foots the bill, in the case of donated goods and transport). Moreover, there is a risk of importing food inappropriate to local conditions. Just as the introduction of new medical intervention strategies (such as for tuberculosis) is risky, so the introduction of new technologies or products may have harmful consequences. Here again, this does not mean that anything new should automatically be rejected; but a distinction must be made between what is appropriate and what is not. The introduction of inappropriate resources (too expensive, or unsuited to needs) is contrary to humanitarian ethics.

#### The Employment of Health-Care Professionals

The dispatch of Western medical teams has several disadvantages, notably the high cost (transportation, salaries) and the Westerners' cultural unsuitability (ignorance of the local language and social customs).

Using local professionals circumvents these problems, but presents other risks. They may be in danger in conflict zones due to their nationality, which links them to one or the other of the parties to the conflict; they may lack technical knowledge in certain specific aspects of armed conflicts (notably, war surgery); and, finally, the attraction of local personnel to emergency operations may be detrimental to the local health services ("brain drain").

The two options can be combined by using teams of outside experts, reduced to the minimum, to train and supervise local personnel during the course of the mission.

## 4. Program Evaluation

Evaluation consists in measuring the performances of an intervention program. It is also, however, a kind of steering device for the intervention itself.

There are two levels of evaluation: monitoring and impact evaluation

### 4.1 Monitoring

#### Monitoring the Aid Provided to the Victims

The aid provided to the victims can be monitored in different ways. The humanitarian agencies can ascertain whether the victims indeed have access to routine services (health, water, law, etc.), or they can verify that the supply distributions (food, drugs) that they finance or provide do indeed get to the victims who need them.

All humanitarian agencies accept the necessity of monitoring aid. This is why some of them, including the ICRC, make the assistance they provide conditional on their being allowed to supervise it themselves:

"When emergency assistance is required and the ICRC is particularly well placed to play a useful role by virtue of its specific mandate, it sets three conditions before undertaking any relief action, namely that it be allowed access to the persons requiring assistance, to observe their situation and to evaluate their needs; that it be present when the aid is brought in; and, finally, that it be allowed to exercise administrative supervision in order to prepare reports on distributions made."[10]

If the authorities will not give advance consent to the monitoring of humanitarian assistance, the humanitarian agencies can either withhold assistance until they receive a guarantee that they will be able to supervise it, or provide the aid in the hope that the authorities will eventually yield.

The crucial point here is how urgent the victims' needs are. If the situation is critical, postponing humanitarian assistance is ethically questionable. If conditions are less drastic, it is then possible to temporize while trying to obtain permission to supervise the operation. In the time required to conduct such negotiations, however, the victims' condition may deteriorate dramatically, and the humanitarian agency again faces the same problem, now compounded by the accusation that it did not act early enough to prevent the crisis.

This type of situation is, unfortunately, not uncommon. Consequently, relief agencies must take into account both the necessity of supervision and the importance of not penalizing the victims who need the aid.

## 4.2 Evaluating the Impact of the Intervention on the Victims

The inputs mobilized should furnish a certain number of services, such as medical examinations, food distributions, and surgical interventions. Evaluation is a means of verifying whether the services provided correspond to what had been anticipated quantitatively and qualitatively. Accordingly, the quantity and quality of the services must be assessed. This involves making a value judgment concerning the quality of medical and surgical activities. For health-care professionals, then, the issue becomes one of medical ethics.

## 4.3 Impact Evaluations

Evaluating the impact of an intervention is essential. "[The ICRC] also seeks authorization to return to the scene in order to assess the impact of its work on the condition of the population (health, food, clothing, hygiene, etc.) in relation to the targets set."[11]

Humanitarian organizations have a responsibility to carry out evaluations on a systematic basis. Objections may arise on the grounds that:

- it is too difficult;

[10] Marion Harroff-Tavel, *op. cit.*: 215.
[11] *Ibid.*

- it is not a priority (the first priority is feeding, treatment, etc. — if there is any time left over, evaluate);
- it is better not to know the impact of the intervention.

All these arguments can be refuted.

*Difficulty*:
The institution of a surveillance system is certainly not easy, but it is not impossible.

*Priority*:
The purpose of analyzing the impact of an intervention is not to satisfy the intellectual curiosity of the program managers. It is an essential tool for orienting the operation.

*Fear of value judgments*:
There are so many constraints in situations of armed conflict that interventions often have a limited impact. It would be tendentious to reject evaluation on this ground, for fear of having to face questions concerning the lack of impact of the program evaluated.

Once the necessity of impact evaluation has been acknowledged, what should be evaluated?

- **Impact on Victims' Health Status**

For health-care professionals, a program's impact is measured in relation to the objective established at the beginning of the operation (we will not review the details of measurable health indicators here).

- **Impact on Vital Needs**

The concept of "comprehensive needs" developed previously is appropriate here. A situation may arise where the food distributions have achieved their stated purpose (for example, to return malnutrition to its normal level) but in the meantime have generated perverse effects (such as increased tension between those who receive food aid and those who do not). Arrangements should be made to measure this type of harmful effect on the same basis as malnutrition rates.

- **Impact on All the Victims**

Evaluation will indicate whether the aid is uniformly distributed among all members of the target population.

- **Impact of One Program on Another**

What one program does may have negative consequences for what another is doing. For example, distributing food tends, in the long run, to make victims irresponsible, fostering a mentality characteristic of chronic aid recipients. Moreover, it may destabilize the local market. Then, if agricultural rehabilitation programs are offered, there will be few takers, since the general feeling will be: "Why grow anything? We are given food, and, in any case, what we produce won't be worth much on the market."

"Ideally, any aid input even in times of emergency should attempt to reduce rather than increase vulnerability. In Lesotho there exist many local coping-strategies, and although clearly compromises, nevertheless provide some protection to individual households. One may, therefore, legitimately inquire whether or not the kind of emergency-response in Lesotho helped to support these local strategies in, for instance, increasing transfer of income between households and providing added social security measures guaranteeing some degree of protection for the destitute. Agricultural practice has its own mechanisms for distributing food and cash and any intervention which blocks these life-saving mechanisms is necessarily counter-productive." [12]

Evaluating the impact of humanitarian interventions is essential both for the conduct of operations in progress and as an instrument of operational research to achieve a better approach to future operations. To reject the principle of evaluation for the sake of other priorities is unethical.

# II. Code of Conduct for Relations between Humanitarian Agencies

Humanitarian interventions have evolved over the last twenty years. The era of amateurism has given way to the professionalization of the big humanitarian agencies. Although this change may have resulted in a loss of spontaneity, humanitarian operations have, in exchange, gained in efficiency. It should therefore be possible to develop a joint code of conduct for the humanitarian agencies, based on accepted professional principles — although each agency has different interests depending on its mandate, its level of development, the nature of its relations with the States, and its financial means.

## 1. Relations between Agencies

Relations between humanitarian agencies are complex. They depend on the factors described below, as well as the kind of situation involved.

### 1.1 Concentration

Major humanitarian emergencies, especially those receiving heavy media coverage, are flooded with humanitarian organizations (governmental, non-governmental, UN, etc.).

[12] Frances D'Souza, Famine: social security and an analysis of vulnerability, case study: Lesotho 1983-85, edited by G.A. Harrison, Oxford University Press, 1988.

## 1.2 Confusion

Confusion often arises, especially at the beginning of humanitarian operations, when numerous agencies arrive on the terrain without any precise mandate or objectives. The confusion is greatest concerning the responsibilities that each agency is entitled or obligated to undertake, unless one of them is able to impose a modicum of order.

## 1.3 Consultation

Before undertaking a humanitarian action, the potential actors should consult one other to find out their respective plans for a given situation. Unfortunately, it is still all too common for such contacts not to take place until after the humanitarian operations have begun, when participants meet to exchange information about operations in progress.

## 1.4 Conferring

Conferring goes further than mere consultation. It allows the agencies to outline general spheres of action, without actually defining structured plans.

## 1.5 Coordination

At this stage, each agency must fit its own operations into the framework of a global strategy, and define objectives that will permit a distribution of intervention programs based on each agency's skills and resources.

## 1.6 Cooperation

In the field, cooperation may manifest itself in the sharing of resources or services. Thus, the World Food Programme (WFP) often puts food supplies at the disposal of other organizations; similarly, the ICRC offers logistic assistance to facilitate the work of other agencies.

## 1.7 Contribution

Some of the humanitarian organizations have no operational capacity. Their role is to provide other agencies with the financial, human, or logistic resources needed for a given operation.

The United Nations Department for Humanitarian Affairs has suggested launching consolidated appeals incorporating all the demands of all the agencies for a given situation. This procedure involves obvious dangers. It slows down the intervention process in emergencies, limits the agencies' independence, and risks confusing the donors concerning the respective mandates of the agencies.

**Types of Relations between Humanitarian Agencies**

- Concentration
- Confusion
- Consultation
- Conferring
- Coordination
- Cooperation
- Contribution
- Coercion
- Competition
- Contest
- Confrontation
- Conflict

## 1.8 Coercion

Contribution should not become a means of coercion. It is easy to imagine the case of resource supply agencies which try to impose relief operations favoring specific groups of victims to the detriment of other groups in equally critical conditions. There is a clear risk here that agencies will be forced to intervene according to criteria unrelated to their mandates.

## 1.9 Competition

Several agencies work in the same field and find themselves in competition with each other. Each will try to do better than the others. The competition is even fiercer if the field involved is one with public impact — that is, one that generates resources.

It is not uncommon for the headquarters of different humanitarian agencies to compete over the definition of their respective mandates. In a given situation, this competition between identical programs (nutritional rehabilitation, medical care) leads to genuine anarchy and a waste of resources.

## 1.10 Contest

A contest is a form of competition, cultivated as a sport. Not only does each agency want to be the best, but it must also get to the scene of action first!

Some agencies are particularly attracted by competition, to the point where it may become their main objective. In this case, the victims' interests come second, which in the end results in interventions that are badly targeted, useless, or even dangerous for the beneficiaries.

## 1.11 Confrontation

Not infrequently, agencies clash over intervention strategies or the line to take with local authorities. Confrontation is desirable except in the acute phases of operations, for it involves an exchange of opposing points of view which ultimately develops the approach to humanitarian situations.

### 1.12 Conflict

A conflict between agencies is apt to ensue when there is confusion over their respective mandates.

**Of course, relations between agencies can move rapidly from one stage to another, depending on circumstances. Consultation favors coordination, whereas confusion may lead to conflict.**

The advantages of coordination between different humanitarian agencies are obvious. However, although all the agencies recognize the need for coordination, few of them are willing to accept the resulting constraints: the obligation to respect the mandates of others or the commitments made towards others, joint decision-making, etc.

This last point is crucial for the ICRC, since its role as a neutral, independent intermediary obliges it to preserve complete autonomy in its decision-making. In large-scale interventions, the ICRC may coordinate its intervention with those of other agencies; but it cannot be coordinated by them.

This intransigence, founded on the demands of neutrality and independence, is not the sole preserve of the ICRC. Each agency has its own criteria for intervention and its own way of operating in the field. Nonetheless, humanitarian interventions must maintain a certain coherence. To achieve it, a model for interagency relations may be proposed. Such a model should be based not on a rigid coordination, but rather on a flexible system of mutual conference.

## 2. A Code of Conduct Based on “Good Relations” between Agencies

A practical code of conduct will help to harmonize the interaction of humanitarian interventions in a given situation.

### 2.1 Problems and Priorities: The Decision to Intervene

When events call for a humanitarian intervention, the humanitarian agencies will assess the problems and priorities. Their decision to intervene will depend on the nature of the problems identified and the nature of their mandate. When the one coincides with the other, the agencies will consult together to find out what each plans to do, while respecting one another’s independence and neutrality. This approach does not entail any formal undertaking between the agencies, but is a way to consolidate support for the actual principle of intervening and to determine the forms that intervention could take.

## 2.2 Determining Objectives and Dividing Responsibilities between the Agencies

The method for defining a humanitarian intervention's operational objectives has already been reviewed several times. As mentioned, it includes:

- a definition of the health problem targeted;
- a definition of the group for whom the intervention is intended, by category (displaced populations, refugee populations, resident civilian populations, detainees, wounded, etc.) and locality;
- a statement of the expected outcome;
- the length of time anticipated to achieve this outcome.

The definition of objectives can serve as a basis for coordination between agencies. After all, if one agency defines an objective clearly in terms of the criteria listed above, other agencies will know what problems are being treated, for which group of victims, and for how long.

This coordination of objectives, however, is not really satisfactory, since inasmuch as each agency remains in control of its own objectives, there is a risk of competition, of rivalry, even of conflict.

Although planners might contemplate creating some mechanism of coordination to define the objectives of each organization, this would be difficult because:
- if one agency agreed to exercise this responsibility, it would come into conflict with all the others' vague desires for independence;
- the institution of a cooperative system including several agencies with an equal power of decision would hinder their ability to respond quickly enough to emergency situations;
- delegating the responsibility to the authorities would challenge the principle of neutrality, which is indispensable in situations of armed conflict.

This brings us back to a flexible coordination mechanism in which each agency defines its own objectives and harmonizes its own interventions with those of the other agencies. If an agency is to be effective, it must observe a certain discipline, which involves at the same time respect for:

- mandates;
- intervention strategies;
- operational commitments undertaken during the definition of objectives.

Practically speaking, in any given situation this last point is important. To achieve an objective, several organizations will often mobilize for different but complementary activities which are all directed towards the same goal. In this process, if one of the agencies does not fulfill its obligations, the entire operation will suffer.

Coordination may be based on programs, geographical regions, or intervention phases.

### Programs

The distribution of programs is itself a mode of technical coordination. Essentially, it is important to avoid two agencies setting up the same kind of program in the same regions, which would result in duplication with perverse effects (such as the victims' using services furnished by both organizations at the same time). Agencies' attempts to outbid each other translate into a tendency to more sophisticated services which are both inappropriate and costly.

### Geographical Regions

The geographical distribution of programs depends mostly on the respective mandates of the different agencies. For example, areas of intense conflict where insecurity is dominant are the first priority for the ICRC.

### Phases of the Intervention

Coordination based on the phase of intervention permits the establishment of a link between emergency relief and programs for rehabilitation and development — for example, insuring a transition from a food-aid distribution program to a program for agricultural assistance (seeds, tools, etc.).

The analytical study of the impact of interventions is useful for identifying deficiencies. The purpose is not to stigmatize those responsible, but to allow agencies to judge how far they can rely on each other in coordinating subsequent operations.

**Informal coordination combines program effectiveness with the flexibility necessary to insure that the various mandates of the different agencies are respected.**

## 2.3 Resource Mobilization and Cooperation between Agencies

The constraints involved in situations of armed conflict do not always allow relief agencies to conduct their activities at the pace they would like. In the field, the usual practice is for agencies to help each other as current necessity dictates, whether by lending supplies, expert advice, or logistic support (transport). This form of cooperation does not challenge individual mandates, nor program coordination.

Cooperation in respect to material assistance is prepared for in advance, being based on the standardization of drugs and medical supplies. As for human resources, cooperation may be reflected in the training of health-care personnel so that they have a common approach in emergency situations:

"Apart from the very specific co-operation already established in a number of operations particularly with UNICEF, UNHCR and many non-governmental organizations, the ICRC would also like to stress the importance of its general co-operation with the World Food Programme (WFP) for the supply and delivery of relief, as well as with the World Health Organization (WHO) in training medical personnel in situations of armed conflict (the annual HELP course organized in Geneva in co-operation with the Faculty of Medicine of the University of Geneva)."[13]

This code of conduct for relations between agencies is a means of promoting harmony between all the pieces of the puzzle constituting a humanitarian intervention. It must guarantee both respect for the special mandate of each intervening agency and coordination between their programs.

"The need to reinforce coordination between the very numerous protagonists of humanitarian action at work today in the battlefield seems to me an obvious one: The aim is both to avoid duplications and to increase the effectiveness of each one. To this end, two distinct aspects must, in my view, be considered more particularly. On one hand, there is the importance of instituting flexible mechanisms for consultation which do not slow down the decision-making process and which do not complicate life for those working in the field. Indeed, the particular characteristics of each conflict make it impossible to contemplate instituting rigid procedures expected to work in all interventions. On the other hand, and more important in my opinion, is the necessity of developing principles of action to make partnerships compatible while preserving the impartial character of every authentically humanitarian action. In this respect, it might be useful to define a common framework of ethical and operational principles for the use of numerous non-governmental organizations whose actions are not defined by Conventions or by clearly specified mandates recognized by the international community."[14]

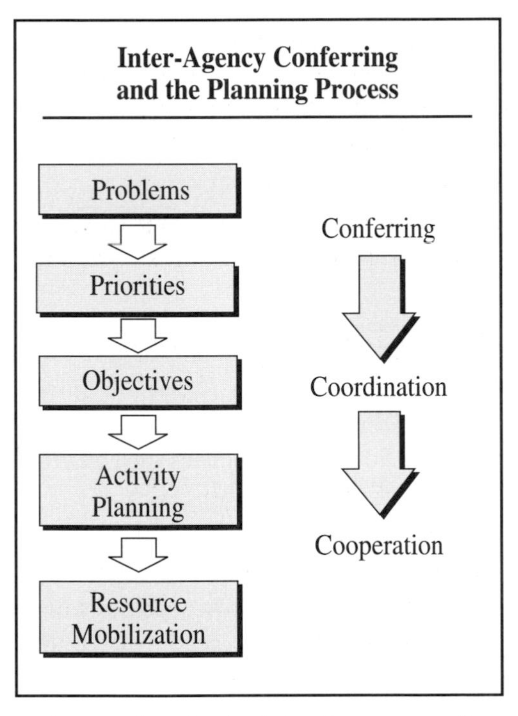


[13] "Strengthening of the Co-ordination of Humanitarian Emergency Assistance of the United Nations," statement by the International Committee of the Red Cross in the United Nations General Assembly, 46th session (New York, 5 Nov. 1991), p. 2.

[14] Cornelio Sommaruga, "Action humanitaire et opérations de maintien de la paix: une complémentarité à définir," *Arès, Paix et Sécurité Internationale* XIV/1 (1993): 64.

There are many codes of conduct. One is the code of conduct for the International Red Cross and Red Crescent Movement and Non-Governmental Organizations (NGOs) in disaster relief.

# III. Humanitarian Organizations

To understand the possibilities of consultation, coordination, and cooperation between the different humanitarian agencies, we must be familiar with the characteristics of each. This section briefly describes the mandate and the *modus operandi* of the humanitarian organizations most involved in the health field and in situations of armed conflict. Each example is representative of a certain type of humanitarian organization.

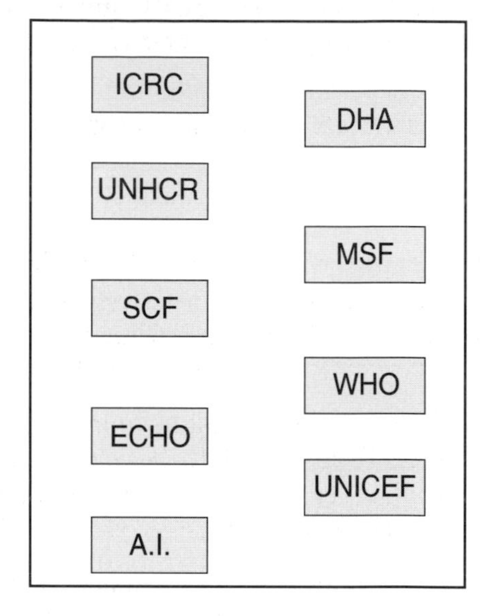


## 1. The International Red Cross and Red Crescent Movement

The International Red Cross and Red Crescent Movement comprises all the recognized National Red Cross and Red Crescent Societies, the International Federation of Red Cross and Red Crescent Societies (which is their central secretariat), and the ICRC.

The activities of the Movement's components are described in the Statutes of the International Red Cross and Red Crescent Movement. Moreover, a 1989 agreement between the ICRC and the International Federation specifies which tasks fall to which institution. Thus, the ICRC has the lead role in the Movement's international activities in armed conflicts and other situations requiring the presence of a specifically neutral and independent organization, whereas the Federation coordinates the relief efforts of the National Societies in the wake of major disasters. These rules make the Movement more efficient and strengthen its unity.

### 1.1 The International Conference of the Red Cross and the Red Crescent

The International Conference is the highest deliberating body of the Movement. As such, it decides the Movement's major options with respect both to doctrine and to actions and organization. Through the dialogue that it promotes with the signatory States of the Geneva Conventions, the International Conference is a forum for debating problems arising from the application of international humanitarian law, a forum in which States can be brought to confront the responsibilities this law imposes on them.

The International Conference can pass resolutions, make recommendations, assign mandates to the ICRC and the Federation, and formulate draft proposals for the development of international humanitarian conventions.

## 1.2 The International Committee of the Red Cross (ICRC)

### *History*

On 24 June 1859, the battle of Solferino took place, in the course of which Henry Dunant was horrified to see wounded men abandoned to their fate. After returning to Geneva, in 1862 he published the book *Un Souvenir de Solferino* (A Memory of Solferino), which had a profound impact in Europe.

In February, 1863, the "International Committee for Relief to Wounded Soldiers" was created. In October of the same year, an international conference was organized in Geneva with representatives from 16 States. It adopted the distinctive sign of the red cross on a white background.

In 1864, the Swiss Federal Council convoked another international conference at which the plenipotentiaries of the States drew up the Geneva Convention of 22 August 1864 for the Amelioration of the Condition of the Wounded in Armies in the Field. In 1880, the International Committee for Relief to Wounded Soldiers changed its name to "International Committee of the Red Cross."

### *Status and structure*

By virtue of the mandate conferred on it by the international community in the Geneva Conventions and their Additional Protocols, the ICRC has a specific status. Although non-governmental, its international tasks and responsibilities give it a stature which goes beyond that of a simple NGO. It is recognized as an international legal entity, and the many headquarters agreements it has concluded with States puts it on a par with intergovernmental organizations. As such, the ICRC benefits from several privileges and immunities, and its personnel usually has diplomatic status. These advantages guarantee that the ICRC can act in total independence. The specific status of the ICRC was confirmed in 1990 when the United Nations General Assembly granted it observer status.

The ICRC has its headquarters in Geneva. Its governing body is the Committee, composed of up to 25 members, all of Swiss nationality and elected by co-option.

The Committee meets in an Assembly, which decides matters of general policy and the acting principles of the institution. The Executive Board is in charge of the conduct of affairs. It meets once a week and, like the Assembly, is chaired by the President of the ICRC.

### *Role*

The ICRC's role is defined in Article 4 of its Statutes:

"1. The role of the ICRC shall be in particular:

a) to maintain and disseminate the Fundamental Principles of the Movement, namely humanity, impartiality, neutrality, independence, voluntary service, unity and universality;
b) to recognize any newly established or reconstituted National Society, which fulfils the conditions for recognition set out in the Statutes of the Movement, and to notify other National Societies of such recognition;
c) to undertake the tasks incumbent upon it under the Geneva Conventions, to work for the faithful application of international humanitarian law applicable in armed conflicts and to take cognizance of any complaints based on alleged breaches of that law;
d) to endeavour at all times — as a neutral institution whose humanitarian work is carried out particularly in time of international and other armed conflicts or internal strife — to ensure the protection of and assistance to military and civilian victims of such events and of their direct results;
e) to ensure the operation of the Central Tracing Agency as provided in the Geneva Conventions;
f) to contribute, in anticipation of armed conflicts, to the training of medical personnel and the preparation of medical equipment, in co-operation with the National Societies, the military and civilian medical services and other competent authorities;
g) to work for the understanding and dissemination of knowledge of international humanitarian law applicable in armed conflicts and to prepare any development thereof;
h) to carry out mandates entrusted to it by the International Conference of the Red Cross and Red Crescent (the International Conference).

2. The ICRC may take any humanitarian initiative which comes within its role as a specifically neutral and independent institution and intermediary, and may consider any question requiring examination by such an institution."

Of these tasks, a closer look should be taken at the ICRC's "legal role". The institution is required to "work for the faithful application" of the Geneva Conventions (letter c above). These means that it reminds the parties to armed conflicts (governments, but also, in internal conflicts, armed opposition groups) of their legal obligations. It is also the promoter and custodian of humanitarian law. In practice, ICRC delegates oversee the application of the Geneva Conventions and their Additional Protocols through their presence in the field, for example when visiting prisoners of war. They forward their observations to the parties in conflict and make recommendations.

The ICRC is also charged with ensuring the protection and assistance of the victims of armed conflicts and internal disturbances (letter d above). It has many activities in this respect, in particular relief operations for the civilian population (food, medical care, shelter, drinking water, etc.). Its Central Tracing Agency forwards messages between the members of families separated by war, traces the missing and makes it possible for families to be reunited.

The ICRC has a broad right of humanitarian initiative (paragraph 2 above) which enables it to offer its services when the presence of a specifically neutral and independent institution and intermediary may help resolve humanitarian issues. For example, the ICRC has access to political detainees.

The ICRC's protection and assistance activities are also conducted for people displaced within their own countries who, during armed conflicts, are protected by humanitarian law. Refugees also come under the ICRC's mandate when they are protected by humanitarian law, when they face major security problems, or when UNHCR is unable to come to their aid.

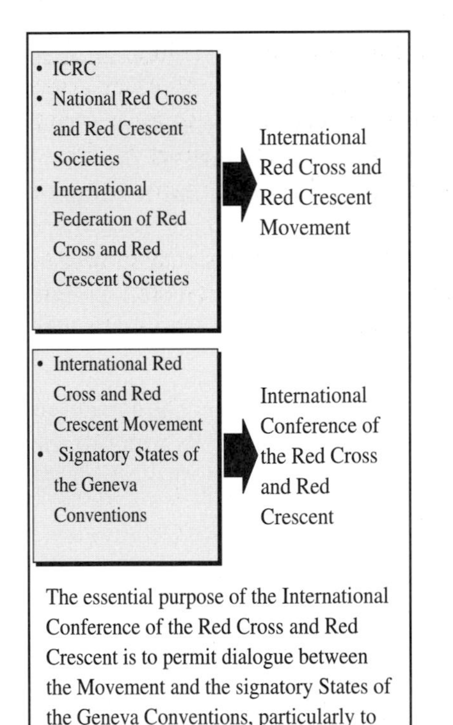


The essential purpose of the International Conference of the Red Cross and Red Crescent is to permit dialogue between the Movement and the signatory States of the Geneva Conventions, particularly to remind them of their responsibility to apply — and insure that others apply — international humanitarian law.

## 1.3 The National Red Cross and Red Crescent Societies

In peacetime, the National Societies' activities are generally concentrated in sectors such as health, health education, and natural-disaster relief.

In situations of armed conflict, the National Societies are called to come to the aid of the victims. The ICRC has a preponderant role as intermediary in such situations, and as such it works together with the National Societies of the parties to the conflict. The ICRC can also recruit health-care personnel in countries that are not involved in the hostilities.

### 1.4 The International Federation of Red Cross and Red Crescent Societies

Created in 1919 to help the National Societies develop their peacetime activities, the International Federation of Red Cross and Red Crescent Societies[15] is their central secretariat. It promotes the humanitarian activities of the National Societies among vulnerable people. By coordinating international disaster relief and encouraging development support, it seeks to prevent and alleviate human suffering.

## 2. The United Nations Office of the High Commissioner for Refugees (UNHCR)

### 2.1 History

UNHCR was created at the behest of the United Nations General Assembly, and has been protecting refugees since 1 January 1951.

### 2.2 Statute

The UNHCR Statute was established by Resolution 428 (V), adopted by the UN General Assembly on 14 December 1950.

"The United Nations High Commissioner for Refugees, acting under the authority of the General Assembly, shall assume the function of providing international protection, under the auspices of the United Nations, to refugees who fall within the scope of the present Statute and of seeking permanent solutions for the problem of refugees by assisting Governments and, subject to the approval of the Governments concerned, private organizations to facilitate the voluntary repatriation of such refugees, or their assimilation within new national communities."[16]

The 1951 Convention applies to those people who became refugees as a result of events occurring before 1 January 1951. The Protocol of 1967 Relating to the Status of Refugees eliminated that deadline, extending the protection of UNHCR to people who became refugees after 1 January 1951.

### 2.3 Operation

The Executive Committee of UNHCR is composed of 50 States. The organization is largely financed by government contributions. UNHCR works in close cooperation with the other UN agencies, such as the World Food

[15] Formerly called the League of Red Cross Societies.
[16] Statute of the United Nations Office of the High Commissioner for Refugees, Chapter 1, Article 1.

Programme and WHO, as well as with non-governmental organizations (NGOs). UNHCR has in fact begun a series of talks with the NGOs to discuss operational relations and ways of establishing a more constructive, concrete partnership. A plan of action was adopted in June, 1994, in Oslo, at the close of the PARINAC ("Partners in Action") world conference. It represents a synthesis of proposals made in this respect, and takes the form of recommendations to be put into practice at the operational level.

### 2.4 Role

Up to 1990, UNHCR fulfilled its mandate to guarantee the protection of refugee populations and to find permanent solutions to their situation. Since then, its mandate has been expanded to include action to prevent refugee movements. As a result, UNHCR may be obliged to intervene in conflict situations on behalf of civilian populations who are victims of the hostilities, whether they have remained in their original homes or have had to flee and are displaced. The ICRC protects these same victims by virtue of humanitarian law (Fourth Convention and Additional Protocol I for international armed conflicts; common Article 3 and Additional Protocol II for internal armed conflicts).

## 3. The World Food Programme (WFP)

### 3.1 History

The World Food Programme (WFP) was created in 1961 by resolution 1714 (XVI) of the UN General Assembly.

### 3.2 Mandate

The purpose of the WFP is to provide food aid to developing countries, both in the framework of economic development programs and in emergency situations.

### 3.3 Structure

The headquarters of the WFP are in Rome, and its field operations are directed from there.

### 3.4 Role

The WFP is active in development programs in which food distribution serves as support for agricultural or reforestation projects. In emergency situations, the WFP assists refugee and displaced populations by means of food distribution.

# 4. United Nations Children's Fund (UNICEF)

## 4.1 History

The United Nations Children's Fund (UNICEF) was created in 1946 by resolution 57(1) of the UN General Assembly to provide assistance to children in Europe and China after the war. Its mandate was subsequently expanded to include the support of permanent programs to benefit children.

## 4.2 Mandate

UNICEF's mandate is to protect children and to promote, all over the world, the application of the Convention on the Rights of the Child, adopted by the UN General Assembly in 1989 (resolution 44/25). As early as 1924, the League of Nations had adopted the Geneva Declaration on the rights of children.

In the health field, UNICEF activities involve nutrition, education, water supply, immunization, etc.

Children's right to enjoy the best health possible is specified in Article 24 of the Convention on the Rights of the Child.

## 4.3 Structure

The Executive Board of UNICEF is constituted by representatives of 41 countries (as of November, 1994), elected by the UN Economic and Social Council. The executive director is appointed by the Secretary-General of the UN.

## 4.4 Role

Most of UNICEF's activities fall into the category of development programs. However, the organization also intervenes in emergency situations.

To achieve its goals, UNICEF collaborates with the other UN organizations, such as WHO for expanded programs of immunization and UNESCO for education.

# 5. The United Nations Department of Humanitarian Affairs (DHA)

## 5.1 History

The Department of Humanitarian Affairs (DHA) was created in March, 1992, to reinforce the coordination of UN emergency humanitarian assistance (resolution A/46/182, adopted by the UN General Assembly on December 19, 1991). The

DHA assumed in particular the functions previously exercised by the Office of the United Nations Disaster Relief Coordinator.

### 5.2 Structure

The DHA is run by an emergency relief coordinator appointed by the UN Secretary-General. Its seat is in New York and it maintains offices in Geneva.

### 5.3 Role

The DHA's functions are to:
- advise the Secretary-General on emergency situations;
- reinforce the coordination of UN agency responses to emergencies;
- mobilize the international community in cases of natural disaster.

To direct this coordination, the DHA created an Inter-Agency Standing Committee. Other organizations, such as the ICRC and the International Federation of Red Cross and Red Crescent Societies, are represented on this Committee as observers.

The DHA coordinates the financial appeals of the agencies. The ICRC, while invoking its independence and underlining the absolute necessity of making its own financial appeals, agrees to make its emergency appeals jointly with those of the DHA.

## 6. *Médecins sans frontières* (MSF)

### 6.1 History

The organization *Médecins sans Frontières* ("Doctors without Borders") was founded in 1971 in Paris. Today it has seven sections (France, Belgium, Netherlands, Switzerland, Luxembourg, Spain, and Greece).

### 6.2 Structure

Each section is directed by a president and a director-general. The International Council, which meets every three months, comprises the seven presidents and the seven directors-general, as well as the secretary-general of MSF International. The board defines the main policy lines of the organization.

### 6.3 Role

MSF acts in all emergency situations, whether they are caused by natural disasters or armed conflicts. Its sphere of action is essentially health. Assistance to refugees is a major part of its programs.

MSF actions are based on a charter which defines the context and structure of its interventions. Under the charter, MSF volunteers undertake neutral, impartial action in the name of universal medical ethics and the right to assistance. MSF also implements long-term rehabilitation programs, particularly for hospitals.

## 7. The European Community Humanitarian Office (ECHO)

### 7.1 History

The European Community Humanitarian Office (ECHO) was created in 1992 in order to increase the effectiveness and visibility of the European Union's humanitarian efforts. In addition, the European Commission wanted to concentrate its various emergency-relief instruments within a single organization.

### 7.2 Mandate

ECHO reflects the desire of the European Union to provide more rapid and effective assistance to the victims of conflicts taking place in third countries.

### 7.3 Role

ECHO intervenes primarily by obtaining funding for the activities of its operational partners (international and non-governmental organizations, the ICRC). ECHO also implements its own operations as a subsidiary activity.

## 8. A New Organization: the Geneva Foundation

### 8.1 History

The Geneva Foundation was established in 1994 in Geneva. It was born of the perceived need to rationalize the humanitarian response, given the disproportion between the needs of war victims and the resources made available to the organizations working to help them.

### 8.2 Structure

The Geneva Foundation is composed of 12 members: the 4 founding members, 2 members nominated by the ICRC, 2 from the academic world, and 4 proposed by the Swiss cantonal and federal authorities. It is financed by private donations.

## 8.3 Role

The pooling of field experiences and the creation of a multidisciplinary framework for reflection will facilitate a better understanding of health problems in armed conflict situations and foster the development of new and original solutions. The Foundation will collect information, create documentation, and organize international seminars and meetings, as well as study units to examine health matters related to armed conflicts.

**Many other organizations could have been cited (SCF and OXFAM as NGOs, USAID and OFDA as governmental agencies). The purpose here is not to draw up an exhaustive list of all humanitarian agencies, but rather to illustrate their role through a few examples.**

**In situations of armed conflict, needs are not limited to health care, but also include measures to protect the victims. The intervention of humanitarian agencies is occasionally made difficult by the complexity of the political environment, which in many cases restricts access to the victims.**

**Respect for a humanitarian ethic is essential, despite the constraints inherent in situations of armed conflict. Under no circumstances should the difficulties encountered serve as an excuse for interventions that are third-rate or even dangerous for the victims.**

**Consultation, coordination, and cooperation between agencies are the basis for a code of conduct governing the relations between them. However, these forms of collaboration must respect the specific mandate and/or intervention strategies of each humanitarian organization.**

***Mention the word "war", and our thoughts turn at once to those most directly affected: the dead and wounded, prisoners, those who have gone missing or been separated from their families, those who have been forced to flee. Their plight is dramatic and requires immediate humanitarian action, but it is merely the tip of the iceberg, the most visible manifestation of all the perverse effects of war, which can be analyzed from two points of view.***

# CONCLUSION

For **war victims**, **health** most often means survival, which in turn depends on access to those essentials of life which are food, water and medical care. In many cases this access is a challenge that people already have to meet every day in time of peace. In time of war, the lack of security and the political interests involved can suddenly make the search for the basic essentials vastly more complicated.

War does not affect just people; the damage done to the economic sector (agriculture in particular) and the social sector (degradation and even destruction of health systems) has an immediate effect on the population. In the long term, the socio-economic destabilization directly due to war cancels out the development efforts of the past 20 years.

In the area of health, the aim of humanitarian agencies is to protect and assist war victims. They may act directly in behalf of the victims, providing them with food, water, vaccinations and medico-surgical care. Such activities must, however, be accompanied by emergency rehabilitation of local services, providing support for agriculture, health services and the usual water supply system. By adopting this strategy, humanitarian agencies will generally help to establish a more direct link with the resumption of the development process, the impact of which will of course be more lasting than that of emergency humanitarian operations.

The application of this strategy is nevertheless subject to a number of constraints, the most serious of which is undoubtedly poor security, both for the victims and for the teams from humanitarian organizations. These difficulties hold up or slow down relief operations and very often limit their effectiveness.

When the lack of security is used as a means of exerting pressure on the civilian population, the already fragile balance between the people and their basic resources, such as food and water, is upset. When the lack of security is too widespread or the imbalance created too great, flight is the only way out. By the same token, access to health services is seriously hampered when health facilities are impossible to enter or attacks are directed against them.

Security conditions are even more precarious in countries where armed conflicts have led to the disintegration of the State: the absence of responsible authorities or their loss of control over armed bands are the main factors of risk for the medical staff of humanitarian organizations.

The search for innovative intervention strategies in the area of health must remain a priority for humanitarian organizations, but it must not serve as an excuse to by-pass increasingly difficult constraints. Parallel action must be taken to eliminate those constraints so as not to be hampered by them.

In armed conflicts, the strict application of IHL, through the protection afforded to non-combatants and the possibility of intervening when necessary, will make it possible to deal with the victims' health problems promptly and efficiently.

The most elaborate form of preventive medicine that the ICRC has at its disposal is the improved application of international humanitarian law.

We may well consider the possibility of going beyond this form of prevention — which basically consists in limiting the effects of war — and ask the following question:

**Can war be prevented ?**

To prevent war, the fundamental causes of tension and underlying violence must be analyzed. We know that, although these causes are sometimes rooted in territorial claims, they are primarily:

- socio-economic inequalities
- cultural and religious intolerance
- ethnic discrimination

These problems can be solved through development, the word "development" being used here in its broadest sense, that is to say, including reduction of poverty, elimination of all forms of discrimination and promotion of tolerance.

Humanitarian action in behalf of the victims of armed conflicts also helps to promote peace, by maintaining in the midst of war a humanitarian enclave of dialogue and understanding between the parties which in some cases can serve as a starting-point for the resumption of the peace process. "War" and "development" are *a priori* antonyms, the one seeking to destroy and the other to construct. A return to peace is the essential condition for the resumption of a real development process after a war.

MISSION

The International Committee of the Red Cross (ICRC) is an impartial, neutral and independent organization whose exclusively humanitarian mission is to protect the lives and dignity of victims of war and internal violence and to provide them with assistance. It directs and coordinates the international relief activities conducted by the Movement in situations of conflict. It also endeavours to prevent suffering by promoting and strengthening humanitarian law and universal humanitarian principles. Established in 1863, the ICRC is at the origin of the International Red Cross and Red Crescent Movement.